The Neonate

CURRENT TOPICS IN CLINICAL CHEMISTRY

Series Editor

J. STANTON KING, Ph.D.

Sponsored by the American Association for Clinical Chemistry

THE NEONATE

Clinical Biochemistry, Physiology, and Pathology

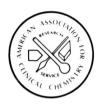

Edited by

DONALD S. YOUNG, M.B., Ph.D.
Chief, Clinical Chemistry Service
Clinical Pathology Department, Clinical Center
National Institutes of Health
Bethesda, Maryland

JOCELYN M. HICKS, Ph.D.
Director, Clinical Laboratories
Children's Hospital National Medical Center
Washington, D.C.
Associate Professor of Child Health and Development and Pathology
George Washington University School of Medicine
Washington, D.C.

A WILEY MEDICAL PUBLICATION

John Wiley & Sons, New York • London • Sydney • Toronto

Library of Congress Cataloging in Publication Data:

Symposium on the Clinical Biochemistry of the Neonate,
  Washington, D.C., 1974.
    The neonate.

   (Current topics in clinical chemistry; v. 2). (A
Wiley medical publication)
   "Sponsored by the American Association for Clinical
Chemistry."
   Includes bibliographical references and index.
   1. Infants (Newborn)—Physiology—Congresses.
2. Infants (Newborn)—Diseases—Congresses. 3. Fetus—
Physiology—Congresses. I. Young, Donald S. II. Hicks,
Jocelyn M. III. American Association for Clinical
Chemistry. IV. Title. [DNLM: 1. Infant, Newborn—
Congresses. W1 CU82ED/WS420 S9925n 1974]

RJ252.S95 1974   618.9'201   76-6157
ISBN 0-471-97982-1

Printed in the United States of America

10 9 8 7 6 5 4 3 2 1

Contributors

GORDON B. AVERY, M.D., Ph.D., Chairman, Department of Neonatology, Children's Hospital National Medical Center, and Professor of Child Health and Development, George Washington University School of Medicine, Washington, D. C. 20006

RICHARD E. BEHRMAN, M.D., Professor and Chairman, Department of Pediatrics, College of Physicians and Surgeons of Columbia University, 630 West 168th Street, New York, New York 10032

JOSEPH A. BELLANTI, M.D., Professor of Pediatrics and Microbiology, Georgetown University School of Medicine, 3800 Reservoir Road, Washington, D.C. 20007

NORMA F. BESCH, Ph.D., Assistant Professor, Department of Obstetrics and Gynecology, Baylor College of Medicine, and Assistant Director, Reproductive Research Laboratory, St. Luke's Episcopal Hospital, Houston, Texas 77025

PAIGE K. BESCH, Ph.D., Professor, Department of Obstetrics and Gynecology, Baylor College of Medicine, and Director, Reproductive Research Laboratory, St. Luke's Episcopal Hospital, Houston, Texas 77025

THOMAS BLUMENFELD, M.D., Assistant Professor, Departments of Pediatrics and Pathology, College of Physicians and Surgeons of Columbia University, and Babies Hospital, The Children's Medical and Surgical Center, 630 West 168th Street, New York, New York 10032

ROSCOE O. BRADY, M.D., Chief, Development and Metabolic Neurology Branch, National Institute of Neurological Disease and Stroke, Bethesda, Maryland 20014

LAURENCE I. BURD, M.D., Research Fellow, Division of Perinatal Medicine, Department of Obstetrics and Gynecology, University of Colorado Medical Center, 4200 East Ninth Avenue, Denver, Colorado 80220

RONALD A. CHEZ, M.D., Chief, Pregnancy Research Branch, National Institute of Child Health and Human Development, Bethesda, Maryland 20014

JULIO O. CUKIER, M.D., Research Fellow in Neonatology, Department of Pediatrics, The Johns Hopkins University School of Medicine, Baltimore, Maryland 21205

PAUL A. DI SANT'AGNESE, M.D., Sc.D. (Med.), Chief, Pediatric Metabolism Branch, National Institute of Arthritis, Metabolism, and Digestive Diseases, National Institutes of Health, Bethesda, Maryland 20014

JOHN M. DRISCOLL, JR., M.D., Department of Pediatrics, College of Physicians and Surgeons of Columbia University, and the Babies Hospital, The Children's Medical and Surgical Center of New York, 630 West 168th Street, New York, New York 10032

PHILIP M. FARRELL, M.D., Ph.D., Pediatric Metabolism Branch, National Institute of Arthritis, Metabolism, and Digestive Diseases, National Institutes of Health, Bethesda, Maryland 20014

v

ANNE B. FLETCHER, M.D., Associate Professor, Newborn Service, Children's Hospital National Medical Center, Washington, D. C., 20009, and Associate Professor of Child Health and Development, George Washington University School of Medicine, Washington, D. C. 20037

RONALD L. GUTBERLET, M.D., Associate Professor of Pediatrics, Department of Pediatrics, University of Maryland Hospital, Baltimore, Maryland 21201

WILLIAM C. HEIRD, M.D., Assistant Professor of Pediatrics, Department of Pediatrics, College of Physicians and Surgeons of Columbia University, and the Babies Hospital, Columbia-Presbyterian Medical Center, 630 West 168th Street, New York, New York 10032

JOCELYN M. HICKS, Ph.D., Director, Clinical Laboratories, Children's Hospital National Medical Center, Washington, D. C. 20009, and Associate Professor of Child Health and Development and Pathology, George Washington University School of Medicine, Washington, D. C. 20006

REBA MICHELS HILL, M.D., Associate Professor of Pediatrics, Baylor College of Medicine, Chief of Newborn Research, The Linda Faye Halbouty Premature Nursery and Newborn Research Center of St. Luke's Episcopal and Texas Children's Hospitals, St. Luke's Episcopal Hospital, Houston, Texas 77025

MARJORIE G. HORNING, Ph.D., Professor of Biochemistry, Baylor College of Medicine, Institute for Lipid Research, Houston, Texas 77025

L. STANLEY JAMES, M.D., Professor, Department of Pediatrics, College of Physicians and Surgeons of Columbia University, 630 West 168th Street, New York, New York 10032

MELVIN E. JENKINS, M.D., Department of Pediatrics and Child Health, Howard University College of Medicine, Washington, D. C. 20059

APOLO C. MAGLALANG, M.D., Research Fellow in Neonatology, Department of Pediatrics, The Johns Hopkins University School of Medicine, Baltimore, Maryland 21205

FLORENCE MOOG, Ph.D., Professor, Department of Biology, Washington University, St. Louis, Missouri 63130

JOHN F. NICHOLSON, M.D., Associate Professor of Pediatrics, Department of Pediatrics, College of Physicians and Surgeons of Columbia University, and Director, Clinical Laboratories, Babies Hospital, The Children's Medical and Surgical Center of New York, 630 East 168th Street, New York, New York 10032

GARY K. OAKES, M.D., Clinical Associate, Pregnancy Research Branch, National Institute of Child Health and Human Development, Bethesda, Maryland 20014

DONOUGH O'BRIEN, M.D., F.R.C.P., Professor of Pediatrics, Department of Pediatrics, B. F. Stolinsky Laboratories, University of Colorado Medical Center, 4200 East Ninth Avenue, Denver, Colorado 80220

GERARD B. ODELL, M.D., Professor of Pediatrics, The Johns Hopkins University, and the Harriet Lane Service of the Children's Medical and Surgical Center of the Johns Hopkins Hospital, Baltimore, Maryland 21205

MARILYN RENFIELD, M.D., Clinical Assistant Professor, George Washington University School of Medicine, Washington, D. C. 20006, and Fellow in Behavioral Pediatrics, Georgetown University School of Medicine, Washington, D. C. 20007

ALLEN W. ROOT, M.D., Professor of Pediatrics, University of South Florida College of Medicine, Tampa, and Ed Wright Pediatric Endocrinology Research Laboratory, All Children's Hospital, St. Petersburg, Florida 33701

PEDRO ROSSO, M.D., Assistant Professor of Pediatrics, Department of Pediatrics, and Institute of Human Nutrition, College of Physicians and Surgeons of Columbia University, 630 West 168th Street, New York, New York 10032

S. JAIME ROZOVSKI, Ph.D., Institute of Human Nutrition, and Department of Pediatrics, College of Physicians and Surgeons of Columbia University, 630 West 168th Street, New York, New York 10032

IRWIN A. SCHAFER, M.D., Associate Professor of Pediatrics, Case Western Reserve University School of Medicine at Cleveland Metropolitan General Hospital, Cleveland, Ohio 44109

CHARLES R. SCRIVER, M.D., Professor of Pediatrics, Department of Pediatrics, McGill University, Montreal, Canada

MICHAEL A. SIMMONS, M.D., Associate Professor of Pediatrics, Division of Perinatal Medicine, University of Colorado Medical Center, 4200 East Ninth Avenue, Denver, Colorado 80220

ELBA VELASCO, M.D., Institute of Human Nutrition, and Department of Pediatrics, College of Physicians and Surgeons of Columbia University, 630 West 168th Street, New York, New York 10032

MARCIA WASSERMAN, M.S., Institute of Human Nutrition, and Department of Pediatrics, College of Physicians and Surgeons of Columbia University, 630 West 168th Street, New York, New York 10032

ROBERT W. WINTERS, M.D., Department of Pediatrics, College of Physicians and Surgeons of Columbia University, and the Babies Hospital, The Children's Medical and Surgical Center, 630 West 168th Street, New York, New York 10032

DONALD S. YOUNG, M.B., Ph.D., Chief, Clinical Chemistry Service, Clinical Pathology Department, Clinical Center, National Institutes of Health, Bethesda, Maryland 20014

CARL ZELSON, M.D., Professor, Department of Pediatrics, New York Medical Center, and Metropolitan Hospital Center, New York, New York 10029

Human biological potential is established, in large measure, in its experiences in prenatal life and in the early postnatal years. This tender period is beset by a host of possible difficulties; unfavorable outcome, in many cases, can mean serious permanent limitation in both physical and mental health and potential. This phase of human life is receiving increasing scientific attention, yet there are few areas where clinical capabilities are so limited by fundamental understanding. An intensive investigative effort directed at elucidation of the events and mechanisms of normal conception, pregnancy, parturition, and postnatal development is of overriding importance.

Clearly all information descriptive of development in other species is relevant to equivalent events in human development. Each month there appear reports of human disorders which find their origins in the events of early life. It is the changing patterns of mortality and morbidity, largely the consequence of the minimization of infectious diseases, which have brought these health problems into new focus as primary hazards to health and happiness.

From *Biology and the Future of Man*, P. Handler, Ed.,
Oxford University Press, New York, 1970, p. 698 (by permission).

Preface

Our intent in organizing this book is to make available to the clinical chemist appropriate background data on the physiological and biochemical development of the neonate necessary for the understanding of normal and abnormal laboratory test results. For the pediatrician we hope to reiterate the importance of the clinical laboratory in the diagnosis of disorders in the neonate, the management of their treatment, and the monitoring of the development of the newborn infant. The symbiotic relationship between pediatrician and clinical chemist already exists in many leading medical centers. We would like to see it accepted in all hospitals for children.

The book is divided into four sections, to cover the biochemistry, physiology, and pathology of the neonate. It is arranged so that it will follow the development of the infant from birth to the end of the neonatal period. The first papers concern the biochemical and physiological development of the fetus. These are followed by the adjustment to extrauterine life. The normal neonate is discussed and then the major medical problems of the newborn are considered. Obviously, it was not possible to cover all aspects of the growth and development of the neonate, yet we believe that this collection of papers does bring together the information needed for understanding the problems of the newborn infant. Throughout the book we have emphasized that the neonate is a unique individual and not a miniature adult. The book emphasizes the need for a strong interaction between neonatologist and clinical chemist, to ensure that the special resources required to monitor the biochemical and physiological development of the infant are made available at the most demanding time in his life.

This collection of papers was presented at a Symposium on the Clinical Biochemistry of the Neonate held in Washington, D.C., December 5–7, 1974. Although the symposium was sponsored by the American Association for Clinical Chemistry, it was intended to be interdisciplinary in character, and indeed it was attended by almost equal numbers of pediatricians and clinical chemists. The symposium was modeled after the May 1973 symposium on Amniotic Fluid, sponsored by the Chicago Section of the American Association for Clinical Chemistry together with the Chicago Gynecological, Immunological and Pediatric Societies. That symposium was volume 1 in this series; thus this is the second volume on perinatology to be presented by the Association.

We are especially grateful to Dr. Gordon B. Avery, who provided great assistance in the planning of this symposium, and we would also like to acknowledge the help of the other members of the planning committee who contributed to making the symposium a very valuable forum for the exchange of ideas between clinical chemists and pediatricians.

We especially thank Drs. David Uddin, Henry Nipper, and Col. Edward C. Knoblock for their contributions in organizing the meeting, as well as Drs. Allen Calvert and William Neeley and Ms. Irma Campbell, who were the other members of the organizing committee.

DONALD S. YOUNG, M.B., PH.D.

JOCELYN M. HICKS, PH.D.

Contents

Section III   The Neonate

Section IV   Medical Problems of the Newborn

Biochemical and Physiological Development of the Fetus

Obstetric History, Placental Folklore, and Neonatal Models

PAIGE K. BESCH, Ph.D.*

NORMA F. BESCH, Ph.D.

4000–400 B.C.: OBSTETRICS IN THE ANCIENT WORLD

Mystery, magic, religion, and medicine originally were one and the same. Healing methods that sprang up thousands of years ago and were developed by various groups of primitive people were all essentially the same. In principle their methods were the same as those practiced today by aborigines in remote or uncivilized regions. We can trace the historical development of medical practice from these earliest times. Some individuals among the savages of the tribes were shrewder or more clever men than the others; perhaps they were not quite as "normal"—a little more eager to look, listen, and learn. At any rate, they were not well understood by the other group members, who came to believe that these men had power over the spirits, those mysterious forces that would send the sunshine and rain, that would bring game to the hunter and give success to the man in combat. Such an individual was the one to whom the others turned for relief from the spirits that brought disease and pain. He became the "medicine man." Unfortunately, but reasonably, these early healers were expected not only to heal their friends but to cast sicknesses upon their enemies as well. They came to practice what we might call both white (healing) magic and black (destructive) magic.

As centuries passed and tribal organizations grew into communal states with appointed, elected, or inherited leaderships, these early medicine men, who were priests as well as doctors, became part of a special group that only the elite might join. These men held all manner of ceremonies and established customs and rites, all to set the stage of development for the healing priest of early civilization. We will examine briefly how the primitive healing priests carried out their duties as physicians.

---

* I dedicate this chapter to my late scientific mentor, Professor Leonard R. Axelrod (1927–1975), who spent many hours teaching a young scientist to have an appreciation for the historical aspects of our profession.

The basic philosophy of primitive medicine was the same throughout almost all of the tribes of early people. It was believed that supernatural forces caused disease. Many different tribal areas simultaneously developed various ceremonies for overcoming these supernatural forces. The remnants of these rites are seen in the various superstitions that have persisted to this day. We should, however, recognize that these practices were not regarded as superstitions in early days. They have become so only since we have gained knowledge about many of the natural forces. Perhaps the most general practice of the medicine man was a crude version of what we now would call psychotherapy. For example, in treating his patient, the healing priest often tried to frighten away spirits by putting on a bizarre and fantastic costume and chanting prayers, dancing around singing to a higher being, or shouting as he shook a rattle before his patient. If the patient believed sincerely that the medicine man was driving away the spirits, the pain was eased and the anxiety dispelled. The patient felt better and in many cases was actually cured. As time passed, these faith-healing priests began to specialize in different types of conditions. As we will discuss later, one of the many Egyptian healing priests would be so specialized as to concentrate only on the left eye or the left leg and leave the right eye or leg to the attention of another specialist. Further, as the store of knowledge grew with civilization, many healers specialized in the use of various herbs and plants for their cures, while others began to use compounded medications that contained salt, mercury, sulfur, and some of the other early known chemical compounds.

Other healing priests with a more physical approach began to study the sun, the stars, and the moon. They believed that the moon influenced bodily functions (whence our word lunatic, which reflects only one of many aspects of the moon's presumed influence). Medicines and various healing rites were given or withheld according to the phase of the moon. The symbolism connected with the moon's periodicity of waxing and waning affected many sorts of human undertakings as well as beliefs about disease. It was, therefore, a logical step to schedule sowing of crops, waging of war, marrying, bleeding, and administering medicines according to the phases of the moon. The 28-day menstrual cycle was also believed to be a phenomenon influenced by the moon. Such ancient beliefs strongly influenced medical practice until the middle of the nineteenth century. The sun and stars likewise played their part in medical practice, giving us almost innumerable superstitions, many of which have persisted for centuries. As recently as two or three hundred years ago, physicians commonly made diagnoses by casting the horoscopes of their patients. Perhaps the ℞ that appears on the top of the physician's prescription pad is a remnant of a once widely prevalent astrological belief. According to some scholars, it is an abbreviation for the Latin word *recipe*, meaning "take"; others hold that it is the astrological sign of Jupiter, under whose protection medicine was generally placed. As such, it is a written charm or invocation to the gods to ensure the efficacy of the medication.

From astrology it is only a step to the magic attributed to other symbols, numbers, colors, and the like. Some superstitions that were held by ancient man to be vital truths in medical matters persist even today. Seven, four, and thirteen were particularly potent numbers, it was thought. A child born in the seventh month of the calendar was supposed—and still is by some people—to have a better chance of living than one born in the eighth month. There were critical days in the course of a disease: three, seven, and nine. Many medicinal seeds or leaves were given according to number, such as seven pieces of ergot rye or three digitalis leaves. As now, in ancient times medicine was commonly to be taken "three times a day."

In this presentation we shall limit ourselves to a discussion of recorded history and folklore surrounding the birth process, with emphasis on the placenta. The earliest references to obstetrical and gynecological events are contained in the Kahun Medical Papyrus (2000–1800 B.C.), the Ebers Papyrus (1500 B.C.), the clay tablets of Mesopotamia (1100–600 B.C.), the Veda (1500–500 B.C.), the biblical books, the Iliad (1300 B.C.), and Chinese writings (600 B.C.). The stage of development reached by the Egyptians was not attained by any of the other civilizations, even though in a few places a unique understanding of some aspect of obstetrics and gynecology may have existed. The influence of the Egyptian culture, including its medicine, was felt in most of the other civilizations, its greatest influence being that on Greek medicine of the sixth century B.C. As an example of the degree to which obstetrics had advanced in the Egyptian culture, a college for midwives existed in the city of Sais. However, without exception in these early cultures, the midwife and not the male physician or priest administered to the parturient woman. While the Egyptians described the female reproductive tract in anatomical terms and discussed prolapse, leukorrhea, menstruation, and fertility, no mention was made of the placenta in relationship to birth, although the placenta was used in their pharmacological treatments. The retained placenta was first described by the Indians during the Brahmanic era (500 B.C.–A.D. 1000).

The Mesopotamian civilization and its medicine developed simultaneously with and independently of the Egyptian—at least in the beginning. The Sumerian Age (about 4000–2400 B.C.) is notable primarily for the invention of pictorial writing and the development of astronomy. To the knowledge of Mesopotamia, regarded as an Oriental civilization, the Babylonians and Assyrians were undoubtedly the principal contributors.

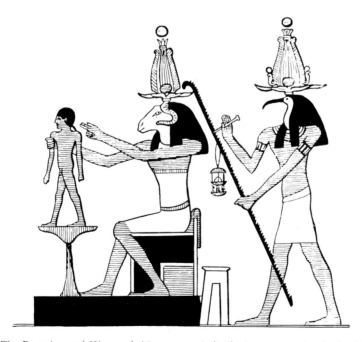

Figure 1. The Egyptian god Khnum fashions a new individual on a potter's wheel, while the god Thoth holds the "Staff of Life." From the general Introductory Guide to the Egyptian Collections in the British Museum, p 205, Harrison and Sons, Ltd., London, 1930.

They were skilled in mathematics and astronomy, originated the decimal system, weights and measures, and established the divisions of time from a 12-month calendar. They were skilled in music, architecture, pottery, glassblowing, weaving, and astrology. Thus astrology and the interpretation of omens merged into prognosis and, as with all early civilizations, the first Babylonian physician was a priest (or, if you prefer, the first priest was a physician).

As early as 2250 B.C., in the Code of Hammurabi, the medical profession in Babylon had advanced far enough in public esteem to be rewarded with adequate fees, carefully prescribed and regulated by law. Internal medicine was mainly concerned with endeavoring to cast out demons of disease. Inasmuch as women had always been considered the least important of mankind, and birth construed as a natural process exhibited by all animals, little if any medical attention was directed toward obstetrics, although very stringent laws were written concerning women during their menstrual period, birth, and the puerperium; these laws were primarily concerned with the isolation of the woman. The Babylonians developed outstanding achievements in public hygiene. They understood the proper disposal of sewage, the need for expulsion of lepers from the community, and they described the pollution of streams by dead animals.

The Persians did little to advance obstetrics. In fact they may have added to the misery of complicated childbirth by prohibiting incantations directed to the obstetrical patient. The main features of their approach were directed toward cult cleanliness, with particular ritual emphasis on the uncleanliness of menstruating women. The idea that contact with a corpse was unclean did much to hinder the progress of medicine. The corpse was exposed to the elements on high places to prevent its burial, which might pollute the sanctity of the earth. This may have been the basis for considering the placenta to be unclean, in that during the gestational period the menstrual flow was thought to accumulate to form the placenta.

Closely connected with Mesopotamian medicine was the medicine of the Hebrews, primarily as a consequence of their Assyrian captivity (722 B.C.) and Babylonian captivity (604 B.C.). The ancient Hebrews were, in fact, the founders of prophylaxis and the high priests were true medical police. They had a definite code of ritual hygiene and cult cleanliness, gradually expanded from contact with different civilizations. The Book of Leviticus contains the sternest mandates about touching unclean objects, the proper food to be eaten, the purifying of women after childbirth, the hygiene of the menstrual periods, and many other sanctions relating to such matters as bestiality and other sexual perversions. During this period we find reference to the professional midwives and particularly the striking reference to the obstetrical chair used in labor (Exod. 1:16), where Pharaoh commands the slaying of all Jewish infants of the male sex, "When ye do the office of a midwife to the Hebrew women, and see them upon the stools." Although the Talmud contains many references to the esophagus, larynx, trachea, the membranes of the brain, pancreas, liver, spleen, kidney, spinal cord and others, the placenta is never mentioned. Further, very few obstetrical and gynecological references are found—with the exception of cardiac shock in precipitate labor (1 Sam. 4:19), uniovular twins (Gen. 38:27), and gonorrhea and leukorrhea (Lev. 13:15). The Hebrews were aware of the existence of the cesarean section, but it is not clear whether or not they utilized it.

As the Hebrews attained the highest eminence in hygiene, so the ancient Hindus excelled all other nations of their time in operative surgery. However, in the earliest Sanskrit documents—the Rig-Veda (1500 B.C.) and the Atharva-Veda—we find the first fragmentary evidence relating to the placenta, and remarks on obstetrics. The Hindus evi-

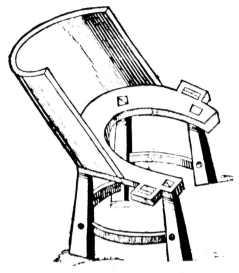

Figure 2. Obstetrical chair used from early recorded Biblical history (700–600 B.C.), until as late as early nineteenth century A.D. See general reference number 3, p 271.

dently connected the products of conception, the fetus and placenta, with copulation. It is also stated that the menstrual blood, absent during gestation, was stored in the body to form milk in the postpartum period. Included in an obstetrical chapter by the Susruta is an admirable section on infant hygiene and nutrition, unexcelled by anything before the time of Aurelius Celsus or Soranus of Ephesus of the second century A.D. There we also find the first known reference to the retained placenta, with a warning that pressure should be externally applied and if this is not successful in promoting its delivery, the patient is to be shaken, and if this is not successful, dropping the patient should be considered. Podalic version appears to have been practiced by the Hindus, but in a primitive manner.

Dystocia was recognized by nearly all of the early civilizations. During labor, various positions were assumed by women of different peoples. According to her build and the shape of the pelvis, a woman would stand, kneel, or lie upon her abdomen, varying these positions in various stages of labor according to the position of the child's head in the pelvis. Dystocia was handled by force rather than manipulation and consisted of squeezing the abdomen, jouncing the woman about, and even sitting or standing on her abdomen. Sometimes sudden fright was provoked to stimulate flagging labor. An important feature of delivery seems to have been that the hand was never inserted into the vagina. If an arm presented, it was seized and pulled. The third stage of labor seems always to have been managed by manual expression of the body.

460–136 B.C.: OBSTETRICS AT THE TIME OF HIPPOCRATES

Throughout the era referred to as the Hippocratic period, midwives dominated obstetrics, and physicians were only consulted when the case was difficult. Even if the midwife sought aid, the physician never actually examined the patient; the midwife related her findings to him. Abnormal postures of the fetus were described in the writings of Hippocrates. All deliveries in which the head did not present were considered abnormal.

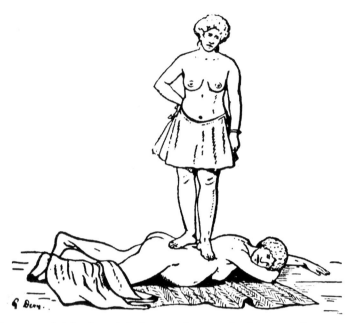

Figure 3. Recommended for dystocia in Loango. See general reference number 9, p 14.

Retention of the placenta was discussed and various ways of promoting expulsion were described, methods less traumatic than those proposed during the earlier times. One method was to seat the mother on a chair that was used for delivery (i.e., one with a hole in the seat), and place the umbilically attached infant on large bags filled with water. The bags were then punctured and as the water slowly escaped, the infant descended and pulled

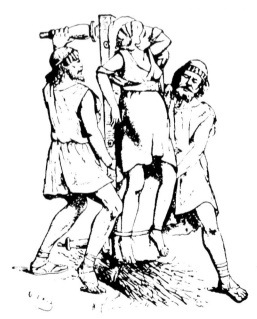

Figure 4. Vikings approach to slowness of labor. See general reference number 2, p 39.

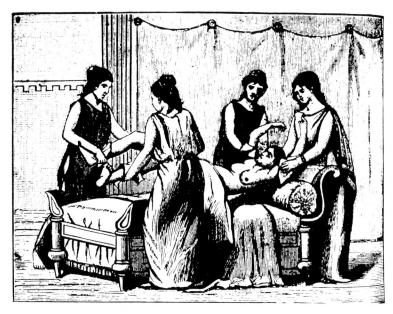

Figure 5. Approach recommended by Hippocrates during dystocia. See general reference number 2, p 57.

the placenta after him. The description goes on to state that if this did not remove the placenta, it was left inside the patient and was said to decompose in about a week.

In the case of extreme dystocia or severe contracted pelvis, craniotomy and thoracotomy were recommended if external version failed to result in delivery. Although Hippocrates' writings were extensive, the precise technique of delivery is described in none of his works. From other sources we know that women of ancient Greece were generally in labor upon stools that had an opening in the middle of the seat.

Although physicians of the day did not examine their obstetrical patients, they felt no hesitancy about writing on the subject, and the following is a quotation from one of the medical texts by Hippocrates:

> "In the third month commences the differentiation into the various parts of the body, legs, arms, and head; in the fourth month follows the distinct development of the body parts and heart; in the fifth are added the flesh and blood; in the sixth are developed hair, nails, bones, sinews, veins, and in the seventh month the embryo is finished with all that is necessary for its existence; in the eighth month the vital force is drawn, now from mother to child, now from child to mother; on account of this to and fro movement the child born in this month is not viable. The hard parts of the body are derived from the father, the soft from the mother. Nourishment is carried on through the vessels which lead chyle from the mother to embryo. During pregnancy, the fetus occupies the uterus, turned toward the mother's back, the head up, the hands folded across the forehead, lying on the right side of the mother, if of the male sex, on the left side if of the female sex; before birth, version occurs."

The first pregnancy test originated during this time, described as follows:

> "If you wish to ascertain if a woman be with child give her hydromel [a mixture of honey and water] to drink when she is going to sleep, and has not taken supper, and if she be siezed with pain in the belly, she is with child, but otherwise she is not pregnant."

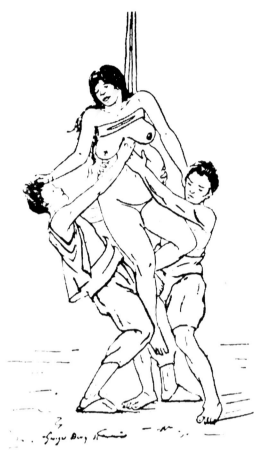

Figure 6. Delivery of a Siamese native from an under-the-arms–hanging position. See general reference number 9, p 18.

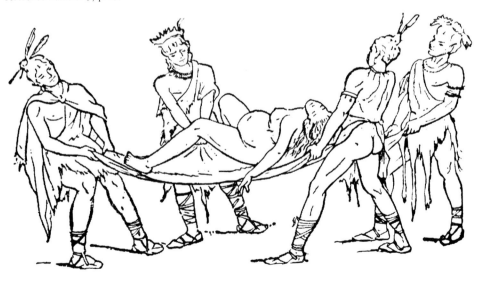

Figure 7. American Indians tossing squaw in a blanket to help "shake" baby out. See general reference number 9, p 11.

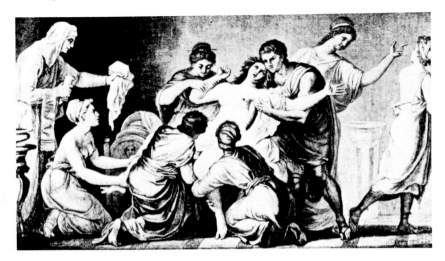

Figure 8. Greeks and Romans of noble birth were attended by many trained midwives during labor. See general reference number 10, p 52.

During this same period the Hindus and the Egyptians likewise left the business of delivery to midwives. Customarily, the expectant mother would be assisted by four individuals. Treatment for sluggish delivery of the placenta had medically advanced to the point that emetics, external pressure, and shaking were now the prescription of the day. The infant was breast-fed on the third day and mother was up and about on the tenth. During this time the Indians, who generally had developed their surgical skill far beyond that of other physicians elsewhere, were acquainted with embryotomy and cesarean section after the death or near death of the mother. However, their knowledge of breech and foot presentations was inadequate compared to that of the Greeks. Meanwhile, in Rome, male practitioners of obstetrics seem to have been commonplace, even in the case of uncomplicated pregnancies, and they assisted at childbirth. Within Rome there existed a popular obstetrical cult that is sometimes mentioned in connection with the history of the field. Lucina was a term applied to Juno and Diana in their duties pertaining to childbirth. Thus this obstetrical cult became known as Lucina. It is generally assumed that the name applied to Juno (in her obstetric aspect, the result of bringing forth the infant into the worldly light). The cult of Lucina was involved with the usual complexities of quasi-magical rituals and mysticisms associated with the obstetrical folklore of these early civilizations. Many of the rich and idle Roman women would occupy themselves rather completely during their pregnancy by discharging the menusica specified by the cult of Lucina, specific ritualistic involvements that seem to have changed with the passage of time. There are no references to these superstitions in later formal medical works.

A very strange law existed, attributed to Numa Pompilius, the second legendary King of Rome (715–672 B.C.). Before the city was formally established, the law (Lex Regina) existed as a custom and was sanctified by time. It provided that no pregnant woman dying in childbirth could be buried without abdominal section to remove the products of conception. The noun *caeso* (presumably derived from the verb *caedere*: to cut, amputate, or prune) was used for a person delivered in this manner from a dead mother. Some say that the first of the Caesars got his name from the surgical operation performed upon his mother. However, other historians have pointed out that this operation was never performed on a living patient, but only after death, thus rendering the existence of a living fetus impossible. Moreover, Julius Caesar's mother was alive at the time of the Gallic wars. The first evidence of the performance of an abdominal extraction on a living woman dates from the sixteenth century, and the Lex Regina probably exerted no more influence on the history of obstetrics than did the cult of Lucina.

After Alexandrian times, obstetrics slowly progressed in the understanding of the anatomical and physiological components of pregnancy. Briefly, it is said the physician of this day believed that the cervix altered at the onset of pregnancy, regulated menstruation as an essential prerequisite for the pregnancy, and was responsible for different types of dystocia such as transverse lie, incomplete dilatation, failure of the membranes to rupture, uterine inertia as well as hemorrhage, the presence of obstructing growths, and ultimately, fetal death. Thus in these early times it was believed that the cervix and the fetus jointly played an active role in the process of labor. Accordingly, the obstetrician would place his hand in the vagina and digitally dilate the cervix until the hand could be placed within the uterus. After delivery of the child the placenta was manually extracted rather than expressed. From this presumably followed the development of the procedure of decapitation in the case of death in utero. A hook was devised, sharpened in the curve, and this was used in the above procedure. In extracting the placenta with this hook, the operator was cautioned not to engage parts of the uterus. A very strange practice, that of causing a woman in labor to sneeze repeatedly, continued to be one of the most frequently used obstetrical aids, although no clear medical explanation of its usefulness was ever given in the medical writings of these periods.

SORANUS, THE FATHER OF OBSTETRICS AND GYNECOLOGY

Soranus of Ephesus (A.D. 98–177) was the leading authority of his time on obstetrics, gynecology and pediatrics. His treatment of pediatrics is the finest contribution to the subject from this period and contains the most rational precepts as to infant hygiene and nutrition, with separate chapters on diseases of infants, including a recognizable account of rickets. Before moving to Rome, he had practiced medicine in Alexandria. His main written work, *On The Disease of Women*, was an outstanding textbook, which remained in use for *15 centuries*. He was the first of the ancients to adequately describe the female genital tract in detail; he likened the uterus to a cupping instrument that opened during coitus and the menstrual period. He also advised on various forms of contraception by means of cotton, ointments, or fatty substances but disapproved of abortion by various mechanical means. He described menstruation, conception, and amenorrhea for the first time. He was the first to promote the idea that these physiological changes might have a cause-and-effect relationship to childbearing and breast-feeding. He recognized the significance of symptomatology in certain pathological conditions such as infection of the genital tract and prescribed treatment for dysfunctional uterine bleeding and for dysmenorrhea. He paid particular attention to the difficulties that could occur at childbirth. These, he stated, could be due to defects in the mother, such as a contracted pelvis, lordosis, and tumors. He was the first to advise emptying the bladder before delivery by means of a reed catheter.

Further, Soranus recognized that difficulties with childbirth could also be due to the position of the fetus, which might be too large or in an abnormal position. In these cases he stated that the physician must intervene. Soranus illustrated various abnormal positions and explained how to maneuver the fetus into a suitable position in the birth canal in order to deliver the infant. If manual assistance was to no real avail, the physician was advised to use forceps or hooks to extract the fetus. His notations concerning contraception probably were the first to have any scientific basis. He stated that contraceptive measures could be brought about by use of various substances which could be introduced into the vagina before coitus:

". . . to prevent conception, the woman before coitus should smear her cervix with rancid oil, or with honey, or with a concoction of cedar oil, or she should push into the os a sharp strip of lint, or introduce into the vagina an astringent pessary."

The pessary most frequently used was a halved or peeled pomegranate soaked in vinegar.

He is the first obstetrician to extensively discuss version. He felt that if there was difficulty with the delivery in the usual obstetrical chair, the patient should then

". . . be placed in bed in a prone position, bending her knees upon her thighs, in order that the womb, being carried to the abdomen, may present with its mouth direct."

By means of the fingers, the mouth was to be smeared with cerates or fatty substances, and gently dilated.

"And if there be any complaint in the parts it must be previously attended to; and hardened feces when retained be expelled by an emollient clyster. The membranes may be divided either by the fingers, or by a scalpel concealed within them, the left hand directing it. And some of the fatty liquids may be thrown up into the uterus by a syringe. When the fetus is in an unnatural position, we may restore the natural position, by sometimes pressing it back, by sometimes drawing it down, sometimes pushing it aside, and sometimes rectifying the whole."

Soranus further stated

". . . if a hand or foot protrude, we must not seize upon the limb and draw it down, for thereby it will be more wedged in, or may be dislocated, or fractured; but fixing the fingers upon the shoulders or hip joint of the fetus, the part that has protruded is to be restored to its proper position. If there be a wrong position of the whole fetus, attended with impaction, we must first push it upward from the mouth of the womb, then lay hold of it, and direct it properly through the mouth of the uterus."

Again, the problem of removal of the placenta is manifested and treatment recommended in the following statement:

". . . often, after the removal of the fetus, the placenta (which is also called the secudines) is retained in the uterus. When the mouth of the uterus is dilated and the placenta separated and rolled into a ball in some part of the uterus, the extraction is most easy. But if they adhere to the fundus uteri we must introduce the hand in and grasp them and pull them along, not straight down for fear of prolapse nor with great violence, but they are to be removed gently, at first from this side to that and afterwards somewhat more strongly, for thus they will yield and be freed from their adhesions."

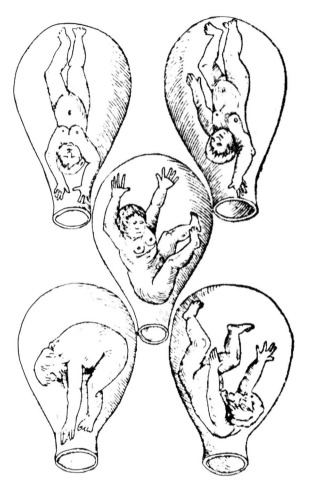

Figure 9. Various positions of the fetus as drawn by Soranus and reprinted in *The Boke of Children*, by Thomas Phayre, 1545.

OBSTETRICS IN THE MIDDLE AGES

Obstetrics and gynecology both suffered as a result of the intellectual twilight that preceded the Renaissance. After the downfall of Rome, Europe was left practically nationless and at the mercy of wandering barbarians. In the great struggle between individualism and collectivism, intellectual independence was seriously hampered. This period of feudalism and ecclesiasticism was associated with a resurgence of superstitious practices and religious sanctions. The social and medical climate of Europe for several centuries can be characterized as a regression from the stage of development reached by preceding civilizations.

The church emerged as the most powerful institution during this period, due in large part to the instability of the political structure. Thus it may be seen as responsible for both the progress and the regression seen in medicine. Obstetrics and gynecology as a field fared the worst under the influence of the church. The practice of obstetrics made a full return to the unskilled hands of the midwife and remained there. Abortion was forbidden and cesarean surgery was recommended in its place. Surgery, without anesthesia, was not performed by physicians but by barber-surgeons or sow gelders. The church's primary concern was with the soul of the infant; at this time an instrument was developed for the baptism of the infant in utero. Turning now to progress, in the interest of alleviating suffering, the church established hospitals for care of the ill. Because of the poor hygienic practices of those times, these hospitals soon became known as houses of death, particularly for the parturient woman. In summary, there were no notable advances in obstetrics and gynecology during the period from A.D. 600 to A.D. 1450, as was also the state of affairs for other fields of endeavor during this same period.

THE RENAISSANCE

In the transition of mankind from the beginning of the Renaissance through the revival of learning and into the Reformation (1452–1600), undoubtedly the most potent events were the inventions of gunpowder, leading to the demise of feudalism and the rise of nationalism, and of printing, leading to great advances in the dissemination of knowledge. Other important influences were the waning power of the church, the discovery of the New World, and the acceptance of new concepts in astronomy.

One of the earliest books printed (1477) was a popular medical text called *Artzneibuch*, by Ortollf of Bavaria. His *Das Frauenbuchlein* (*Little Book of Women*), which was a popular handbook for lying-in women, was published in 1500. The major value of Ortollf's theses was that they were written in the language of the day and were thus valuable in the guidance of the midwife. In this small publication, a stern warning is given the midwife concerning retention of the placenta in the following passage:

> "If the afterbirth is late or slow in coming make the woman sneeze but never shall it be drawn out by force; be gentle in order not to tear it or not to leave behind a part in the woman's body; repeat the sneezing again and again. The afterbirth if left behind begins to spoil, spreads its rotten vapors to the heart, liver, and stomach and makes the woman surely perish."

Essentially, this book was only a written version of the midwife folklore of the day and contained very little new medical information or knowledge.

During this period the influence of several important men seemed to change the whole course of obstetrics. Vesalius (1514–1564) and his pupil, Fallopius (1523–1562), did extensive anatomical descriptions of the ovaries and the fallopian tubes, and named the vagina and placenta. Although the placenta had been described in somewhat less detail by Hippocrates, who gave it the name of cotyledon, which means cuplike, Fallopius felt the proper name of the "afterbirth," as it was commonly referred to, should be placenta or platelike organ. Fallopius did his research at Padua and received the first recorded Doctor of Philosophy degree from that university.

Another very important contributor to obstetrics was Ambroise Paré (1517–1590). Both his father and his uncle were barber-surgeons, which represented the lowest grade in the medical hierarchy. The barber-surgeons wandered from place to place, treating wounds by cauterization, lancing abscesses, and applying ointments and plasters. However, many of these men performed major operations and, besides shaving their customers when not operating, let blood by application of leeches or cupping vessels. Because Paré

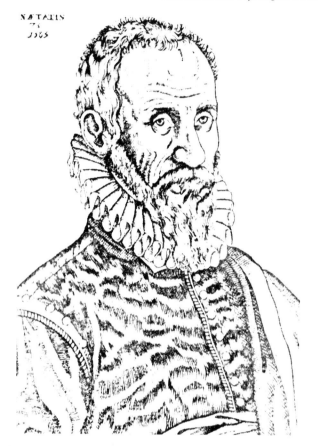

Figure 10.   Ambroise Paré. See general reference number 9, p 145.

had little or no schooling and thus was ignorant of Latin and Greek, a requisite to a university education, he became a barber-surgeon. Paré learned the art of surgery from extensive experience, initially with his relative, who was a barber-surgeon in Paris, then as a house surgeon at the Hôtel Dieu, an old hospital that had been founded by monks in the Middle Ages, and then later on as an army surgeon during the long wars of Francis I with Charles IV and Philip II and the wars of the Reformation. This humble barber-surgeon rose to become a Counselor of State and surgeon to four kings of France. All of his books were written in the vernacular rather than in Latin. Some of the most popular books of the period were those he wrote on the subject of obstetrics and pediatrics, and these went into hundreds of translations and editions and were standard texts until centuries later. He popularized the work of Vesalius and made it accessible to surgeons because he wrote it in colloquial French. Paré is best known for the re-introduction of podalic version and his convincing demonstration of its importance.

During this same period, one of the most successful textbooks to be published was entitled *Der Swangern Frauen und Hebannen Rosengarten* (*The Rose Garden of Pregnant Women and Midwives*), which was written by Eucharius Roesslin, a physician who practiced medicine at Worms and later at Frankfurt. *The Rosengarten*, as it became known, was essentially a collection of Greek and Latin works on obstetrics, rewritten in German

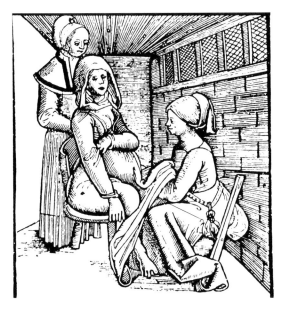

Figure 11. Typical wood cut by Konrad Merkel to illustrate obstetrical techniques, in Roesslin's book of 1513. See general reference number 10, p 76.

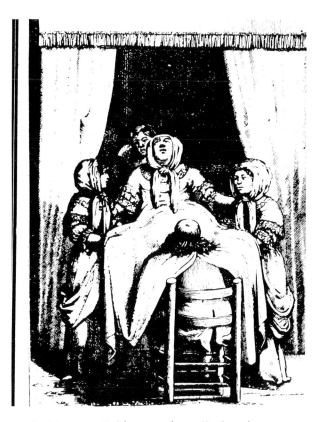

Figure 12. When a physician was called because of complications, he was never permitted directly to visualize his patients when he examined them. See general reference number 10, p 68.

and illustrated with 20 or more woodcuts by Konrad Merkel. The use of the popular language and the inclusion of illustrations most likely account for the enormous success of Roesslin's work. It was translated into several languages in several editions until as late as the eighteenth century. An English version appeared, published in 1540 by Richard Jones, called the *Byrth of Mankynd*. These books combined the Hippocratic principles with material from Soranus but did not recommend podalic version. The publication of practical books on obstetrics was matched during this period by a growing number of works on the subject of pediatrics, many of them written in the vernacular. The first English contribution was the *Boke of Children* by Thomas Phayre, published in 1545.

The publication in 1596 of a major obstetrical book by Scipione Mercurio represents the peak of the writings of the Renaissance. He described the Braxton Hicks procedure two and a half centuries before Hicks' own description. He described the cesarean section in accurate and minute detail and recommended its use in cases of contracted pelvis.

The practice of obstetrics probably represented the worst medical practice of the period. In normal labor, a woman had an even chance if she did not succumb to puerperal fever or eclampsia; historians estimate that approximately half of the women delivering during this period died from puerperal fever. In difficult labor, the woman was usually butchered to death if attended by a barber-surgeon. As a rule, only midwives attended in labor. In 1580 a law was passed in Germany preventing shepherds and herdsmen from attending obstetrical cases. The typical lying-in room was crowded with people bustling in every direction, giving the general impression of a busy marketplace. The obstetrical abuses were remedied to some extent by city ordinances governing midwives, notably those of Ratisbon (1555), Frankfort-on-the-Main (1573), and Passau (1595). Despite the lack of significant improvement in the lot of the parturient woman during the Renaissance, the foundation was laid for progress in obstetrics by advances in the

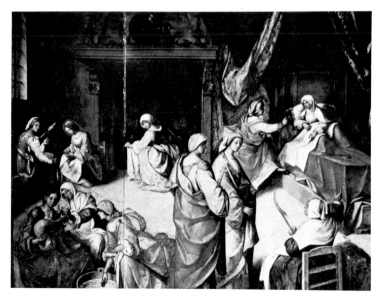

Figure 13. A typical lying-in room of the sixteenth century. See general reference number 4, vol. I, p 153.

L. I B. F R

LIBER QVARTVS.

D E V A R I E T A T I B V S N O N N A-
turalis partus, & earundem curis.

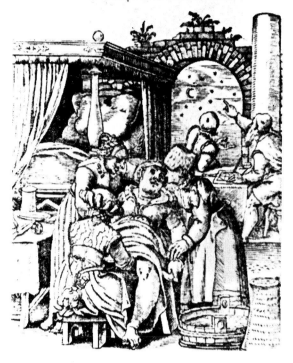

Figure 14. Midwives and astrologers, charting the obstetrical progress by the moon and the stars. From Jacob Rueff's *De Conceptu* et *Generatione Hominis*, 1587. See general reference number 10, p 108.

field of anatomy and the publication and widespread use of obstetrical writings giving a more rational basis to the field.

THE SEVENTEENTH CENTURY

Anatomy was further advanced in the seventeenth century by building upon sixteenth century progress, but was also due in large part to the discovery of the microscope by Leeuwenhoek. Among the major contributions to anatomy in the field of obstetrics and gynecology were descriptions of nabothian cysts of the cervix, the round ligament, the corpus luteum (as distinguished from an ovarian cyst), the graafian follicle, the hydatid mole, cervical polyps, and Bartholin's gland. More importantly, the seventeenth century marked the beginning of the field of physiology, the single most important event being Harvey's discovery of the circulation of blood, which occasioned revolutionary changes in the nature of subsequent medical thinking and concepts. The seventeenth century was also the occasion for a number of other firsts in clinical obstetrics and gynecology. The hypothesis was advanced that hydatidiform mole developed from placental tissue. In addition Peu recommended the immediate removal of retained placenta; it only remained for Credé, in 1853, to show how removal could be accomplished. Tubal and ovarian pregnancies were first described by Peu.

Forceps for delivery of a living child came into use in the seventeenth century, but knowledge of use of this instrument was not widespread until the eighteenth. Although forceps were used in antiquity to remove the dead fetus, the invention of the modern forceps is credited to Chamberlen I, the Elder, in 1598. It was a closely guarded family secret until the late 1700s. The invention and the development of the design and use of the forceps are correctly regarded as events of major importance in the field of obstetrics. As knowledge grew about the mechanisms of labor, there were corresponding changes and improvements in the design of forceps, changes that continued to occur into the twentieth century.

THE EIGHTEENTH CENTURY

The eighteenth century, a relatively quiet time, saw the widespread creation of hospitals and medical schools in both the Old and New World. Some advances were made in obstetrics related to the establishment of pelvimetry and increased understanding of the mechanisms of labor. The circulation of the placenta was described by Hunter. While new surgical techniques were developed in gynecology in the eighteenth and early nineteenth centuries, real progress awaited the discoveries of asepsis and anesthesia.

THE NINETEENTH CENTURY

During this century, great scientific advances were made that affected all fields of medicine. In mid-century, anesthesia was discovered in the United States, making surgical intervention a reasonable method of treatment rather than a procedure of last resort. Simpson, a Scottish obstetrician who, subsequent to the discovery of ether, used chloroform to relieve the pain of childbirth, was violently opposed by the Scottish clergy, who argued from the Scripture (Gen. 3), "Unto the woman He said, I will greatly multiply their sorrow and thy conception; in sorrow thou shalt bring forth children." Simpson had learned the Bible by rote as a child and could effectively counter each religious argument as it arose. He published a pamphlet entitled *Answer to the Religious Objections Advanced Against the Employment of Anesthetic Agents in Midwifery and Surgery*, but perhaps his best-known defense is his quote (Gen. 3): "And the Lord God caused a deep sleep to fall upon Adam and he slept, and he took one of his ribs and closed up the flesh instead thereof." Six years later, Queen Victoria received anesthesia for the birth of Prince Leopold; this effectively ended the battle against the use of anesthesia in obstetrics in England and Scotland. The same type of resistance occurred in the United States and in France against two other pioneers in obstetrical anesthesia, Channing and Fournier-Deschamps, respectively.

The names of Pasteur and Lister are associated with the understanding of the cause and prevention of infection. However, these men were preceded by men who recognized that infection was contagious and that it could be prevented by various means. Puerperal fever was, in most cases, the infection being considered. Oliver Wendell Holmes in 1843 presented *The Contagiousness of Puerperal Fever*, which he published in 1855 as *Puerperal Fever as a Private Pestilence*. In the Vienna Lying-In Hospital, Semmelweis observed that the mortality rates in the First Clinic, which was the one used for medical-student training, were considerably higher than in the Second Clinic, which was used for midwife training. Among pertinent observations that he made was that the medical students came directly from the dissection laboratory to the First Clinic. In 1847 he instructed the students to wash their hands with chlorinated lime before examining a patient, and by 1848 this simple measure had significantly lowered the mortality rate, thereby conclusively demonstrating the contagious nature of puerperal fever. In his book, *The Cause, Concept, and Prophylaxis of Puerperal Fever*, published in 1861, Semmelweis wrote that puerperal fever was a resorption fever, produced by the resorption of decomposed animal organic material, and that in most cases the material that produced childbed fever was brought to the individual from without. The abuse heaped upon Semmelweis and Holmes was greater than that suffered by the proponents of anesthesia and was, in part, due to the fact that both men suggested that the major source of the infection was the unclean hands of the examining physician. Even with the subsequent discoveries of Lister, Pasteur, and Koch, the elimination of puerperal fever as an epidemic disease was slow in coming. As late as 1914, 4664 women in the United States died from puerperal sepsis. Clearly, the contribution of these men to medicine was more apparent in the conquest or prevention of such dread diseases as tuberculosis, rabies, cholera, typhoid, diphtheria, and yellow fever.

The combined effect of the acceptance of anesthesia and asepsis led to rapid progress in dealing with problems in obstetrics and gynecology that could be attacked by surgery. However, in obstetrics cesarean section did not become widely practiced or safe until well into the twentieth century.

THE TWENTIETH CENTURY

We are of the twentieth century, and rather than recounting significant events to make us aware of the progress made, the same purpose may be served by discussing the studies conducted during this period on the placenta or the fetoplacental unit. By way of introduction, a brief discussion of the folklore surrounding the placenta will be presented.

While there is little historical evidence to indicate that physicians considered the placenta an important organ, a rather rich folklore developed concerning it, dating from antiquity. The folklore very likely derived in large part from observations of animal behavior. Many female animals eat their placenta. The female chimpanzee, during labor and following it, has been observed to drink her urine. At the turn of the century, many ranchers in the southwestern part of the United States believed that depriving a cow of her placenta rendered her infertile.

One of the earliest beliefs, which can be found in mythology and was widely held during the Middle Ages, is that a child born "with a caul"—that is, born in the amniotic sac—was supposed to be immune to death from drowning. Porters at dockside maternity hospitals today still strip the membranes from normal placentas and sell them to sailors.

As mentioned earlier, the placenta was considered unclean by many primitive tribes as well as by the people of several early civilizations. The North American Indian shared this belief. Their tribal rules called for burial of the placenta in an area where rainwater would not wash over the burial site and flow onto their croplands, because it was believed it would spoil the crops.

Several other practices that have appeared in widely separated parts of the world bear certain similarities to each other. Hungarian peasant women bite their own placentas to restore their strength lost during labor. Many Chinese women are given dried placenta to eat during a long labor to help speed up contractions. The Chinese are also known to have administered dried placenta from its own birth to a child when the child became ill later in life. The Chinese woman also had great faith in the medicinal properties of a boy's urine and used it after extended labor. Javanese women ate the placenta to increase their already proven fertility. In Iceland the placenta was held firmly on the newborn baby's head while being washed in the mother's urine. In Kalotaszeg, Russia, a woman who desired no more children would burn her placenta and place the ashes in her husband's drink. (Should we look for antispermatic compounds in ashed placentas?) These practices remind us of the abundance and diversity of hormones found in urine (particularly pregnancy urine), amniotic fluid, the cord, and the placenta.

Until the last two decades, the placenta was the least-studied organ in the human. Except in the cases of gross anatomical abnormality, the placenta was discarded in the hospital; only when pathological features were encountered was the placenta sent to the pathology laboratory. The first recognition of its value was the discovery that it contained large amounts of gamma globulin, whereupon freezers appeared on the labor and delivery floor. The gamma globulin manufacturers supplied the freezers and the residents were paid 50 cents apiece for frozen placentas. Yet the biochemistry and physiology of the placenta were relatively unknown compared to other tissues.

In 1898, Holzapfel probably made the first attempt at any physiological measurements in the placenta when he filled the membranes with water, to study the distention of the fetal sac so that he could obtain some qualitative number to correlate with various pathophysiological studies of shape and volume. This type of study did not gain any popularity until 1950, when Colmeiro-Laforet, using similar methods, reported 100 cases. In the first five decades of the twentieth century, few if any biochemical studies of the normal or pathological placenta were being done. Although it is the fastest growing nonmalignant tissue, very few investigators appeared to be interested in its synthetic properties. It was as if the taboo from antiquity had spanned the centuries to reach into the modern laboratories of the twentieth century.

In the early 1960s, a sudden change occurred in academic attitudes toward birth, delivery, and overpopulation. The basic scientist in the medical school became more aware of his clinical colleagues in the hospital across the campus. One of the few remaining virgin areas for investigation was the physiological, pharmacological, and biochemical aspects of the human fetoplacental unit. Reproductive research in all forms became the vogue rather than the unusual for yet another reason—funding! One could not study contraception alone; to help prevent overpopulation of our planet, one had to understand reproduction in general. Thus, the interest in normal and pathophysiological biochemical studies was spawned.

In 1962, after the first International Hormonal Congress in Milan, the first international meeting concerned with the biochemistry of the placenta was held. It was jointly organized by Professor Egon Diczfalusy of Sweden and Dr. Ralph Dorfman of the United States. Very soon after this meeting, various model systems began to be devised to study not only the placenta but the fetoplacental unit. Many of the well-established facts concerned with this physiological unit will be discussed in other chapters and thus we shall present only a few figures and remarks to illustrate some of the models used to elucidate biochemical questions related to the unit.

It has long been recognized that there is indeed a species difference between placentas. Even the placenta of the baboon, one of the great primates, does not closely resemble that of the human. Thus it was quickly realized that there was a need for human placental material in order to study the fetoplacental unit. In the United States in the early 1960s, few abortions were being done—primarily in cases in which the pregnancy was life threatening or for psychiatric reasons. Thus it became obvious that sufficient material for these types of studies would not be available in the United States. There were two countries at this time that not only allowed therapeutic abortions but also voluntary abortions. These countries were Sweden and Japan. Obviously, if English-speaking scientists were to travel to these countries and have these materials available, it would be far easier to communicate in Sweden than in Japan, because in Sweden English is a second language to almost everyone. A second reason that brought scientists from all over the free world to Sweden was that Professor Diczfalusy had set up a reproductive research institute at the Karolinska Sjukhuset in Stockholm. The institute was well supported; funds came from NIH, WHO, and from a private source, the Ford Foundation. These institutions not only provided the money for the research but also provided various fellowship grants to investigators during their tenure at the institute. During the decade that followed, hundreds of individuals visited and studied in Professor Diczfalusy's laboratory for periods ranging from several days to several years. The work of these investigators resulted in several hundred publications. It was the work of this large, well-coordinated team of investigators that provided much information that appears in this book.

Very early the question was raised as to why steroids such as progesterone and estriol increase during the period of human gestation. What was the precursor of these compounds? Of what physiological significance was this increased excretion of these steroids? All of these questions were investigated and, therefore, a series of model systems was devised specifically to answer them. One of the earliest systems, which had been reported at the first placental conference in Milan, was that of in vitro incubation of normal and pathological placentas. This involved removing the placenta, either mincing or homogenizing various portions, and incubating them with various radiolabeled precursors such as androstenedione to determine the percentage conversion to various estrogens. As we look back, these were the simplest forms of the investigations that were conducted, and from these evolved the more sophisticated physiological approaches to the fetoplacental problem. As knowledge accumulated, it soon became evident that the placenta and the fetus worked as a unit, in harmony, one having very specific enzyme systems not available to the other component of the unit, and vice versa. Many of these basic studies were essential in leading investigators into more analytic approaches.

A second very early model system was one devised and used extensively in Stockholm. When women were admitted to the hospital and brought to the operating room for hysterotomies, the abdomen would be opened and the umbilical cord removed through the abdominal opening. At this time a labeled substance—or several substances with different labels—was injected into the blood vessels between the placenta and the fetus. In the meantime, an indwelling catheter had been placed in the patient. After a predetermined time had passed (which allowed the free coursing of the labeled compounds between the fetus and placenta), the hysterotomy was completed. The entire conceptus was taken to the laboratory where the various metabolites and their concentration were determined in most organs and glands of the fetus. These types of experiments with use of radiolabeled compounds were done on patients who were having a hysterotomy followed by a sterilization procedure. Obviously, this type of information would lead to understanding the location of metabolism and synthesis of various compounds of interest.

Another approach used extensively was to remove the placenta after a normal birth and then perfuse it in the laboratory. Here, various compounds could be used with single or dual labels in such a manner as to study their metabolism under such conditions as hypoxia, increased temperature, altered blood flow or pH, and the like. Many of these early experiments were influential in designing model systems in later years that more nearly approached physiological conditions.

Perhaps the earliest approach to a more physiological model was that carried out by the group at the Karolinska Institutet. Here the entire conceptus was removed and perfused in the laboratory. Under these conditions, various physiological alterations, as described above, could be investigated. Early in these studies, it was noted that the presence or absence of the adrenal was significant in the type of metabolites formed. This type of in vitro experiment with the fetoplacental unit led investigators to recognize that some of the well-understood pathways for estrogen synthesis in other tissues such as the ovary and adrenal, were not being followed in the fetoplacental unit; an entirely new approach to the production of estrogens from a precursor was being used and had to be elucidated. These now well-established biosynthetic pathways will be presented in the chapters that follow.

Yet another system was devised in the United States (with the assistance of many NIH dollars) that more nearly approached a physiological system than any of those previously discussed. This was the extracorporeal perfusion apparatus: Full-term, vaginally delivered placentas, free of any abnormalities, could be put into a perfusion apparatus and perfusion of both circulatory systems—that is, from the maternal surface and from the cord—could be established within 10 minutes of parturition. Additionally, the previable, intact fetoplacental unit recovered at the time of hysterotomy could be placed in the perfusion apparatus and perfused only from the maternal surface of the artificial uterus. Normal intervillous space pressures of 3.2–3.7 kPa (24–28 mmHg) could be achieved. This would afford fetal circulation in the range of 80–100 ml/min and develop umbilical arterial pressures of 9.3–17.8/40–80 kPa (70–120/30–60 mmHg).

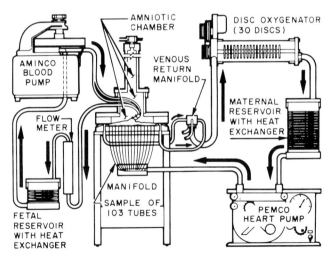

Figure 15. Overall system used in the extracorporeal perfusion apparatus. From Krantz, K. E. et al., *Am. J. Obst. Gynec.* 83, 1214 (1962).

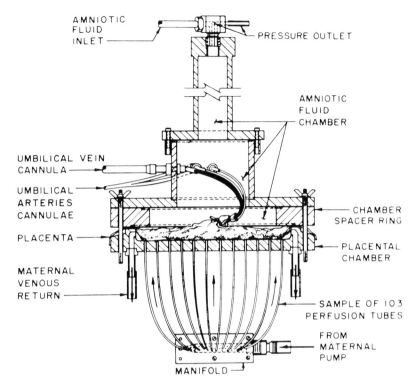

Figure 16. Detail design of the placental perfusion chamber. From Krantz, K. E. et al., *Am. J. Obst. Gynec. 83*, 1214 (1962).

During the perfusion period, recordings and correction of the pH, p_{CO_2}, p_{O_2}, temperature, gas flow, arterial pressure, and flow rate could be made. The pH, p_{CO_2}, and p_{O_2} were checked with Beckman electrodes which were set into a specially designed electrode container and read on a Beckman Model 160 physiological gas analyzer. The pH on the maternal side was maintained at 7.25 to 7.4, that on the fetal side at 7.4 to 7.3. Blood glucose and blood urea nitrogen were likewise sequentially monitored.

Yet another approach to a greater understanding of the physiology of the fetoplacental unit was to study the metabolism of a labeled compound by the in situ placenta after normal vaginal delivery of the infant. Rather easily delivered multiparous patients, in whom no oxytocics were used and who were to have a BPS after delivery, were used in these studies. Immediately after delivery of the infant, the umbilical cord was clamped and, with aseptic technique, the fetal membranes were stripped from the cord, the umbilical vessels exposed, and an 18-gauge needle was secured in each umbilical artery with a ligature and arterial clamp. A French feeding tube was inserted into the umbilical vein and secured with a suture. The cross-matched blood containing various anticoagulants and labels such as tritiated dehydroepiandrosterone (DHEA) were allowed to run into the umbilical arteries under hydrostatic pressure. As much blood as possible was allowed to drain from the cannulated venous side. The placenta was delivered spontaneously and normally after this procedure, then taken to the laboratory, where it was inserted in one of the above-described types of extracorporeal perfusion apparatus. It was then perfused under as nearly normal as possible physiological conditions—except that the blood perfusing the placenta from the fetal side was changed and the isotope likewise changed (perhaps, e.g., to [^{14}C] DHEA). These studies were carried on to compare in situ metabolism of a labeled substance with those values obtained by in vitro perfusion of the same placenta with the same substance differently labeled.

Many variations of the techniques described above were used in various institutions during the mid- and late-sixties. Eventually support was withdrawn from this type of experiment, because many considered it to be another step toward the *Brave New World* of Aldous Huxley. Although this form of artificial placenta or extracorporeal perfusion apparatus could take over oxygenation, acid-base balance, and nutritional regulation, it never seemed to enjoy widespread acceptance by those individuals concerned with physiologically significant experimentation. By the beginning of the 1970s, these types of experiments completely disappeared from the medical literature. However, during this brief period of five to eight years, some very significant data were assembled. One can easily think of research that has no comparable physiological basis, yet continuous support is forthcoming. Thus the critical cries of "unphysiological" for use of the fetoplacental unit may only be a smokescreen for a much more fundamental reason. Is it that we are experiencing a return to the Dark Ages concepts, with perhaps thoughts of experimenting with life, death, and the soul?

In closing we would like to point out that the process of birth has not changed, only the surroundings in which it takes place, the knowledge of it, and preparation for it— nor have the fears and joys to which it gives rise.

SUMMARY

A decade ago the least understood human organ was the placenta. It was usually discarded without careful examination, and very little was known concerning its many biochemical systems. Throughout history the placenta has been concealed in the shroud of superstition and folklore. To some extent, the birth process contributed to this apprehensiveness that had its origin in rudimentary facts and fiction. This still extends to modern times. The history and folklore are reviewed. Physiological and biochemical models used in the past decade are discussed in order to present a review of concepts concerning the fetoplacental unit. These include in vivo and in vitro systems, the latter designed to mimic in utero conditions.

REFERENCES

1. Guthrie, D., *A History of Medicine*, J. B. Lippincott Co., Philadelphia, Pa., 1946.
2. Garrison, F. H., *An Introduction to the History of Medicine*, W. B. Saunders Co., Philadelphia, Pa., 1913.
3. Neuburger, M., *History of Medicine*, **I** and **II**, Oxford University Press, New York, N.Y., 1910.
4. Baas, J. H., *Outlines of the History of Medicine*, **I** and **II**, R. E. Krieger Pub. Co., Inc., Huntington, N.Y., 1971.
5. Mettler, C. C., *History of Medicine*, The Blakiston Co., Philadelphia, Pa., 1947.
6. Haggard, H. W., *The Doctor in History*, Yale University Press, New Haven, Conn., 1934.
7. Haggard, H. W., *Devils, Drugs and Doctors*, Harper and Bros., New York, N.Y., 1929.
8. Margotta, R., *An Illustrated History of Medicine*, Paul Hamlyn Pub. Group, 42 The Centre, Feltham, Middlesex, U.K., 1970.
9. Cianfrani, T., *A Short History of Obstetrics and Gynecology*, Charles C Thomas, Springfield, Ill., 1960.
10. Graham, H., *Eternal Eve. The History of Gynecology and Obstetrics*, Doubleday & Co., Inc., Garden City, N.Y., 1951.

Normal Physiological Development of the Fetus

MICHAEL A. SIMMONS, M.D.

Maintenance of fetal life depends entirely on normal placental function. The placenta functions as the fetal organ of respiration, excretion, and—to a still largely unknown extent—as a primary metabolic organ. Satisfactory placental function is directly related to: (*a*) uteroplacental blood flow, (*b*) umbilical blood flow, and (*c*) membrane properties of the placenta (Figure 1).

Major differences in circulatory patterns exist between fetal and postnatal life, among them the large blood flow required to supply the placenta (i.e., the umbilical circulation). Figure 2 depicts the anatomical arrangement of the fetal circulation. In contrast to post-natal life, where the two ventricles work in series, in fetal life the ventricles are arranged in parallel, pumping blood from the great veins to the pulmonary artery and to the aorta. Total cardiac output is about 8.4 ml·kg^{-1} per second (525 ml/kg/min) (1), with 55% of this output via the left ventricle (2). The umbilical blood flow averages 3.3 ml·kg^{-1} per second (200 ml/kg/min), or nearly 40% of the total cardiac output.

In the human, the umbilical arterial blood is supplied through paired umbilical arteries, except in occasional developmental abnormalities where a single umbilical artery exists, often in association with other congenital anomalies. After perfusing the capillary bed of the intervillous space of the placenta, the blood returns to the fetus from the placenta via a single umbilical vein. Obviously, those substrates and substances passing from fetus to mother will be in higher concentration in the umbilical artery than in the umbilical vein, while substrates crossing from mother to fetus will be in higher concentration in the umbilical vein than in the umbilical artery.

The umbilical vein continues into the inferior vena cava of the fetus via the ductus venosus, a structure that functions only during fetal life and usually closes soon after birth. The ductus venosus effectively shunts most of the umbilical venous return away from the substance of the liver (3). The blood in the inferior vena cava then courses toward the right atrium. It is an unusual and quite striking feature of fetal life that there is incomplete mixing of the blood returning to the right atrium from the superior and inferior venae cavae. The more oxygenated inferior vena caval blood tends to stream directly across the foramen ovale, a small window between the right and left atria, and

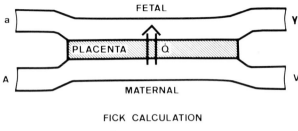

FICK CALCULATION

$\dot{Q}$ = Flow ([A]−[V])

Fetal Uptake = ([Y] − [a]) · Umbilical Flow

Figure 1.   Diagram of the placenta, showing the two perfusing blood streams (*A*, maternal: *a*, fetal), and the placental membrane.

thus into the left ventricular outflow, which supplies the cerebral and coronary circulation (*4*). The blood returning from the superior vena cava follows the usual course: right atrium to right ventricle to pulmonary artery. However, because of the high pulmonary arterial resistances existing in fetal life (in large part owing to nonexpanded lung), there is little perfusion of pulmonary tissue via the pulmonary artery; most of the pulmonary artery flow is shunted through the ductus arteriosus to the abdominal aorta.

Figure 3 is a schematic representation of the streaming that occurs in the right atrium, which selectively diverts inferior vena caval blood toward the left ventricular output and the superior vena caval blood toward the right ventricular output. Figure 4 depicts the shunt of the major portion of the pulmonary artery flow away from the lungs through the ductus arteriosus to the abdominal aorta.

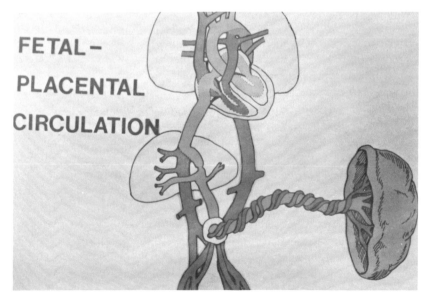

Figure 2.   The normal fetal circulatory pattern, with the most highly saturated blood returning from placenta to fetus via the large umbilical vein (larger of the two vessels to the placenta).

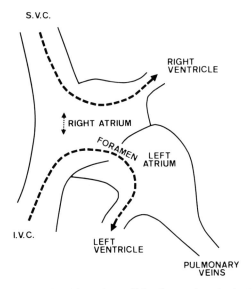

Figure 3. Preferential streaming in right atrium of blood returning via the inferior vena cava (*IVC*) and superior vena cava (*SVC*).

The specific nature of the streaming and shunting described above has important sequelae in terms of oxygen content of the perfusing blood for various regions. Figure 5 illustrates the percentage oxygen saturation to be expected in various fetal streams. The most nearly saturated blood is in the umbilical vein, where the saturation of 80% corresponds to a p_{O_2} of 4.0 kPa (30 mmHg). This blood is diluted in the inferior vena cava by venous blood returning from below the liver, so that the blood returning toward the

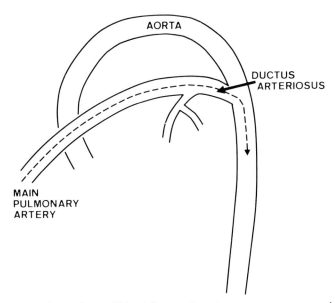

Figure 4. Ductus arteriosus shunt of blood from main pulmonary artery to aorta during fetal life.

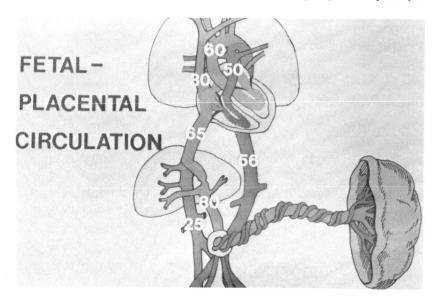

Figure 5.   Oxygen saturations in various fetal streams.

right atrium from the inferior vena cava has a saturation of ∼65%. Because of streaming of inferior vena caval blood through the foramen ovale, little mixing occurs with the less-saturated superior vena caval blood in the right atrium, and the oxygen saturation of the left ventricular outflow is ∼60%. This blood perfuses the coronary and cerebral circuits, and is much more saturated than the blood perfusing all other organs, except for the liver, which is partially perfused with umbilical venous blood.

In contrast, the superior vena caval blood proceeds through the right ventricular out-flow tract and is 50% saturated. As this flow is shunted through the ductus arteriosus, it is mixed with the outflow from the left side, with its higher oxygen saturation, so that the saturation in the abdominal aorta is ∼56%.

Although reliable data on primates are difficult to obtain, it is clear in ruminant species that the distribution of cardiac output to various organs changes with gestational age. Near term, umbilical blood flow continues to represent 40% of cardiac output, with 2% going to kidneys, 5.5% to the gastrointestinal tract, 3.5% to the myocardium, and 3.0% to the brain (1). These flows, when expressed in terms of tissue weight, show that at term, cerebral blood flow is ∼1.25 ml/g of brain, myocardial blood flow ∼2.90 ml/g of heart, and gastrointestinal blood flow ∼0.70 ml/g of tissue. The values change markedly immediately after birth, the most striking change being the removal of the placental circuit. Because of the relatively low resistance of the placental circuit, there is an associated increase in blood pressure at birth from a mean fetal pressure of ∼5.3 kPa (40 mmHg) to ∼6.7 kPa (50 mmHg) after birth.

The study of fetal uptake and excretion of substances has relied on the development of chronic animal preparations and the application of the Fick principle to the umbilical circulation. Figure 1 also illustrates the application of the Fick principle to the measurement of fetal uptake of various substances. The difference between the concentrations of a given substance in the umbilical vein and umbilical artery multiplied by the umbilical blood flow gives the net fetal uptake for that substance.

Applying such an approach to the measurement of oxygen uptake by the fetus, fetal oxygen consumptions average $\sim 0.1 \, \text{ml} \cdot \text{kg}^{-1}$ per second ($\sim 6 \, \text{ml}/\text{kg}/\text{min}$) (5), a value not far different from oxygen consumptions measured in neonates. The striking difference is, of course, the low p_{O_2} values noted in fetal life. Because of the low p_{O_2} and relatively low oxygen saturations and oxygen contents in the fetus, it has often been assumed that the fetus is "hypoxic." Several facts argue against such a view. First of all, the fetus under normal steady-state conditions is not acidotic, as it would be if true hypoxia existed. In fact, the presence of fetal acidosis has been used as a clinical tool for predicting fetal hypoxia, and thus a compromised infant. Hypoxia cannot be defined by any given absolute value of p_{O_2} or of oxygen content, but rather is more accurately viewed as the condition where oxygen demand exceeds oxygen availability. One would anticipate, then, that a fetus, if it were "hypoxic" and thus had its oxygen consumption limited by inadequate oxygen supply, would increase its oxygen utilization in response to an increased oxygen availability. Table 1 outlines data on oxygen consumption in a fetus when breathing room air as compared to breathing 100% oxygen. Fetal oxygen consumption, with the exception of two fetuses that were not in stable condition and were probably hypoxic, is not affected by increased oxygen availability (6).

The transfer of oxygen across the placenta is largely flow-limited. That is, changes in uterine or umbilical blood flow can markedly alter fetal oxygen uptake. In the previous schematic drawings of the placental circulation, the flow arrangement has been drawn as concurrent. Although there continues to be debate about the concurrent versus countercurrent arrangement of the placenta, all physiological data illustrate that the placenta behaves as a concurrent exchange system (7). Figure 6 demonstrates the relationship

Table 1. Blood Flows and Oxygen Consumption before and after Oxygen

Gest. age, days	Fetal weight, g	Inspired gas	Umbilical blood flow, ml/min	Uterine blood flow, ml/min	q_{O_2}, ml/min	Q_{O_2}, ml/min
131	2034	Air	275	1489	7.6	26.3
		Oxygen	240	1270	8.4	23.4
140	2700	Oxygen	453	549	24.4	30.9
		Air	406	478	18.5	25.4
140	2165	Air	351	632	10.7	18.6
		Oxygen	277	636	12.5	16.5
90	475	Oxygen	62	559	2.6	9.3
		Air	44	530	2.4	8.0
120	1828	Air	357	1128	12.3	27.1
		Oxygen	354	1018	11.3	27.6
120	2233	Oxygen	291	227	13.6	18.7
		Air	373	319	14.1	21.3
Term	3504	Air	546	1323	22.3	30.6
		Oxygen	583	1777	21.8	36.4
Term	4809	Oxygen	724	1613	34.1	*
		Air	539	1373	27.5	

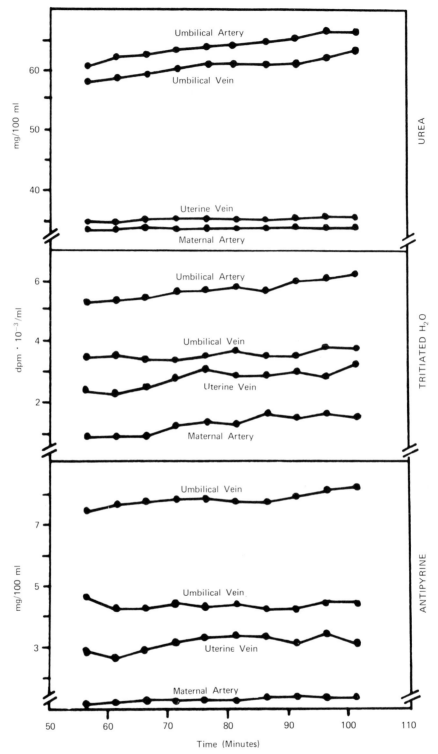

Figure 6. Concentrations of urea, ^3H_2O, and antipyrine in four blood streams during steady-state infusions to the fetus. For flow-limited substances (antipyrine, ^3H_2O), the uterine venous concentrations are slightly lower and directly proportional to simultaneous umbilical venous concentrations. For permeability-limited substances (urea) there is a large concentration gradient between the two venous streams.

between concentrations of three substances (all of which have been infused into the fetus) in the umbilical artery, umbilical vein, uterine artery, and uterine vein. It is clear that, as would be predicted by a concurrent system, the concentrations in umbilical vein and uterine vein approach each other, but never achieve equilibrium.

The relationship between maternal uterine venous p_{O_2} and umbilical venous p_{O_2} is seen in Figure 7. The umbilical venous p_{O_2} is always slightly less than the uterine venous p_{O_2}. This concept has caused much confusion in understanding fetal oxygenation. The arterial p_{O_2} of the mother can be significantly altered by increasing the concentration of oxygen in the inspired air, but such an increase is not proportionally reflected in the mother's venous p_{O_2}, and thus only small increases in umbilical venous p_{O_2} occur. Figure 8 illustrates the relationships between p_{O_2} in the uterine artery, uterine vein, umbilical vein, and umbilical artery during oxygen or air breathing. The large increase in maternal arterial p_{O_2} is not proportionally reflected in the umbilical venous p_{O_2}, which is itself directly proportional to the p_{O_2} in the uterine vein.

Similar approaches have been made to the assessment of fetal carbon dioxide excretion across the placenta (5). Carbon dioxide production (and excretion) is about $0.087 \text{ ml} \cdot \text{kg}^{-1}$ per second (5 ml/kg/min) near term gestation. Figure 9 shows steady-state data for p_{CO_2}, illustrating the constantly higher p_{CO_2} in the fetal artery than in the maternal artery. Fetal arterial p_{CO_2} averages 6.1 kPa (46 mmHg) in the absence of maternal hyperventilation, but changes in direct proportion to maternal p_{CO_2}. The pH of fetal blood is always slightly lower than is the pH of the mother's blood, although standard bicarbonate

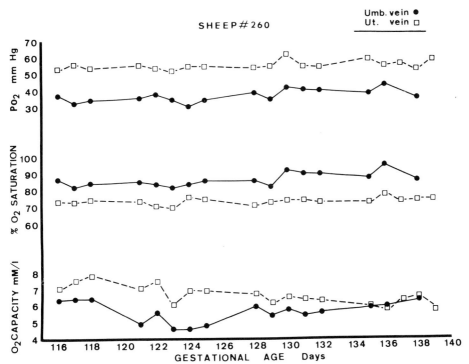

Figure 7. Relationship of oxygen saturations and p_{O_2}'s in the umbilical venous and uterine venous blood streams. Umbilical venous p_{O_2} is always less than simultaneous uterine venous p_{O_2}. Umbilical venous O_2 saturation is higher because of fetal hemoglobin.

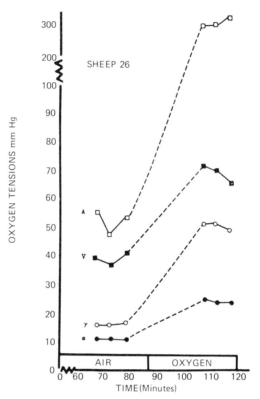

Figure 8. Effect of maternal oxygen breathing on the p_{O_2} in four blood streams (A, maternal artery; V, maternal uterine vein; γ, fetal umbilical vein; a, fetal umbilical artery). The close relationship between uterine vein p_{O_2} and umbilical vein p_{O_2} is again demonstrated. Note the relatively small increase in maternal venous p_{O_2} as compared to that in arterial p_{O_2} obtained with high oxygen breathing.

concentrations are similar. Acute changes in maternal respiratory acidosis or alkalosis are directly represented in the fetus, but because of the slow diffusion of HCO_3^- there may be paradoxical responses of fetal blood pH in the presence of acute maternal metabolic acidosis or alkalosis.

It follows from the above data on oxygen consumption and carbon dioxide production that the fetal respiratory quotient is nearly one (R.Q. = 1). Several studies in the early literature suggested that, on the basis of an R.Q. of one, the primary fetal oxidative substrate must be glucose; glucose was regarded universally as the sole significant fetal fuel (8). Recent studies have disproved this hypothesis, with data now available from chronic animal preparations.

By use of metabolic quotients (defined as the amount of a given substrate utilized, divided by total oxygen consumption), it can be clearly shown that glucose uptake by the fetus—even assuming complete oxidation of all the glucose to CO_2—can account for only 45% of oxygen consumption. Total glucose uptake approximates 0.37 μmol·kg^{-1} per second (4 mg/kg/min).

In contrast to previous assumptions, it has now been shown that amino acid catabolism comprises a significant proportion of total oxidative metabolism in the fetus. If one uses fetal urea production rates (which average 0.15 μmol·kg^{-1} per second [0.54 mg/kg/min])

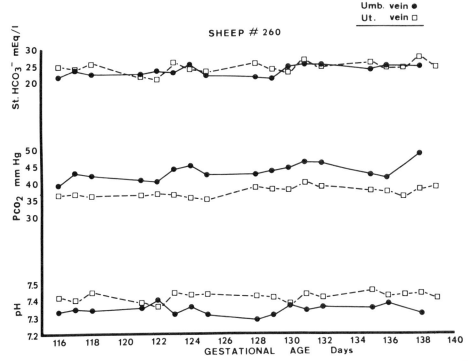

Figure 9. p_{CO_2}, pH, and HCO_3^- in the umbilical vein and uterine vein. Umbilical venous p_{CO_2} is always slightly higher than uterine vein p_{CO_2}. Fetal blood pH is usually slightly lower than maternal blood pH, but in the presence of acute maternal metabolic acidosis or alkalosis it may show a paradoxical effect.

and assumes the catabolism of amino acids from a protein of "average" composition, amino acid catabolism can be shown to account for ∼25% of fetal oxygen consumption (9).

Studies of glycerol, fructose, and fatty acid utilization by the fetus have shown that they make an insignificant contribution to total oxidative metabolism (10, 11).

Recent studies have demonstrated a significant umbilical uptake of lactate; lactate/oxygen quotients demonstrate that ∼25% of fetal oxygen consumption can be accounted for by lactate catabolism.[1] Table 2 summarizes the fetal oxidative metabolism balance sheet as it is currently perceived.

In the presence of maternal starvation, there is an even smaller contribution of glucose to total catabolism (11). Recent studies suggest that, at least in the initial stages, catabolism of amino acids may account for as much as 75% of oxygen consumption during starvation (12).

Although substrate/oxygen quotients are useful for approximating the potential contributions of various substrates to catabolism, a growing organism is obviously accumulating substrate, as well as catabolizing it. Table 3 outlines the nature of carbon balance in the sheep fetus. Although there is a net positive balance of carbon uptake, given the nature of physiological measurements, these numbers are in satisfactory agreement. The

[1] Burd, L. I., Personal communication.

Table 2.   Contributions of Various
Substrates to Fetal Oxidative Catabolism

Glucose	0.45
Amino acids	0.25
Glycerol	0.01
Fructose	0.01
Free fatty acids $(C > 5)$	0.01
Lactate	0.25
	1.00

striking feature is the amount of amino acid carbon crossing from mother to fetus. Not only is amino acid important as a catabolic substrate, but it supplies the bulk of total carbon for growth. It is also significant that the contribution of carbon from lactate is of the same magnitude as the glucose contribution; glucose is thus by no means the primary fetal fuel or anabolic substrate.

Table 3.   Carbon Balance in the Sheep Fetus

	$g \cdot kg^{-1}$ per day
Carbon accumulating in carcass	3.2
Carbon excreted as carbon dioxide	4.4
Carbon excreted as urea	0.2
	7.8
Carbon from amino acid uptake	6.7
Carbon from glucose uptake	1.8
Carbon from lactate uptake	1.3
	9.8

Similar data for nitrogen balance are presented in Table 4. There is an excess of nitrogen uptake that currently cannot be explained by accumulation or excretion. Alternative nitrogen excretion products are among the possibilities currently under investigation. If one calculates the carbon/nitrogen ratio for the excess of carbon and nitrogen, the ratio of 1:5 is unusual for any biological compound that might serve as an excretory source.

Table 4.   Nitrogen Balance in the Sheep Fetus

	$g \cdot kg^{-1}$ per day
Nitrogen accumulating in carcass	0.6
Nitrogen excreted as urea	0.36
Other nitrogen excretion products	?
	0.96
Nitrogen uptake from amino acids	2.3

Regardless of the specific substrate utilized, fetal nutrition is characterized by the provision of nutrients whose concentrations have been "buffered" by a series of organ systems. Substrate concentrations in the mother are modulated by her own hormonal and metabolic controls, primarily in the liver. Fairly stable concentrations are presented to the placenta, which itself can modulate any unusual concentration variations. Before substrates are distributed in the fetal circulation, the fetal liver can further modify their concentration in the umbilical venous drainage.

Investigation into specific organ physiology in the fetus is really just beginning. Recent work on fetal cerebral metabolism has confirmed that the glucose/oxygen quotient across the brain is 1.0, with no significant lactate production by the fetal brain. This confirms that, in the fed steady state, only aerobic catabolism of glucose occurs to any degree (13). Fetal cerebral glucose utilization is $\sim$4.6 nmol·g^{-1} per second ($\sim$5 mg/100 g/min) (14), which implies an absolute glucose utilization of 2.3 nmol/s (2.5 mg/min). Thus less than 20% of transplacental glucose uptake need be diverted to meet cerebral metabolic requirements. Even in total maternal starvation, when transplacental glucose uptake declines to 25% of normal, there is a margin of safety for cerebral glucose needs. Cerebral oxygen consumption averages 0.67 μl·g^{-1} per second (4.0 ml/100 g/min), a value comparable to that for the adult (14). Oxygen and glucose requirements of fetal brain, which are similar to those in the adult, must be met with significantly smaller quantities of the substrate in the in-flow arterial stream; cerebral uptake is critically dependent on adequate cerebral blood flow.

Fetal renal function is characterized by the excretion of large amounts of hypo-osmolar urine. Fetal urine flows average 2.4 μl·kg^{-1} per second (8.5 ml/kg/h) (15), which compares to neonatal flow rates of $\sim$0.56 μl·kg^{-1} per second ($\sim$2.0 ml/kg/h) (16). These flow rates are achieved despite low renal blood flow and a low glomerular filtration rate, and are accounted for by the decreased tubular reabsorption of water. In comparison to neonatal life, there is a significant renal sodium loss. It is clear that fairly drastic alterations in fetal renal function are required to adapt to conditions imposed by extrauterine life.

SUMMARY

In summary, dramatic changes must occur in fetal circulation, nutrition, metabolism, and organ function at the time of birth. These changes from the physiological pattern existing during intrauterine life have been named "birth shock."

REFERENCES

1. Rudolph, A. M. and Heymann, M. A., Circulatory changes during growth in the fetal lamb, *Circ. Res.* **26**, 289 (1970).

2. Dawes, G. S., *Foetal and Neonatal Physiology*, Yearbook Medical Publishers, Inc., Chicago, Ill., 1968, p. 95.

3. Lind, J. and Wegelius, C., Human fetal circulation, *Cold Spring Harbor Symposium on Quantitative Biology* **19**, 109 (1954).

4. Barclay, A. E., Franklin, K. J., and Prichard, M. M. L., *The Foetal Circulation and Cardiovascular System and the Changes They Undergo at Birth*, Blackwell Scientific Publications Ltd., Oxford, England, 1944, p. 36.

5. James, E. J. et al., Fetal oxygen consumption, carbon dioxide production, and glucose uptake in a chronic sheep preparation, *Pediatrics* **50**, 361 (1972).

6. Battaglia, F. C., Meschia, G., Makowski, E. L., and Bowes, W., The effect of maternal oxygen inhalation upon fetal oxygenation, *J. Clin. Invest.* **47**, 548 (1968).

7. Meschia, G., Battaglia, F. C., and Bruns, P. D., Theoretical and experimental study of transplacental diffusion, *J. Appl. Physiol.* **22**, 1171 (1967).

8. Dawes, G. S., *Foetal and Neonatal Physiology*, Yearbook Medical Publications, Inc., Chicago, Ill., 1968, p. 210.

9. Gresham, E. L. et al., Production and excretion of urea by the fetal lamb, *Pediatrics* **50**, 372 (1972).

10. James, E., Meschia, G., and Battaglia, F. C., A-V differences of free fatty acids and glycerol in the ovine umbilical circulation, *Proc. Soc. Exp. Biol. Med.* **138**, 823 (1971).

11. Tsoulos, N. G. et al., Comparison of glucose, fructose, and O_2 uptakes by fetus of fed and starved ewes, *Am. J. Physiol.* **221**, 234 (1971).

12. Simmons, M. A., Meschia G., Makowski, E. L., and Battaglia, F. C., Fetal metabolic response to maternal starvation, *Pediatr. Res.* **8**, 830 (1974).

13. Jones, M. D. et al., Cerebral metabolism in the sheep: A comparative study of the adult, the lamb, and the fetus, *Am. J. Physiol.* **229**, 235 (1975).

14. Makowski, E. L. et al., Cerebral blood flow, oxygen consumption, and glucose utilization of fetal lambs in utero, *Am. J. Obstet. Gynecol.* **114**, 292 (1972).

15. Gresham, E. L. et al., An evaluation of fetal renal function in a chronic sheep preparation, *J. Clin. Invest.* **51**, 149 (1972).

16. Jones, M. D., Jr., Gresham, E. L., and Battaglia, F. C., Urinary flow rates and urea excretion rates in newborn infants, *Biol. Neonate.* **21**, 321 (1972).

Present Techniques for Assessing Fetal Well-Being: An Overview

GARY K. OAKES, M.D.

RONALD A. CHEZ, M.D.

Obstetricians, like all physicians, have been searching for the ideal test to reassure themselves and their pregnant patients that all is well. Unlike other physicians, obstetricians are dealing with and caring for two patients simultaneously, mother and fetus. The mother is readily available for examination, but the fetus is relatively inaccessible. Because of this inaccessibility and a lack of technology, an ideal test for fetal assessment does not exist.

The ideal test would meet several criteria: If it is to be used to screen all patients, a test must be quite safe, noninvasive, and relatively inexpensive. To be dependable, the test must be accurate, sensitive, and reproducible. To aid in clinical decision-making, the test should be reasonably simple and, more importantly, the result should be rapidly obtainable.

In starting to develop the ideal test, we first have to see which materials are available for assay and for what purpose the assay is being designed. Both now and in the past, the principal substances used for antepartum examination have been urine and blood from the mother, and the amniotic fluid. However, biophysical approaches are currently receiving considerable investigation.

The goal of fetal assessment is threefold. First, after pregnancy is confirmed, we want to be assured that fetal growth is progressing normally. Secondly, even with a normal growth pattern, it is essential to know about fetal well-being. Thirdly, the maturity of the fetus should be defined to help determine the duration of gestation and to aid in the prognostic evaluation of the neonate.

HORMONES

Human Chorionic Gonadotropin (Choriogonadotropin)[1]

This peptide hormone, produced by the placenta, was first recognized in 1927. Its molecular weight is 46 000 and the molecule is composed of two subunits, designated A and B. It is biologically and immunologically similar to luteinizing hormone (lutropin); apparently only the B subunits differ. Recently, radioimmunoassays specific for the B subunit have allowed measurement of this hormone and the consequent diagnosis of pregnancy at 24 days, even before the first menstrual period is missed (*1*).

In normal pregnancy, the concentration of the hormone increases to a maximum at 8 to 11 weeks of gestation, then decreases somewhat and is maintained at a lower but constant value to the end of pregnancy, except for a possible slight peak at 33 to 36 weeks of gestation. Because the concentrations in blood (or in urine) are unrelated to size of fetus or placenta, measurement of this hormone has been of little help in managing high-risk pregnancy, but it does have two clinical applications. First, determination of the presence of this gonadotropin is the basis of all the immune-type pregnancy tests. Secondly, trophoblastic disease can be effectively managed chemotherapeutically according to the concentration of the gonadotropin in serum.

Large amounts of progesterone are produced by the placenta during pregnancy, and plasma progesterone concentrations increase progressively throughout gestation. Similarly, the urinary excretion of pregnanediol, the principal metabolite of progesterone, gradually increases.

Because the mother's plasma cholesterol is the principal precursor for the placental production of progesterone, an intact or functional fetus is not required for the progesterone value to be normal; only an intact, functional placenta is required. Thus measurement of progesterone is of little benefit in fetal assessment.

Measurement of another hormone produced by the placenta, human chorionic somato-mammotropin (choriomammotropin)—also called human placental lactogen—has been more helpful. It also is a protein hormone, with a molecular weight of 21 500. It shares similar chemical, biological and immunological properties with both prolactin and growth hormone (somatotropin). It functions as an insulin antagonist and may be the agent responsible for the relative glucose intolerance found during normal pregnancy.

This hormone can be measured in the mother's serum as early as the fifth week of gestation; its concentration increases progressively with advancing gestation, and values found for it significantly correlate with both placental and fetal weights (*2*). The correlation with placental weight is better and thus more significant. Certain high-risk complications of pregnancy are associated with low values. Those conditions that affect placental function—such as hypertension, severe diabetes mellitus, postmaturity, and idiopathic placental failure with its associated intrauterine fetal growth retardation—can be evaluated by this test (*3*).

In these disease states, concentrations of this hormone may abruptly decrease before fetal death occurs. Other high-risk conditions such as Rh sensitization and mild or mod-

---

[1] *Ed. note*. The names given parenthetically are those recommended by the IUPAC-IUB Commission on Biochemical Nomenclature (1974). Use of abbreviations (such as ACTH) is being discouraged, and these generally shorter and more internally consistent names are proposed to replace the nonevocative abbreviations that have proliferated.

erate diabetes mellitus are not well reflected by such measurements, because it is placental function that is really being assessed, rather than fetal condition. If the placenta is compromised to the extent that little reserve exists, then abnormal values may be seen. In addition, values for this hormone are statistically predictive of 1-min Apgar scores and intrapartum release of meconium, but cannot be correlated with 5-min Apgar scores or fetal heart rate patterns.

Estrogens

One of the most commonly used measures of fetal status is the determination of estrogen concentrations in the mother's serum or urine. This is useful because normal placental production depends on the interaction of both fetus and mother (4). The placenta cannot synthesize estrogen from simple precursors such as acetate or cholesterol; estriol production requires both placental and fetal function, in that the placenta produces pregnenolone from circulating cholesterol. Most of the pregnenolone is converted into progesterone by the placenta, but a substantial amount reaches the fetal circulation, where it is sulfated. The fetal adrenal produces dehydroepiandrosterone sulfate from the pregnenolone sulfate, some being converted by the placenta into estradiol and estrone, but most being hydroxylated at the 16 position by the fetal liver to 16-hydroxydehydroepiandrosterone sulfate. The placenta rapidly and efficiently converts this compound into estriol.

Of the major estrogens, estriol is quantitatively the most important in pregnancy. In the urine, estriol accounts for about 80% of the measurable estrogen, all of which is conjugated to sulfate or glucuronate. In contrast, no particular estrogen is predominant in plasma.

In most clinical correlations with estrogen determinations, urinary estriol is what is measured. Assay of urinary estriol has its advantages and disadvantages. The advantages include the easily determined amounts of hormone that are present, measurement of a single entity, and a partial elimination of circadian variations when a 24-h urine specimen is used. The major disadvantage is the difficulty in obtaining an accurate 24-h urine specimen. Determinations of estrogen in plasma are currently being investigated and may well replace urinary assays in the future, even though profound and frequent fluctuations in values from specimen to specimen are so common, making interpretation a problem.

There are many steps in estriol formation, and a defect in any of these can lead to low values for urinary estriol. For instance, anencephaly is associated with fetal adrenal hypoplasia, and therefore low estriol values. Subnormal 16-hydroxylation or placental sulfatase activities have been reported and are associated with low estriol values. Administration of corticosteroids to the mother causes low estriol values because of fetal adrenal suppression. Similarly, spurious estriol values can result after use of certain antibiotics by the mother. Ampicillin, phenoxymethyl penicillin, or neomycin alters the intestinal flora and inhibits normal portal recirculation of the conjugated estriol. Mandelamine®, on the other hand, destroys urinary estrogens because of its own conversion to formaldehyde (5).

In normal pregnancy, estriol concentrations in the mother's serum progressively increase during gestation. Each laboratory should establish its own mean, as well as 10th and 90th percentiles, for following such a change. If the previously mentioned factors that can cause estriol values to be low are eliminated, the fetus in greatest jeopardy is the one for which the mother's estriol excretion is about half the 10th percentile value, or whose estriol values either fail to increase or actually decrease. Estriol determination is more useful in patients with diabetes mellitus, pre-eclampsia, suspected placental insufficiency, and prolonged pregnancy. It has also been used in patients with Rh incompatibility, third trimester bleeding, and suspected fetal malformation (6).

For estriol measurement to be most effective and helpful, it must be done frequently. Indeed, daily measurements may be required to avoid missing relatively abrupt decreases in estriol values. In any one individual, even if 24-h urines are being assayed rather than plasma, there can be a 20 to 30% fluctuation from one day to the next; thus it is essential to make serial determinations if the interpretation is to be reliable.

ENZYMES

In addition to hormone determinations, many enzyme-activity assays are used, the two most widely studied being heat-stable alkaline phosphatase (EC 3.1.3.1) and diamine oxidase (EC 1.4.3.6).

Alkaline phosphatase is not a single enzyme, but rather a group of isoenzymes that differ according to the organ in which they originate. Alkaline phosphatase activity in maternal plasma progressively increases in late gestation (7), probably as a result of a contribution from the placental isoenzyme. This isoenzyme is stable at 65 °C; in contrast, alkaline phosphatases from other sources are heat labile and are almost entirely inactivated in 30 min at 56 °C. Even though the activities in the mother's plasma progressively increase during gestation, there is a very wide range of presumably normal values. Because of this wide range, the results in abnormal pregnancy states such as toxemia or diabetes mellitus are not consistent from investigation to investigation, and no critical level of enzyme activity has been established that necessarily signals a fetus in distress.

Diamine oxidase is present in plasma in relatively large amounts only during pregnancy (8). Its function is not established, but it appears to participate in the inactivation of histamine. There is a wide range of reported "normal" values, as is the case for alkaline phosphatase, but there is also considerable variation among patients at the same stage of gestation. Measurements of diamine oxidase activity are mostly of use in the first 20 weeks of gestation. In cases of threatened abortion, a progressive increase in diamine oxidase has usually been associated with the continuation of pregnancy, whereas a decrease has been associated with imminent abortion. Difficulty arises when one must interpret minimally increasing or static diamine oxidase values. Both patterns have been associated with normal pregnancy and impending abortion. The interpretation of information on plasma diamine oxidase activity after 24 weeks of gestation is fraught with uncertainty.

Direct monitoring of the fetus during labor has been a significant advance in the past decade. However, we cannot wait until labor begins to determine fetal status. In fact, many fetuses cannot tolerate labor and should not be subjected to it. Labor is a nonsteady state and may not be an appropriate time for evaluation of the basal condition.

OXYTOCIN CHALLENGE TEXT

An outgrowth of intrapartum fetal monitoring has been the development of the oxytocin (vasotocin) challenge test (9).

Uterine contractions can be stressful to the fetus. During a contraction, uterine blood flow decreases. The maternal blood flow through the intervillous space is inversely proportional to the intrauterine pressure. With this decreased blood flow, there can be a disruption in maternal-fetal gas exchange, resulting in a temporary hypoxic state. Depending on its well-being and reserve, the fetus may show a bradycardia.

The test consists of the concomitant observation of uterine contractions and fetal heart-rate pattern as early as 28 weeks of gestation. The test is performed by combining a 10-min baseline recording of fetal heart rate (by use of an external ultrasound monitoring system) with an abdominal tocodynamometer, which assesses uterine activity. If there are spontaneously fewer than three contractions in a 10-min period, 0.5 mU oxytocin/min is given intravenously, and this amount is doubled every 15 to 20 min until contractions last 30 to 80 s.

A positive test is defined as one showing persistent late fetal heart-rate decelerations occurring with most contractions. A negative test reveals no late decelerations and provides assurance that the fetus is likely to tolerate labor if it ensues within six to seven days.

There are three disadvantages of the test. First, the procedure is long and technically demanding; it takes about 2 h and requires either the physician or an associate trained in this area to be with the patient constantly. Secondly, about one of every seven tests is unsatisfactory because of technical problems or hyperstimulation, and the test must be repeated. Thirdly, a borderline or suspicious result occurs in about 5% of tests—a suspicious result consisting of occasional late decelerations in fetal heart rate that are not persistent or consistent from contraction to contraction; this result also requires a repeat test in 24 h.

A positive result, when combined with estriol measurements and maturity assessment can help the clinician decide on the timing of delivery as well as the obstetrical procedure to be used.

A simpler evaluation by use of this system may be made by correlating fetal heart rate with fetal movement: Transient fetal heart-rate accelerations during fetal movement and the presence of good beat-to-beat variability are considered to be a reliable sign of fetal well-being.

BIOPHYSICAL TECHNIQUES

Ultrasound

Pulsed ultrasound consists of short pulses of low-intensity, high-frequency sound. In the clinical application, these pulses are transmitted from a transducer through the maternal abdomen. The sound wave is partly reflected at tissue interfaces and tissue discontinuities. When the ultrasound beam strikes an interface at a 90° angle, the reflected echo is received by the same transducer. The ultrasonic energy is converted into electrical energy and, after amplification, is displayed in a memory-tube oscilloscope.

For clinical application, two different modes of ultrasound are used: A-scan is used for unidimensional measurements, and the echos are displayed as vertical deflections on a horizontal time base; B-scan produces a two-dimensional image by tracing the exact anatomical outline of a structure.

There is a wide range of ultrasound application in obstetrics, because it is simple, noninvasive, nontraumatic, and apparently harmless to fetus and mother. The major disadvantage is cost. Not only the equipment but the personnel time required is expensive. The major current uses of ultrasonography are the following.

Diagnosis of early pregnancy.   The gestational sac may become visible as early as five weeks from the last menstrual period, and consistently at 10 weeks. Embryonic growth can be assessed by serially measuring crown-rump length during the first trimester.

Estimation of fetal size.   Fetal growth is best evaluated by serially measuring the fetal biparietal diameter (*10*). This is done by scanning the fetal head longitudinally, to establish the angle it makes with the vertical axis. A transverse scan is performed at this angle through both parietal eminences. A strong midline echo that bisects the two parietal echos is noted when the transverse section is correct.

The biparietal diameter increases progressively throughout gestation. The accuracy of this measurement is shown by the fact that in 95% of cases, two such measurements made on the same occasion will differ by <1 mm. Because of this accuracy, the measurement is sometimes used to assess maturity and size.

Placental localization.   The location of the placenta can be demonstrated after only 16 weeks of gestation. To do so is essential in patients with late gestational vaginal bleeding and before doing an amniocentesis. In late pregnancy the placenta can be localized with 99% accuracy.

Diagnosis of multiple pregnancy.   Early in pregnancy, a multiple gestation can be recognized by the appearance of more than one gestational sac. After 16 weeks, the diagnosis is made when more than one fetal head or thorax is seen.

Fetal cranial malformation.   The two common cranial malformations, anencephaly and hydrocephaly, can be diagnosed, anencephaly being characterized by an absence of the normal cephalic outline and hydrocephaly by comparing serial values for biparietal diameter with fetal thoracic diameters and noting the discrepancy from normal.

Diagnosis of intrauterine fetal demise.   In gestations of more than 14 weeks' duration, fetal death can be diagnosed 12 to 48 h after it occurs. A coarsening and thickening of the fetal outline in addition to a collapse of the fetal thorax and skull are seen.

Diagnosis of hydatidiform mole.   The ultrasound pattern in hydatidiform mole is extremely characteristic and the diagnosis very accurate. Multiple spicules are seen, which fill the uterine cavity. Each spicule represents a vesicle.

A modification of traditional ultrasound technique, as well as a new frontier in antenatal fetal assessment, is used to evaluate fetal respiration. It had been previously speculated that fetal respiratory movement occurred, but Dawes (*11*) first observed episodic breathing in utero in fetal lambs.

An ultrasonographic A-scan technique has been used in the human (*12*). An ultrasonic beam is directed at the fetal thorax. The anterior chest wall reflection is identified, and changes in this echo can be recorded continuously to give data from which a quantitative measure of respiratory rate and a qualitative measure of the depth are obtained.

Human fetal breathing has been detected as early as 13 weeks of gestation. The rate is irregular up to about 28 weeks. From 28 to 32 weeks, the rate becomes regular. After 32 weeks, fetal breathing is present about 70% of the time, at a rate of 30 to 70/min. It seems to be correlated with fetal rapid-eye-movement sleep. The per cent occurrence of fetal breathing within a measured time period varies with many physiologic indexes, which are now being investigated. It seems to be decreased in high-risk pregnancies, including diabetes mellitus, hypertension, mothers with infants that are small for gestational age, and during labor (*13*).

Occasional sighs and gasps are normal, but when the incidence of gasps exceed 10% of the inspirations, and the overall breathing rate decreases, immediate delivery is indicated.

ELECTROCARDIOGRAPHY

Another biophysical assessment tool that has evolved from fetal electrocardiographic monitoring is the analysis of the individual events within the fetal cardiac cycle. Although still in the preliminary stages of investigation, this work holds much promise.

The fetal electrocardiogram is simultaneously coupled with the arterial pulse and a phonocardiogram. The individual cardiac valvular events are identified by electronic filtration of the signal. .

Many time-periods have been studied, but the pre-ejection period appears to be the most valuable. This period is defined as the interval from beginning of ventricular depolarization (beginning of the Q-wave) to the onset of left ventricular ejection (aortic valve opening). Because the length of the pre-ejection period depends on myocardial contractility as well as on aortic diastolic pressure and ventricular filling pressure, it is a reflection of cardiac function. In the fetus, these factors are sensitive to changes in fetal environment including arterial pressure, p_{O_2} and pH. The period is independent of heart rate (*14*). C. B. Martin et al. (*15*) have found that in rhesus monkeys it increases with gestational age. Their most exciting finding is that the pre-ejection period correlates with fetal pH through the 7.0 to 7.4 range, and increases with progressive acidosis. With this type of evaluation, it may be possible in the future to assess antepartum fetal pH noninvasively.

SUMMARY

None of the tests now used for fetal assessment constitutes a single tool that is ideal and practicable for all patients. At present, it is necessary to have a multitude of tests and procedures available. It would be ideal to perform several serial biochemical and biophysical tests on all pregnant women, but this is not feasible in practice. Therefore, clinical research must continue to be principally directed toward developing a more ideal intrauterine fetal assessment test as well as evaluating various combinations of tests that are now available, to increase the effective yield of information.

REFERENCES

1. Jaffe, R. B., Lee, P. A., and Midgley, A. R., Jr., Serum gonadotropins before, at the inception of, and following human pregnancy, *J. Clin. Endocrinol. Metab.* **29**, 1281–1283 (1969).

2. Spellacy, W. N. et al., Control of human chorionic somatomammotropin levels during pregnancy, *Obstet. Gynecol.* **37**, 567–573 (1971).

3. Spellacy, W. N. et al., Value of human chorionic somatomammotropin in managing high-risk pregnancies, *Am. J. Obstet. Gynecol.* **109**, 588–598 (1971).

4. Beling, C. G., Estrogens. In *Endocrinology of Pregnancy*, F. Fuchs, and A. Klopper, Eds., Harper & Row, New York, N.Y., 1971, pp. 32–65.

5. Tikkanen, M. J. and Adlercreutz, H., Effects of antibiotics on estrogen metabolism, *Br. Med. J.* **ii**, 369 (1973). Abstract.

6. Klopper, A., The assessment of feto-placental function by estriol assay, *Obstet. Gynecol. Survey* **23**, 813–838 (1968).

7. Lee, A. B. H. and Lewis, P. L., Alkaline phosphatase activity in normal and toxemic pregnancies, *Am. J. Obstet. Gynecol.* **87**, 1071–1073 (1963).

8. Weingold, A. B., Enzymatic indices of fetal environment, *Clin. Obstet. Gynecol.* **11**, 1081–1105 (1968).

9. Ray, M., Freeman, R., Pine, S., and Hesselgesser, R., Clinical experience with the oxytocin challenge test. *Am. J. Obstet. Gynecol.* **114**, 1–9 (1972).

10. Campbell, S. and Newman, G. B., Growth of the fetal biparietal diameter during normal pregnancy. *J. Obstet. Gynaecol. Br. Commonw.* **80**, 680–686 (1973).

11. Dawes, G. S., Breathing and rapid-eye-movement sleep before birth. In *Foetal and Neonatal Physiology*, Cambridge University Press, London, 1973, pp. 49–62.

12. Boddy, K. and Robinson, J. S., External method for detection of fetal breathing in utero, *Lancet* **ii**, 1231–1233 (1971).

13. Boddy, K. and Mantell, C. D. Observations of fetal breathing movements transmitted through maternal abdominal wall, *Lancet* **ii**, 1219–1220 (1972).

14. Organ, L. W., Bernstein, A., Smith, K. C., and Rowe, I. H., The pre-ejection period of the fetal heart: patterns of change during labor, *Am. J. Obstet. Gynecol.* **120**, 49 (1974).

15. Murata, Y., Martin, C. B., and Petrie, R. H., Cardiac systolic time intervals in fetal monkeys, *Gynecol. Invest.* **5**, 32 (1974).

Placental Insufficiency Syndromes

LAURENCE I. BURD, M.D.

During its life span of 274 days, the human placenta functions as an organ of nutrient exchange, metabolic conversion, respiration, excretion, hormone production, and immunological protection (Figure 1). The fetus depends on the placenta for normal growth and development; optimal placental performance, in turn, depends on a homeostatic maternal environment. Placental dysfunction occasionally results from intrinsic disease, but more commonly it reflects maternal pathophysiology.

The transfer of substrates from mother to fetus depends on placental blood flow and permeability of the placental membrane. In a discussion of placental insufficiency, these two phenomena must be considered.

Estimates of uterine blood flow in humans (1) indicate that total flow increases throughout gestation; however, because of inadequate mixing of indicator substances, as well as instability of the patient during the period of experimentation due to stress and anesthesia, results among individual investigators vary markedly. Studies of uterine blood flow in sheep (2), made with the use of radio-labeled microspheres, indicate that uterine blood flow increases throughout pregnancy, with a proportionately greater increase in flow to the placental site late in pregnancy, concomitant with the greatest increase in fetal weight.

Studies of factors that control the uterine circulation reveal physiological mechanisms that are unique to this vascular bed. During pregnancy, uterine vessels appear to be maximally dilated and do not respond with further dilatation to the effects of reduced perfusion pressure, hypoxia (3), or hyperoxia (4). Estrogen, which produces marked vasodilatation in the nonpregnant animal (5), has little effect late in pregnancy (6). Furthermore, the uterine vessels show no response to β-adrenergic or parasympathetic nerve stimulation (7). Any reduction of maternal systemic perfusion pressure produces a proportional decrease in uterine blood flow, which demonstrates that the uterine circulation lacks autoregulation (8). Factors that decrease blood flow are: stimulation of sympathetic nerves (9), administration of epinephrine or norepinephrine (10), and myometrial contractions (11). Such controlling factors frequently play a role in the development of acute placental insufficiency.

Placental permeability is determined in part by surface area and thickness. More solute will be transferred by a large placenta with a thin membrane than by a small placenta with a thick membrane. It is important as well to consider the concentration difference

PLACENTAL FUNCTIONS

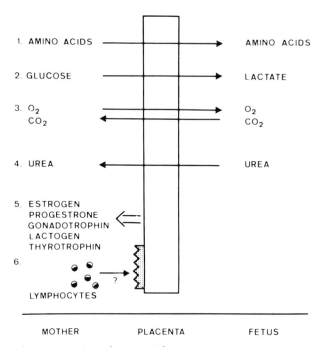

Figure 1. Schematic representation of placental functions: *1*, nutrient exchange; *2*, metabolic conversion; *3*, respiration; *4*, excretion; *5*, hormone production; *6*, immunological protection.

across the placenta. We have found determination of placental clearance to be useful in describing the efficiency with which the placenta transfers various substrates (*12*). Placental clearance, like renal clearance, is a measurement of the excretion of a molecule by an organ versus the concentration of that molecule in the plasma that supplies that organ (Figure 2). The transfer of a molecule across the placenta is determined by the arteriovenous difference in the concentration of that molecule times the rate at which the molecule is delivered to the placental exchange surface (i.e., the blood flow). Concentrations in either the uterine vein or the umbilical artery—and their flow rates—are used, according to the direction of transfer. Figure 3 illustrates the expression of placental clearance when

$$\text{Placental Clearance} = \frac{F(A-V)}{a-A_2}$$

$$\text{Clearance} = \frac{\text{excretion}}{\text{plasma conc.}}$$

$$\text{Renal Clearance} = \frac{U \times V}{P}$$

Figure 2. Two expressions of clearance. F, umbilical blood flow; A, concentration of substance in umbilical arterial whole blood; V, in umbilical venous whole blood; a, in umbilical arterial plasma; A_2, in uterine arterial plasma; U, in urine; V, urine volume; P, concentration of substance in plasma.

$$C_{\text{Placental Clearance}} = \frac{F_{\text{Umbilical Blood Flow}} \times \left(A_{1 \text{ Umbilical Arterial Conc.}} - V_{1 \text{ Umbilical Venous Conc.}}\right)}{A_{1 \text{ Umbilical Arterial Conc.}} - A_{2 \text{ Uterine Arterial Conc.}}}$$

Figure 3. Placental clearance for a compound that is transferred from fetus to mother.

a molecule travels from fetus to mother. Antipyrine and tritiated water (*13*) are substances that have maximum permeability. Like these substances, oxygen is rapidly transported across the placenta, and its clearance is determined primarily by blood flow (flow-limited clearance) (Figure 4). Na^+, Cl^-, and urea cross the placenta less rapidly, and their clearance is determined by permeability (permeability-limited clearance). Changes in placental blood flow will influence their transport little. Recently, it has been found that glucose, a major fetal substrate (*14*), is permeability limited (*15*). These concepts provide insight into the pathophysiology of acute and chronic placental insufficiency syndromes. Fetal growth, which depends on adequate glucose transport, is frequently disturbed when placental permeability is diminished. Intrauterine growth retardation is the hallmark of chronic placental insufficiency. Oxygen clearance, which has been found to be flow limited, decreases markedly when uterine blood flow is diminished. Abrupt disturbances in uterine blood flow result in acute placental insufficiency and produce the classic signs of fetal hypoxia: an altered fetal heart rate and passage of meconium. When placental insufficiency occurs, it may be either chronic or acute; most often, it is a combination of both.

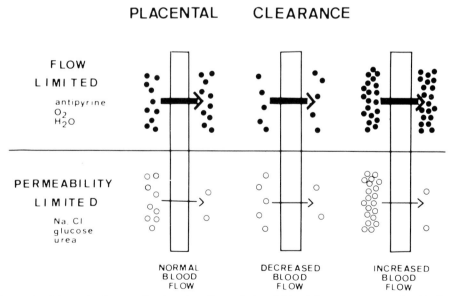

Figure 4. Schematic diagram showing the effects of altered blood flow on compounds with flow-limited clearance or permeability-limited clearance.

PLACENTAL FUNCTION AND NORMAL FETAL GROWTH

The rate of fetal growth evidently decreases late in the third trimester (16). Gruenwald (17) confirmed this finding, noted that placental growth rate slows somewhat earlier than fetal growth rate, and suggested that the decrease in fetal growth rate is caused by a degree of placental insufficiency that occurs in all pregnancies near term. Contrary to this opinion, Aherne and Dunnill (18) demonstrated by placental morphometry that the area of fetomaternal exchange, the chorionic villous surface area, increased progressively until term, suggesting increasing placental function throughout gestation. This finding has been confirmed in our laboratory by Kulhanek et al. (19), who showed that placental urea permeability increased until term although placental growth had been markedly curtailed. Such evidence appears to indicate that the changed fetal growth rate that occurs in normal pregnancies at term is not the result of decreasing placental function.

CHRONIC PLACENTAL INSUFFICIENCY

In certain conditions there is an increased incidence of fetal growth retardation—as well as perinatal morbidity and mortality—which is clearly based on a "preplacental" limitation of substrate. These include maternal malnutrition (20), hypoxia at high altitude (21), and anemia (22). Diseases of purely placental origin, such as chorioangiomas (23), are rare. Although placental pathology has been described in diabetes mellitus (24) and collagen diseases (25), the physiological significance of such pathology is unclear. More cogent evidence of placental insufficiency has been gathered for hypertensive diseases of pregnancy, idiopathic intrauterine growth retardation, and prolonged pregnancy.

Hypertensive diseases of pregnancy.   An examination of the records for all deliveries at Colorado General Hospital from 1958 through 1970 reaffirms the finding of increased perinatal mortality in hypertensive mothers. Low et al. (26) found that intrauterine growth frequently is retarded if the mother is hypertensive, and the degree of growth retardation appears to be related to the duration and severity of hypertension. Evidence for decreased blood flow has been obtained in humans by use of the indicator-disappearance technique (27) and angiography (28). The total placental surface area of exchange is diminished as a result of a decrease in the volume of the intervillous space (18). The frequency with which placental infarction is observed varies among investigators (29).

Idiopathic intrauterine growth retardation.   Newborns who are considered to be growth retarded are those below the 10th percentile for weight at birth. If retardation is severe, there will be a similar decrease in height, head circumference, and in weight/height ratio (30). The increased mortality described for this group of infants was noted in our statistical review (31). Besides the preplacental factors listed above, inadequate intrauterine growth has been associated with fetal infections such as rubella (32) and with chromosomal abnormalities. In more than half of the cases, there is no clear etiological factor.

Studies of multiple gestations by McKeown and Record (33) demonstrate that the degree of growth retardation increases with the number of fetuses contained within the uterus. Limitation of fetal growth by placental size was suggested by finding that monozygotic twins sharing the same placenta were smaller than dizygotic twins of different placentas. Winick (34) supports this hypothesis by finding that growth-retarded infants without major congenital anomalies are born with placentas that weigh less because of a decreased number of cells and not because of a subnormal cell size. Aherne and Dunnill (*18*) report a 40% decrease of trophoblastic surface area in normotensive women with growth-retarded infants. Their studies suggest that placental permeability is limited by reduced placental size.

Prolonged pregnancy. Clifford (*35*) called attention to the problem of the pregnancy that lasts beyond 42 weeks of gestation. He described the "dysmature" infant—born long, thin, with meconium staining of the skin and nails, and decreased subcutaneous tissue—and considered it to be a product of decreased placental function. An increased mortality rate is reported for this group of fetuses (*36–38*); this is so for our population as well. Particular attention has been called to the high incidence of antepartum still-births (*39*). Anatomical or physiological studies of the placenta thus far are unable to demonstrate evidence of decreasing function during this period.

ACUTE PLACENTAL INSUFFICIENCY

Premature placental separation, abruptio placentae, results in a rapid, sudden decrease in placental function. Other causes of acute insufficiency are related to abrupt changes in placental blood flow owing to maternal hypotension produced by hypovolemia, spinal anesthesia, or the supine hypotension syndrome. Because the uterus lacks the ability for autoregulation, a decrease in systemic pressure results in a parallel decrease in uterine blood flow. During labor, tetanic uterine contractions, either occurring spontaneously or induced by uterotonic agents such as oxytocin, will also decrease placental blood flow and result in acute placental insufficiency.

The Clinical Diagnosis of Placental Insufficiency

Measurement of placental blood flow and placental clearance of various substrates would be an ideal way to monitor a pregnancy with suspected placental insufficiency. Because this requires invasive techniques, the assessment of both factors remains beyond the reach of the clinician; however, several laboratory aids have been developed in the last decade that can be used in the management of pregnancies complicated by placental insufficiency.

Traditionally, decreasing placental function is diagnosed when the uterine fundus fails to reach its expected height. Other classical signs are meconium staining of the amniotic fluid after rupture of membranes, fetal bradycardia, or tachycardia upon auscultation between uterine contractions. The use of ultrasound, estriol determinations, amnioscopy, fetal heart-rate monitoring, and fetal scalp-blood sampling have provided techniques to help refine our appraisal of placental function.

Ultrasound. Intrauterine growth retardation is difficult to recognize from clinical criteria alone. During a one-year period in our clinic, only half of such infants were predicted from uterine measurements, and, conversely, 75% of the patients who were thought to have growth-retarded fetuses delivered infants of normal size. Although Treolar (*40*) states that the patient's menstrual history is reliable for the calculation of gestational age, we find it to be invalid for about 20% of the patients followed in our clinic. In cases where the size of the uterus is inappropriate for the calculated gestational age we have found serial ultrasonic measurements of biparietal diameter to be the most helpful in confirming growth retardation or miscalculated dates. The principle of this technique is that ultrasonic waves are generated in a transducer by an electric current striking a piezo-electric crystal. These waves can be focused to a point, and when they strike a tissue inter-face at a 90° angle they are reflected back to the transducer, producing an electrical im-pulse that is displayed on a cathode-ray oscilloscope. In this way the intrauterine contents can be visualized. The transducer head is moved across the patient's abdomen at various angles so that the ultrasonic impulse can be reflected at all interfaces. The position of the fetus and placenta can thus be determined. When the fetal head is identified, the biparietal diameter can be measured. There are tables for correlating consecutive biparietal diameter measurements with gestational age (41). Serial ultrasonic measurements are required to determine the intrauterine growth rate. The value of this technique has been demon-strated by Campbell and Dewhurst (42), who were able to identify 70% of the growth-retarded infants from a selected population.

Estriol.   Production of estriol during pregnancy requires contributions from both fetus and placenta (43). Androgens, predominately dehydroepiandrosterone and 16-hydroxy-dehydroepiandrosterone, as sulfates, are produced by the fetal adrenal. Dehydroepi-androsterone is hydroxylated at carbon number 16 by the fetal liver (44). Arriving at the placenta, these compounds are then desulfated by placental sulfatases and then aromatized to estriol (45). Estriol is conjugated by the maternal liver, principally to the glucuronide, which is excreted in the urine (46). The placenta can metabolize androgens from both mother and fetus to estriol; however, quantitatively, the fetal precursors are more im-portant. The amount of estriol produced by the placenta can be measured in the urine (47), plasma (48), or amniotic fluid (49). Most laboratories evaluate the 24-h urinary excretion of estriol by the mother; however, measurement of concentrations in plasma have proved equally useful (50).

During a normal pregnancy, estriol excretion increases weekly (51). Each laboratory must establish its own normal values for each gestational age. Greene and Touchstone (52) demonstrated abnormally low estriol excretion in patients whose pregnancies were complicated by diseases associated with placental insufficiency. They postulated that estriol formation is decreased if umbilical blood flow is decreased, if there is trophoblastic damage, or if the metabolism or excretion of estriol is abnormal. Decreased uterine blood flow must be considered as well, and may explain why patients with pre-eclampsia have low estriol excretion (53). In cases of prolonged pregnancy, estriol determinations can be used to identify the fetus at risk (54). Values for 24-h urines are usually decreased when there is growth retardation (55). When these clinical problems exist, urine or plasma from the mother should be serially sampled. If normal values are obtained, the pregnancy may be continued without fear of an intrauterine demise; however, if a decreasing curve is plotted for consecutive values, delivery should be considered. An accurate estimation of gestational age is essential, because the detrimental effects of prematurity must be balanced against those of placental insufficiency. Estimation of the concentration of creatinine (56) or bilirubin (57), the percent of fat-staining cells (58), or calculation of the lecithin/sphingomyelin ratio (59) in the amniotic fluid may also be helpful when early delivery is contemplated.

Amnioscopy and amniocentesis.   These techniques can be used to detect meconium in the amniotic fluid before the membranes rupture. The prevalence of meconium-stained amniotic fluid is 1.3% in uncomplicated pregnancies and increases to as high as 20% in pregnancies complicated by placental insufficiency (60). In a series of patients whose amniotic fluid was clear before delivery, the perinatal mortality rate was 0.4%, compared with 6.1% when meconium was found (61). Although the increased incidence of meconium staining has been confirmed in problem pregnancies, a precise explanation of its mechanism is still lacking. It has been suggested from experimental studies in animals subjected to hypoxia that there is an increase in peristalsis and relaxation of the anal sphincter.

Amnioscopes (conical-shaped endoscopes) are inserted into the cervix by direct or indirect application, the amniotic membrane is observed, and the color of the amniotic fluid noted. If there is some question about the color observed, amniocentesis is performed to confirm the diagnosis. Amnioscopy is the preferred technique because it provides less risk to the infant.

In cases of toxemia, or after 36 weeks of gestation, or when pregnancy continues after the 10th day of the expected day of confinement, it has been recommended (62) that amnioscopy be done every other day. The role of this procedure, when fetal growth retardation is suspected, is less well defined. If meconium is identified, the course of action remains controversial. Saling (62) recommends immediate rupture of membranes, fetal scalp-blood sampling, and induction of labor. Others regard this test as a screening procedure to indicate further methods of fetal monitoring.

The fetal stress test. Several procedures have been developed to artificially decrease fetal oxygenation in utero and produce changes in fetal heart rate. These include administration of 10% (by vol) oxygen (63) to the mother, and the Master's two-step exercise test (64). A new technique, the fetal tolerance test (65), also called the "oxytocin challenge test," has recently been developed. As noted previously, myometrial contractions decrease placental blood flow. If the fetus has been exposed to placental insufficiency, small transient decreases in flow will result in further hypoxia, which is demonstrated by altered heart rate and a characteristic pattern of bradycardia. Myometrial contractions are produced by the administration of oxytocin over a 10- to 30-min period. The relationship between fetal heart rate and uterine contractions is displayed on a pen recorder. It has been suggested that if there are no alterations in heart rate there is little likelihood that intrauterine death will occur during the following week. Freeman et al. (66) made the interesting observation that the stress test frequently becomes abnormal before abnormal estriol excretion. This observation attests to the diversity of placental function.

MONITORING THE HIGH-RISK FETUS DURING LABOR

Biophysical measurements. The use of the fetal stress test is an outgrowth of the widespread use of fetal heart-rate monitoring during labor. Auscultation of the fetal heart rate at this time has been practiced in obstetrics since the nineteenth century. Counted between uterine contractions, the normal heart rate is considered to be between 120 and 160 beats per minute. With the development of techniques to obtain the fetal electrocardiogram and by utilizing methods of rate averaging, it has been demonstrated (67, 68) that characteristic changes can occur in the fetal heart-rate pattern during the time of a uterine contraction. Signals from the fetal heart can be obtained from the maternal abdomen by ultrasound, phonocardiography, or electrocardiography. Uterine contractions can be timed by a tocodynamometer, which registers changes in the contour of the maternal abdomen. The most reliable method of obtaining the relationship between fetal heart rate and uterine contractions is by directly applying an electrode to the presenting part of the fetus and inserting a catheter into the amniotic cavity to measure intrauterine pressure. Three types of relationships have been described. Early decelerations (68) or Type I dips (67) occur when there are uniform decreases in the fetal heart rate that correspond in time sequence to increases in intra-amniotic pressure. Late decelerations (68) or Type II dips (67) are uniform decelerations that are out of phase with the increase in intra-amniotic pressure; the nadir of the fetal heart rate occurs well after the peak of the contraction. Variable decelerations are nonuniform and occur at different intervals during a contraction.

The physiological mechanisms involved in producing these heart-rate patterns have been clarified to some degree. Early decelerations appear to be caused by increased intracranial pressure, which results from compression of the fetal head (69). Variable decelerations have been shown to be secondary to compression of the umbilical cord (70). Late decelerations are thought to be caused by myocardial hypoxia (71). Various authors agree that the appearance of late decelerations is an ominous sign that reflects reduced placental blood flow and fetal hypoxia. Severe variable decelerations and late decelerations have been associated with fetal acidosis (72), depression (73), and death. Another important point to be noted is the amount of variability that occurs in the heart-rate pattern. The normal beat-to-beat changes are expected, due to the influence of the central nervous system on the heart (74). Normal variability ranges from 5 to 10 beats per minute; its absence suggests fetal depression (75). The most useful finding during fetal heart rate monitoring is normal beat-to-beat variation in the absence of bradycardia. If no abnormal patterns are present, Schifrin et al. (76) found that 99% of infants will have a normal Apgar score. If ominous patterns are present, the ability to predict fetal outcome falls to 20%. The difficulty appears to be in relating the rate and severity of abnormal patterns to the degree of intrauterine hypoxia. When late or severe variable patterns are present, fetal scalp-blood should be sampled and analyzed (see below), to confirm the diagnosis of fetal distress.

Biochemical monitoring.   Saling (62) first demonstrated that microsampling of fetal scalp-blood during labor provides reliable information regarding fetal well-being, particularly in cases where there are clinical signs of fetal distress. He showed that during labor there was a decrease in O_2 saturation, p_{O_2}, and pH, and an increase in p_{CO_2} and base deficit. These changes were attributed to intermittent decreases in uterine and umbilical blood flow during the period of uterine contractions. Normal values during labor are: O_2 saturation = 30–50%, p_{O_2} = 2.4–2.9 kPa (18–22 mmHg), pH = 7.25–7.35, p_{CO_2} = 5.3–6.7 kPa (40–50 mmHg) and base deficit = 0 to −10 mmol/litre (mEq/litre). In patients with chronic or acute placental insufficiency, more profound changes occur.

Samples are obtained through an amnioscope placed against the fetal head. Following rupture of the membranes, a 2 × 2 mm pre-set blade is used and blood is collected into a pre-heparinized catheter or capillary tube. Saling (62) found that the fetal-blood pH determination provided the best correlation to outcome as judged by Apgar score, and others have confirmed this observation (77). Errors in assessment of the fetal condition are frequently related to sampling-delivery time, amount and duration of maternal anesthesia and analgesia, traumatic delivery, and abnormal maternal acid-base balance. Disadvantages of fetal scalp-blood sampling are that it requires frequent repositioning of the patient and that it does not continuously assess the fetal condition. Most authors agree (78,79) that fetal heart-rate monitoring and fetal scalp-blood sampling should be complementary techniques, used to refine the diagnosis of fetal distress.

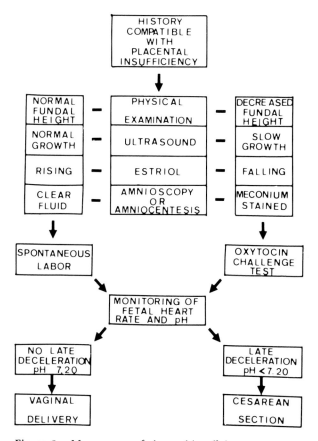

Figure 5. Management of placental insufficiency.

SUMMARY

In summary, use of these laboratory aids in the clinical management of a pregnancy complicated by placental insufficiency can be directed toward determining the optimal time and method of delivery (Figure 5). Prolonging gestation is always the goal. Vaginal delivery is preferred to cesarean section. If by ultrasound the fetus appears to be growth retarded and serial estriol measurements are decreasing or meconium is noted in the amniotic fluid, an oxytocin stress test should be performed. If it is positive, labor may be contraindicated. If induction of labor is attempted, careful attention must be given to the development of abnormal fetal heart-rate patterns. If these patterns persist or if fetal acidosis is found on scalp-blood sampling, delivery must be accomplished by cesarean section.

REFERENCES

1. Assali, N. S., Rauramo, L., and Peltonen, T., Measurement of uterine blood flow and uterine metabolism. VIII. Uterine and fetal blood flow and oxygen consumption in early human pregnancy, *Am. J. Obstet. Gynecol.* **79,** 86 (1960).
2. Rosenfeld, C. R. et al., Circulatory changes in the reproductive tissues of ewes during pregnancy, *Gynecol. Invest.* (in press)

3. Huckabee, W. E., Uterine blood flow, *Am. J. Obstet. Gynecol.* **84,** 1623 (1962).

4. Meschia, G. and Battaglia, F. C., Acute changes of oxygen pressure and the regulation of uterine blood flow. In *Foetal and Neonatal Physiology,* K. S. Comline, K. W. Cross, G. S. Dawes, P. W. Nathanielez, Eds., Cambridge University Press, Cambridge, 1973, pp 272–278.

5. Killam, A. P. et al., Effect of estrogens on the uterine blood flow of oophorectomized ewes, *Am. J. Obstet. Gynecol.* **115,** 1045, (1973).

6. Rosenfeld, C. R. et al., Effect of estradiol-17,β on blood flow to reproductive and nonreproductive tissues in pregnant ewes. (in preparation)

7. Greiss, F. C., Jr., A clinical concept of uterine blood flow during pregnancy, *Obstet. Gynecol.* **30,** 595 (1967).

8. Ladner, C., Brinkman, C. R., Weston, P., and Assali, N. S., Dynamics of uterine circulation in pregnant and nonpregnant sheep, *Am. J. Physiol.* **218,** 257, (1970).

9. Greiss, F. C., Jr. and Gobble, F. C., Jr., Effect of sympathetic nerve stimulation on the uterine vascular bed, *Am. J. Obstet. Gynecol.* **97,** 962 (1967).

10. Greiss, F. C., Jr., The uterine vascular bed: Effect of adrenergic stimulation, *Obstet. Gynecol.* **21,** 295 (1963).

11. Greiss, F. C., Jr., Effect of labor on uterine blood flow, *Am. J. Obstet. Gynecol.* **93,** 917 (1965).

12. Meschia, G., Cotter, J. R., Makowski, E. L., and Barron, D. H., Simultaneous measurement of uterine and umbilical blood flows and oxygen uptakes, *Q. J. Exp. Physiol.* **52,** 1 (1967).

13. Meschia, G., Battaglia, F. C., and Bruns, P. D., Theoretical and experimental study of transplacental diffusion, *J. Appl. Physiol.* **22,** 1171 (1967).

14. Tsoulos, N. G. et al., Comparison of glucose, fructose, and O_2 uptakes by fetuses of fed and starved ewes, *Am. J. Physiol.* **221,** 234 (1971).

15. Simmons, M. A., Jones, M. D., Battaglia, F. C. Makowski, and E. L. Meschia, G., Placental clearance of glucose: Diffusion versus flow limitation. (in preparation)

16. McKeown, T. and Record, R. G., The influence of placental size on foetal growth in man, with special reference to multiple pregnancy, *J. Endocrinol.* **9,** 418 (1953).

17. Gruenwald, P., Chronic fetal distress and placental insufficiency, *Biol. Neonat.* **5,** 215 (1963).

18. Aherne, W. and Dunnill, M. S., Quantitative aspects of placental structure, *J. Pathol.* **91,** 123 (1966).

19. Kulhanek, J. F., Meschia, G., Makowski, E. L., and Battaglia, F. C., Changes in DNA content and urea permeability of the sheep placenta, *Am. J. Physiol.* **226,** 1257 (1974).

20. Smith, C. A., Effects of maternal undernutrition upon the newborn infant in Holland (1944–1945), *J. Pediatr.* **30,** 229 (1947).

21. Lichty, J. A., Ting, R. Y., Burns, P. D., and Dyar, E., Studies of babies born at high altitude, *Am. J. Dis. Child.* **93,** 666 (1957).

22. Beischer, N. A., The effect of maternal anemia upon the fetus, *J. Reprod. Med.* **6,** 262 (1971).

23. Battaglia, F. C. and Woolever, C. A., Fetal and neonatal complications associated with recurrent chorioangiomas, *Pediatrics* **41,** 62 (1968).

24. Driscoll, S. G., The pathology of pregnancy complicated by diabetes mellitus, *Med. Clin. North Am.* **49,** 1053 (1965).

25. Benirschke, K. and Driscoll, S. G., *The Pathology of the Human Placenta,* Springer-Verlag, New York, N.Y., 1965, p. 226.

26. Low, J. A. and Galbraith, R. S., Pregnancy characteristics of intrauterine growth retardation, *Obstet. Gynecol.* **44,** 122 (1974).

27. Johnson, T. and Clayton, C. G., Diffusion of radioactive sodium in normotensive and preeclamptic pregnancies, *Br. Med. J.* **i,** 312 (1957).

28. Bieniarz, J., Julio, W., and Grainer, L. Utero-placental circulation: An angiographic study. In *Perinatal Factors Affecting Human Development,* Pan American Health Organization, Washington, 1969, p. 81–95.

29. Marais, W. D., Human decidual spiral aterial studies, *S. Afr. Med. J.* **37,** 117 (1963).

30. Lubchenco, L. O., Assessment of gestational age and development at birth, *Pediatr. Clin. North Am.* **17,** 125 (1970).

31. Lubchenco. L. O., Searls, D. T., and Brazie, J. V., Neonatal mortality rate: Relationship to birth weight and gestational age, *J. Pediatr.* 81, 814 (1972).

32. Cooper, L. Z. et al., Neonatal thrombocytopenic purpura and other manifestations of rubella contracted in utero, *Am. J. Dis. Child.* 110, 416 (1965).

33. McKeown, T. and Record, R. G., Observations on foetal growth in multiple pregnancy in man, *J. Endocrinol.* 8, 386 (1951–1952).

34. Winick, M., Cellular growth of human placenta, *J. Pediatr.* 71, 390 (1967).

35. Clifford, S. H., Postmaturity—with placental dysfunction, *J. Pediatr.* 44, 1 (1954).

36. Lucas, W. E., Anctil, A. O., and Callagan, D. A., The problem of postterm pregnancy, *Am. J. Obstet. Gynecol.* 91, 241 (1965).

37. Zwerdling, M. A., Factors pertaining to prolonged pregnancy and its outcome, *Pediatr.* 40, 202 (1967).

38. McClure Browne, J. C., Postmaturity, *Am. J. Obstet. Gynecol.* 85, 573 (1963).

39. Gruenwald, P., The fetus in prolonged pregnancy, *Am. J. Obstet. Gynecol.* 89, 503 (1964).

40. Treloar, A. E., Behn, B. G., and Cowan, D. W., Analysis of gestational interval, *Am. J. Obstet. Gynecol.* 99, 34 (1967).

41. Levi, S. and Smets, P., Intra-uterine fetal growth studied by ultrasonic biparietal measurements, *Acta Obstet. Gynecol. Scand.* 52, 193 (1973).

42. Campbell, S. and Dewhurst, C. J., Diagnosis of the small-for-dates fetus by serial ultrasonic cephalometry, *Lancet* ii, 1002 (1971).

43. Diczfalusy, E., Endocrine functions of the human fetoplacental unit, *Fed. Proc.* 23, 791 (1964).

44. Schwers, J., Govaerts-Videtsky, M., Wiquist, N., and Diczfalusy, E., Metabolism of oestrone sulphate by the previable human foetus, *Acta Endocrinol.* 50, 597 (1965).

45. Ryan, K. J., Conversion of androstenedione to estrone by placental microsomes, *Biochim. Biophys. Acta.* 27, 658 (1958).

46. Wilson, R., Eriksson, G., and Diczfalusy, E., Oestriol metabolism in pregnant women. *Acta Endocrinol.* 46, 525 (1958). Abstract.

47. Klopper, A. and Billewicz, W., Urinary excretion of oestriol and pregnanediol during normal pregnancy, *J. Obstet. Gynaecol. Br. Commonw.* 70, 1204 (1963).

48. Jewelewicz, R. and Levitz, M., Plasma estriol levels during normal spontaneous labor and labor induced by oxytocin infusion. *J. Clin. Endocrinol. Metab.* 27, 648 (1967).

49. Berman, A. M., Kalcham, G. G., Chattoraj, S. C., and Scommegna, A., Relationship of amniotic fluid estriol to maternal urinary estriol, *Am. J. Obstet. Gynecol.* 100, 15 (1968).

50. Taylor, E. S. et al., Estriol concentrations in blood during pregnancy, *Am. J. Obstet. Gynecol.* 108, 868 (1970).

51. Scommegna, A. and Chattoraj, S., Gas chromatographic estimation of urinary estriol in pregnancy, *Am. J. Obstet. Gynecol.* 99, 1087 (1967).

52. Greene, J. W. and Touchstone, J. C., Urinary estriol as an index of placental function, *Am. J. Obstet. Gynecol.* 85, 1 (1963).

53. MacLeod, S. C., Mitton, D. M., and Avery, C. R., Relationship between elevated blood pressure and urinary estriol during pregnancy, *Am. J. Obstet. Gynecol.* 109, 375 (1971).

54. Beischer, N. A., Brown, J. B., Smith, M. A., and Towsend, L., Studies in prolonged pregnancy. II. Clinical results and urinary estriol excretion in prolonged pregnancy, *Am. J. Obstet. Gynecol.* 103, 483 (1969).

55. Yousem. H., Seitchik, J., and Solomon, D., Maternal estriol excretion and fetal dysmaturity, *Obstet. Gynecol.* 28, 491 (1966).

56. Pitkin, R. M. and Zwirek, S. J., Amniotic fluid creatinine, *Am. J. Obstet. Gynecol.* 98, 1135 (1967).

57. Mandelbaum, B., La Croix, G. C., and Robinson, A. R., Determination of fetal maturity by spectrophotometric analysis of amniotic fluid, *Obstet. Gynecol.* 29, 471 (1967).

58. Brosens, I., and Gordon, H., The estimation of maturity by cytological examination of the *liquor amnii*, *J. Obstet. Gynaecol. Br. Commonw.* 73, 88 (1966).

59. Gluck, L. et al., Diagnosis of the respiratory distress syndrome by amniocentesis, *Am. J. Obstet. Gynecol.* 109, 440 (1971).

60. Vujic, J., Amnioscopic determination of occurrences of meconial amniotic fluid for no obvious reason at the onset of delivery. In *Intrauterine Dangers to the Fetus*, J. Hursky, Z. K. Stembera, Eds., Exerpta Medica Foundation, Amsterdam, 1968, pp. 400–405.

61. Kubli, F., Amniotic fluid and the early detection of fetal hypoxia. In *Perinatal Medicine*, P. J. Huntingford, K. A. Hüter, E. Saling, Eds., Academic Press, Inc., New York, N.Y. 1969, pp. 4–11.

62. Saling, E., *Foetal and Neonatal Hypoxia in Relation to Clinical Obstetric Practice*, Williams & Wilkins, Co., Baltimore, Md., 1968, pp. 55–56.

63. Wood, C., Hammond, J., and Lumley, J., Effect of maternal inhalation of 10 percent oxygen upon the human fetus, *Aust. N. Z. J. Obstet. Gynaecol.* 81, 361 (1971).

64. Hon, E. H. and Wohlgemuth, R., The electronic evaluation of the fetal heart rate, effect of maternal exercise. *Am. J. Obstet. Gynecol.* 81, 361 (1961).

65. Pose, S. V. et al., Test of fetal tolerance to induced uterine contractions for diagnosis of chronic distress. In *Perinatal Factors Affecting Human Development*, Pan American Health Organization, Washington, 1969, p. 96.

66. Ray, M., Freeman, R., Pine, A., and Hesselgesser, R., Clinical experience with the oxytocin challenge test, *Am. J. Obstet. Gynecol.* 114, 1 (1972).

67. Calderyo-Barcia, R. et al., Control of human fetal heart rate during labor. In *The Heart and Circulation in the Newborn and Infant*, D. E. Cassels, Ed., Grune & Stratton, New York, N.Y., 1965, pp. 7–36.

68. Hon, E. H. and Quilligan, E. J., The classification of fetal heart rate. II. A revised working classification, *Conn. Med.* 31, 779 (1967).

69. Hon, E. H., The electronic evaluation of the fetal heart rate, *Am. J. Obstet. Gynecol.* 75, 1215 (1958).

70. Hon, E. H., Observations on "pathologic" fetal bradycardia, *Am. J. Obstet. Gynecol.* 77, 1084 (1959).

71. Myers, R. E., Mueller-Heubach, E., and Adamsons, K., Predictability of the state of fetal oxygenation from a quantitative analysis of the components of late deceleration, *Am. J. Obstet. Gynecol.* 115, 1083 (1973).

72. Kubli, F. W., Hon, E. H., Khazin, A. F., and Takemura, H., Observations on heart rate and pH in the human fetus during labor, *Am. J. Obstet. Gynecol.* 104, 1190 (1969).

73. Wood, C. et al., Fetal heart rate and acid-base status in the assessment of fetal hypoxia, *Am. J. Obstet. Gynecol.* 98, 62 (1967).

74. Hon, E. H., Additional observations on "pathologic" bradycardia, *Am. J. Obstet. Gynecol.* 118, 428 (1974).

75. Hon, E. H., *An Atlas of Fetal Heart Rate Patterns*, Harty Press, New Haven, Conn., 1969.

76. Schifrin, B. S. and Dame, L., Fetal heart rate patterns. Prediction of Apgar score, *J. A. M. A.* 219, 1322 (1972).

77. Beard, R. W., Morris, E. D., and Clayton, S. G., pH of foetal capillary blood as an indicator of the condition of the foetus, *J. Obstet. Gynaecol. Br. Commonw.* 74, 812 (1967).

78. McCrann, D. J. and Schifrin, B. S., Fetal monitoring in high risk pregnancy, *Clin. Perinatol.* 1, 229 (1974).

79. Freeman, R. K., Intrapartum fetal evaluation, *Clin. Obstet. Gynecol.* 17 (No. 3), 83 (1974).

Effects of Maternal Undernutrition on Placental Metabolism and Function

PEDRO ROSSO, M.D.

MARCIA WASSERMAN, M.S.

S. JAIME ROZOVSKI, Ph.D.

ELBA VELASCO, M.D.

It has been demonstrated in several mammalian species, including man, that maternal undernutrition is associated with fetal growth retardation (1,2). The mechanisms involved in this retardation are still unknown, although it is generally assumed that it is a direct consequence of the abnormally low amounts of nutrients that are available to the fetus.

However, several recent reports indicate that placental growth and metabolism are also affected by undernutrition. Because of the important role of the placenta in fetal growth, changes in this organ as a result of maternal undernutrition suggest the possibility that the fetus is not solely affected by a decreased availability of nutrients but that there also may be a certain degree of placental insufficiency.

Here we discuss available published evidence, as well as our own results, suggesting the existence of placental insufficiency during maternal protein and calorie restriction.

PLACENTAL INSUFFICIENCY: A CONCEPTUAL DEFINITION

Placental insufficiency is considered to be the cause of fetal growth retardation in those situations in which no clear intrinsic fetal abnormalities can be found (3). Generally, maternal factors that presumably may alter placental circulation—such as chronic hypertension or toxemia—are present, but in many cases there is no apparent cause for the syndrome. A frequent finding is a small placenta (3), with fewer cells (4) and a smaller-than-normal villous surface (5) that may have an increased number of vascular lesions (6). What is placental insufficiency in functional and biochemical terms? We do not know.

59

From a purely conceptual point of view, we may define placental insufficiency as a reduced organ "capacity" or a reduced organ "efficiency," or both.

The function of the placenta is to maintain normal fetal growth, which is accomplished by inducing maternal changes through hormonal mediation, the so-called adaptive changes of pregnancy, and by transferring all the nutrients and other substances essential for fetal growth from the maternal circulation into the fetus. To perform these functions, the placenta itself grows and matures, especially near term, at which time its ability to transfer nutrients increases markedly (7). If the placenta is smaller than normal, the total amount of nutrients that can be transferred into the fetus per unit of time will be decreased. Thus its "capacity" to function is decreased.

Because of metabolic alterations, the placenta may also be less "efficient." For example, protein synthesis may be altered and the amount of carriers necessary to maintain a normal transfer of certain molecules may consequently be diminished. In this case placental size may be normal but the ability of the organ to carry out its function is lessened.

Finally, as is likely to happen in vivo, the same stimulus that interferes with placental growth—i.e., vascular insufficiency—may also alter placental metabolism.

Thus, we may have combined subnormalities of placental "capacity" and "efficiency."

MATERNAL UNDERNUTRITION AND PLACENTAL GROWTH

Both placental weight and DNA content, which reflects the number of placental cells, have been found to be subnormal in women who are presumably suffering some degree of undernutrition (8,9). Thus, maternal undernutrition is associated with a smaller placenta. Moreover, there seems to be a rather specific effect of maternal dietary restriction on placental villous surface, as shown by a study (*10*) of poor Guatemalan women as compared with middle-class American women. The peripheral villous surface was found to be significantly smaller in the Guatemalan population. We have found similar effects of maternal undernutrition on placental DNA, RNA, and protein content in the rat (Figure 1).

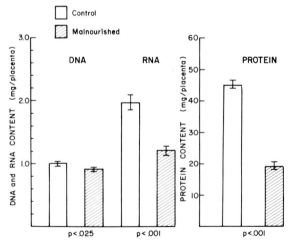

Figure 1. Placental DNA, RNA, and protein content in rats fed a diet containing 66 or 27 (control) g of casein/kg during pregnancy. In each group, values represent means ± SE for 10 samples from five different animals. Statistical significance was calculated by use of Student's *t*-test.

Thus, in both human and rat, maternal undernutrition results in subnormal placental size and, accordingly, in subnormal capacity.

MATERNAL UNDERNUTRITION AND PLACENTAL METABOLISM

Our knowledge of the effects of maternal undernutrition on placental metabolism is still fragmentary and is largely based on experimental data. As Figure 1 shows, the RNA and protein content of placentas of undernourished rats are proportionately more decreased than is DNA. This suggests a subnormal cytoplasmic mass of the placental cells. Such a reduction in the proportion of RNA and protein has also been found in the placentas of low-birth-weight infants from the Guatemalan population (*10*). Another interesting finding of this study was that the polysome/monosome ratio of the poor women was half that of the control group (*11*), which suggests an altered placental RNA metabolism as well as a generally decreased capacity of the organ to synthesize protein. However, incorporation of [^{14}C]leucine per milligram of ribosomal RNA by a cell-free preparation of mixed ribosome pellets was not significantly different in the two groups.

Further studies done in our laboratory have shown that other variables thought to be related to RNA metabolism, such as activity of alkaline (pH 7.8) ribonuclease (RNase, EC 3.1.4.22) and the concentration of polyamines in the placenta are also altered by maternal undernutrition.

Although the specific cellular role of RNase is still to be defined, it has been shown, in rat liver, that the increase in RNase activity during protein malnutrition parallels increments in the rate of RNA turnover (*12*). Increments in RNase activity have been described in brain and liver of rats undernourished early in life (*13*). In a study performed on placentas from a group of underweight low-income Ecuadorian women and a group of well-to-do women, RNase activity was greater in the placentas from the presumably undernourished mothers (Figure 2).

Putrescine is present in subnormal concentrations in placentas of malnourished rats (Figure 3). The exact implication of this finding is still elusive. Polyamines are considered to be related to RNA metabolism, but the nature of this relationship is still under investigation. There is evidence that the concentration of polyamines influences the rate of RNA synthesis. Other evidence suggests that they may stabilize RNA by protecting it from RNA degradation (*14*). As Figure 3 shows, no significant changes were found in the concentration of spermidine and spermine. Because putrescine is the precursor of these two substances, the results suggest that the placenta uses some adaptive mechanisms to maintain a normal concentration of spermidine and spermine in spite of a declining concentration of their precursor.

In the rat, the concentration of placental glycogen is also decreased during maternal malnutrition (Figure 4). Because of our lack of knowledge of the role of placental glycogen, we cannot speculate on the possible implications of this finding, except that it may serve as a general indication that overall placental metabolism is slowed by undernutrition. Decreases in placental glycogen during pregnancy parallel oxygen consumption, the lowest concentration of glycogen and oxygen consumption being found near term (*15*).

From this mosaic of rather disconnected and fragmentary information, we cannot draw any clear conclusion on specific effects of maternal undernutrition on placental metabolism during maternal undernutrition, but collectively the data strongly suggest that it is impaired. Thus, in addition to placental "capacity," placental "efficiency"

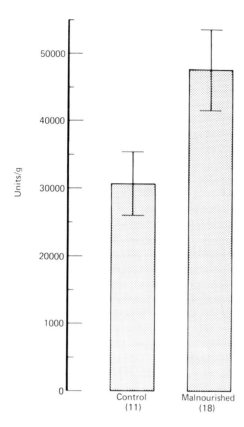

Figure 2. Alkaline ribonuclease activity, expressed as units/g of placental tissue, in women from high and low socioeconomic groups in Quito, Ecuador. Values represent means and SD.

seems also to be affected by maternal undernutrition. Nevertheless, the ultimate proof that maternal undernutrition induces placental insufficiency is to determine whether or not the placental transfer of nutrients from the maternal circulation into the fetus is diminished.

TRANSFER OF NUTRIENTS IN THE MALNOURISHED RAT

Transfer of nutrients from the maternal circulation into the fetus was studied by injecting radiolabeled glucose or radiolabeled α-aminoisobutyric acid into the femoral vein of pregnant rats fed a control or a low-protein diet, and then determining the amount of radioactivity present in the whole fetus and placenta.

We found that the radioactivity reflecting the concentration of labeled glucose, and probably of other metabolic products related to glucose utilization, was smaller in the placentas and fetuses of malnourished rats than in controls 10 min after the substance was injected into the mother (Figure 5). The decreased transfer of tritium into the fetuses of malnourished rats was not due to either a decreased concentration of label in the maternal circulation, a decreased concentration of glucose, or an increased rate of disappearance of the label from the maternal blood.

A similar decrease was found in α-aminoisobutyric acid transfer (16), suggesting that perhaps other amino acids—for which the transport mechanisms are similar to those of

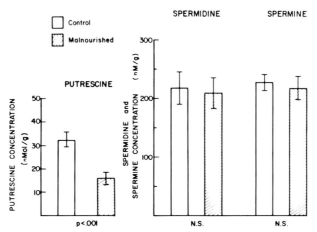

Figure 3. Placental concentration of putrescine, spermidine, and spermine (nmol/g) in rats fed a diet containing 60 or 27 (control) g casein/kg during pregnancy. In each group, values represent means ± SE for 10 samples from five different animals. Statistical significance was calculated by using Student's *t*-test.

α-aminoisobutyric acid—may also be transferred into the fetus at a slower rate during maternal malnutrition.

The rate of blood perfusion of the maternal placenta was not studied in these investigations because of technical problems related to the small size of the rat and to the large number of fetuses, and so we cannot exclude the possibility that a decrease in maternal placental blood perfusion causes the decreased transfer.

In the α-aminoisobutyric acid study, however, it was found that the ratio of fetal concentration to placental concentration of α-aminoisobutyric acid was smaller in the malnourished animals, suggesting that after α-aminoisobutyric acid is taken up from the mother's blood, it remains for a longer period of time in the placentas of the malnourished animals. This clearly suggests that placental transport is altered, but certainly does not

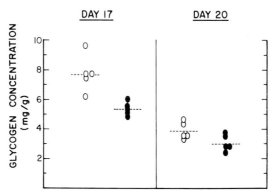

Figure 4. Concentration of placental glycogen (mg/g) at day 17 and day 20 of gestation in rats fed a diet containing 6 (●) or 27 (control) (○) g casein/kg during pregnancy. Each point is the average of the values for three placentas from each different rat. Mean values of each group are indicated. Statistical analysis was performed by using Student's *t*-test $P < 0.002$ at day 17 and $P < 0.05$ at day 20.

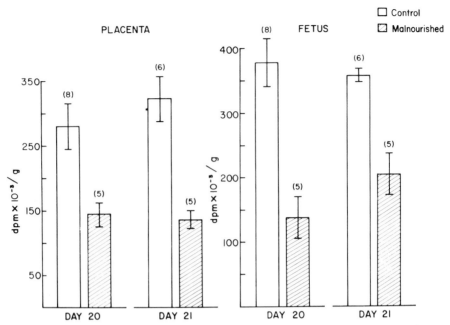

Figure 5. Concentration of tritium (dpm/g × 10⁻³), representing glucose and products of glucose utilization, in placentas and fetuses of control and malnourished rats at day 20 of gestation, 10 min after injection [1-³H]-D-glucose into the maternal circulation. Rats were malnourished as described in previous figures. Values are means ± SE.

rule out a hemodynamic component. Further studies in different species will be required to clarify the situation.

The possibility that there is a certain degree of placental insufficiency during maternal malnutrition changes our present concept of the mechanisms by which fetal growth is affected during this condition.

Some of the possible mechanisms involved are presented in Figure 6. The occurrence of placental insufficiency would also explain why the parasitic capacity of the fetus, based on the higher metabolic rate of its tissues, is limited during maternal undernutrition. From a teleological point of view, this seems to be a mechanism that would tend to preserve maternal health and function so that the mother can better endure the stress of delivery and lactation. In man, where the weight of the fetus at term is about 5% of the maternal weight, this may seem to be an unnecessary and deleterious mechanism for the fetus. However, in other species in which the weight of the fetus at term ranges between 12 and 37% of the maternal weight (*17*) it may be a crucial mechanism for maternal survival when nutrients are in short supply.

SUMMARY

Available evidence indicates that chronically restricting the mother's protein and calorie intake during pregnancy interferes with cellular growth and placental metabolism of both the human and the rat placenta. The functional implications of these placental changes

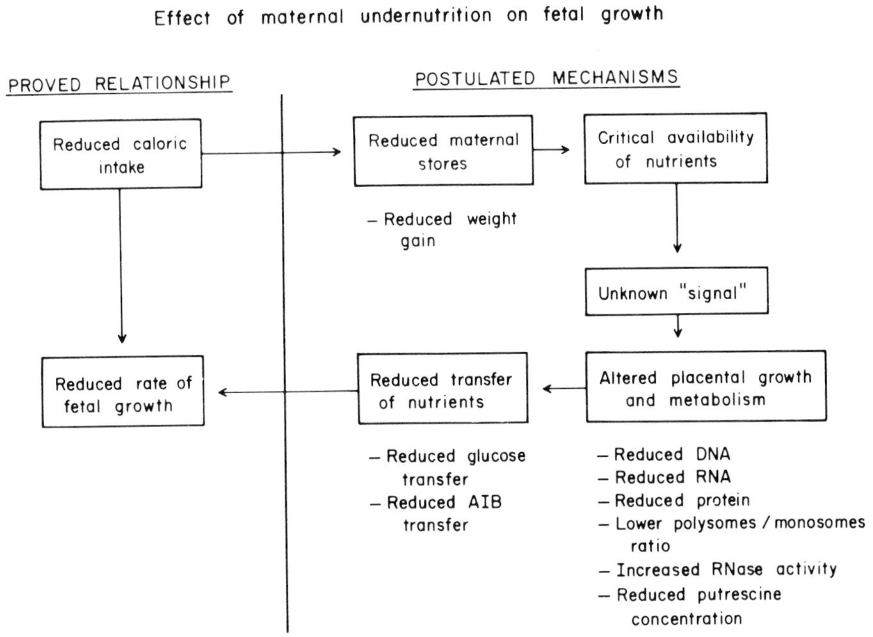

Effect of maternal undernutrition on fetal growth

PROVED RELATIONSHIP   POSTULATED MECHANISMS

```
┌──────────────┐         ┌──────────────┐     ┌──────────────────┐
│ Reduced caloric│ ───→   │ Reduced maternal│ ─→ │ Critical availability│
│    intake    │         │    stores    │     │  of nutrients    │
└──────────────┘         └──────────────┘     └──────────────────┘
                          — Reduced weight                │
                             gain                         ↓
                                              ┌──────────────────┐
                                              │ Unknown "signal" │
                                              └──────────────────┘
                                                        │
                                                        ↓
┌──────────────┐         ┌──────────────┐     ┌──────────────────┐
│ Reduced rate of│ ←──   │ Reduced transfer│ ←─ │ Altered placental growth│
│ fetal growth │         │  of nutrients│     │  and metabolism  │
└──────────────┘         └──────────────┘     └──────────────────┘
                          — Reduced glucose         — Reduced DNA
                             transfer               — Reduced RNA
                          — Reduced AIB             — Reduced protein
                             transfer               — Lower polysomes / monosomes
                                                       ratio
                                                    — Increased RNase activity
                                                    — Reduced putrescine
                                                       concentration
```

Figure 6.   Effect of maternal undernutrition on fetal growth. AIB, α-aminoisobutyric acid.

are unknown. However, recent results suggest that, in the rat, transfer of glucose and α-aminoisobutyric acid to the fetus is decreased during maternal protein malnutrition. We speculate that the growth-retarding effect of maternal undernutrition may be mediated by a certain degree of placental insufficiency.

ACKNOWLEDGMENT

Supported in part by Grant No. 487 from the Nutrition Foundation.

REFERENCES

1.   Naeye, R. L., Blanc, W., and Paul, C., Effects of maternal nutrition in the human fetus, *Pediatrics* **52,** 494 (1973).

2.   Moustgaard, J., Nutritive influences upon reproduction, *J. Reprod. Med.* **8,** 1 (1972).

3.   Gruenwald, P., Chronic fetal distress and placental insufficiency, *Biol. Neonat.* **5,** 215 (1963).

4.   Winick, M., Cellular growth of human placenta. III. Intrauterine growth failure, *J. Pediat.* **71,** 390 (1967).

5.   Aherne, W. and Dunhill, M. S., Morphometry of the human placenta, *Br. Med. Bull.* **22,** 5 (1966).

6.   Scott, J. M. and Jordan, J. M., Placental insufficiency and the small-for-dates baby, *Am. J. Obstet. Gynecol.* **113,** 823 (1972).

7.   Rosso, P., Changes in the transfer of nutrients across the placenta during normal gestation in the rat, *Am. J. Obstet. Gynecol.* **123,** 637 (1975).

8.   Dayton, D. H., Filer, L. J., and Canosa, C., Cellular changes in the placentas of undernourished mothers in Guatemala, *Fed. Proc.* **28,** 488 (1969). Abstract.

9. Winick, M., Velasco, E., and Rosso, P., DNA content of placental and fetal brain, *Pan. Am. Health Org. Scient. Publ.* **185,** 531 (1969).

10. Laga, E. M., Driscoll, S. G., and Munro, H. N., Comparison of placentas from two socioeconomic groups. I. Morphometry, *Pediatrics* **50,** 24 (1972).

11. Laga, E. M., Driscoll, S. G., and Munro, N. H., Comparison of placentas from two socioeconomic groups. II. Biochemical characteristics, *Pediatrics* **50,** 33 (1972).

12. Girija, N. A., Pradhan, D. S., and Sreenivasan, A., Effects of protein depletion on ribonucleic acid metabolism in rat liver, *Indian J. Biochem. Biophys.* **2,** 85 (1965).

13. Rosso, P. and Winick, M., Effects of early undernutrition and subsequent refeeding on alkaline ribonuclease activity of rat cerebrum and liver, *J. Nutr.* 1975. (in press)

14. Bachrach, V., *Function of Naturally Occurring Polyamines.* Academic Press, Inc., New York, N.Y. 1973, p. 47.

15. Longo, L. D., Disorders of placental transfer. In *Pathophysiology of Gestation* **2.** N. S. Assali, Ed. Academic Press, Inc., New York, N.Y. 1972, pp 1–76.

16. Rosso, P., Maternal malnutrition and placental transfer of α-aminoisobutyric acid in the rat. *Science* **187,** 648, 1875.

17. Dawes, G. S., *Foetal and Neonatal Physiology*, Year Book Medical Publishers, Inc., Chicago, Ill. 1969, p 15.

Development of Enzymes
of the Intestinal Surface
in the Fetus and Neonate

FLORENCE MOOG, Ph.D.

THE FUNCTIONAL STRUCTURE OF THE INTESTINAL SURFACE

If the newborn infant is to thrive, its gastrointestinal tract must not only be furnished with enzymes necessary for the digestion and absorption of food, but must also have these enzymes appropriately situated. Whereas it was believed for many years that the enzymes essential to digestion were poured into the lumen of the intestine, with absorption of split products following passively, work culminating within the last decade has demonstrated that at least the terminal phases of digestion are linked to the absorptive function by the localization of key enzymes on the surface membrane of the epithelial cells (1,2). Therefore, to understand how the intestinal lining acquires and maintains its capacity for function, we need to know not only when essential enzymes appear, but also when and how they assume their appropriate spatial orientation.

The epithelium covering the intestinal villi consists of columnar cells bearing at their luminal ends a mass of microvilli measuring approximately $1.0–1.4 \times 0.08$ μm in the jejunum of both large and small species. Their presence increases the area of the surface membrane by a factor of 20 (3). They bear on their outer layer strands of carbohydrate-containing material constituting a dense meshwork (Figure 1) interposed between the wall of the intestine and its contents (4,5). This meshwork, or "glycocalyx," may vary in thickness from cell to cell, and is clearly a product of the individual epithelial cells, not a derivative of goblet-cell secretions (6).

Techniques that make it possible to strip the microvillous border from the bulk of the epithelial cells have demonstrated that alkaline phosphatase (EC 3.1.3.1), both α- and β-disaccharidases, and aminopeptidase are largely restricted to the border (7,8). The electron microscope can also be used to localize alkaline phosphatase, which is found at the outer surface of the microvilli (9). Phosphatase and other enzymes have also been shown to be components of the surface by separating the membrane coat of the microvilli

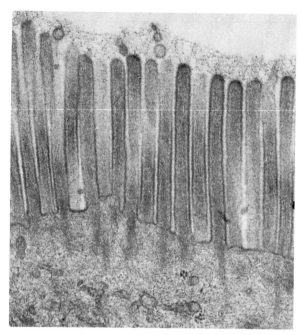

Figure 1. Apical portion of epithelial cell from mouse duodenum, showing microvilli and glyco-calyx. The continuity between the surface membrane and the glycocalyx strands can be seen at several villus tips. $35,000\times$.

from their inner fibrous cores (8,10). However, the enzymes are linked to the membrane in different ways, maltase (EC 3.2.1.20) and sucrase (EC 3.2.1.26) being held by a bond that is readily split by papain (EC 3.4.22.2), whereas phosphatase is more tightly bound to the membrane (11). In the light of the carbohydrate-rich nature of the intestinal surface, it is particularly interesting that the membrane-bound enzymes are glycoproteins (12,13).

The intestinal epithelium undergoes continual replacement. In a variety of mammals, including man (14,15), new cells are formed in the crypts, and glide from the crypts to the villus tip in about two days. On reaching the tip, the cells are extruded, and are thus the predominant source of the alkaline phosphatase and disaccharidase found in the lumen. The enzymes of the brush border are absent deep in the crypts, where the proliferative population resides, but appear near the crypt mouths, as the new cells move out onto the villi. By cross-sectioning frozen villi at right angles to their length, it can be demonstrated quantitatively that the activities of alkaline phosphatase, maltase, sucrase, and leucine aminopeptidase (EC 3.4.11.1) increase progressively to a maximum at or near the villus tip (16,17). It is now well established that protein synthesis goes on in cells in the course of the upward migration on the villus (18), and there is little reason to doubt that new enzyme molecules are being synthesized. That this is so is supported by the fact that the half-life of disaccharidases is substantially less than the transit time (19); moreover, sucrase and maltase are found within the epithelial cells if their transfer to the surface membrane is blocked (20). In addition, [1-^{14}C]glucosamine administered to intact rats is quickly incorporated into the enzyme-rich fraction of the brush-border membrane (12). Synthesis and differentiation of the plasma membrane covering the apical surface of the villus epithelium thus go on throughout life; the component processes must be operating appropriately at birth if the intestine is to play its role in supporting the growth and development of the infant.

DEVELOPMENT OF ENZYMES OF THE INTESTINAL SURFACE IN LABORATORY ANIMALS

Although patterns of intestinal enzyme development have been described in various laboratory and farm animals in both pre- and postnatal stages (*21*), the greater part of the experimental work on the subject has been done on the mouse and rat (*22*). These animals, which have gestation periods of 21 and 22 days, respectively, are very immature at birth, and to some extent exteriorize developmental events that occur in utero in the human and other species. Newborn mice and rats develop rather gradually during the first two weeks but in the third week enter into a brief period of accelerated structural and physiological differentiation that enables them to become independent of the mother during the fourth week.

The first systematic study of the development of an intestinal enzyme showed that alkaline phosphatase activity in the duodenum of the mouse increases between 16 and 19 days in utero to a peak maintained through term; in the neonate a gradual loss of activity is followed, at about 15 days, by a swift upsurge to a maximum above the adult value (*23*). The same pattern occurs in the rat, except that the increase begins two to three days later (*24,25*). Other surface enzymes that are abundant in mature intestine—maltase, sucrase, aminopeptidase—all rise concomitantly with phosphatase in late fetal life, and in the third week of postnatal life, in both mouse and rat (*26–29*).

Attempts to alter the postnatal pattern of alkaline phosphatase accumulation in the mouse led to the observation that separation from the mother, rather than dietary alteration *per se*, could elicit precocious increase of phosphatase activity (*30*). The implication that the pituitary-adrenal system might underlie the change was verified by experiments showing that the great increase in phosphatase activity in the third week could be evoked several days early by administration of cortisone or corticotropin, and it could be prevented by adrenalectomy on the eleventh or twelfth postnatal day (*30*). Exogenous corticosteroids also elicit precocious increase of sucrase (*29,31,32*), maltase (*29*), and aminopeptidase (*28*), the enhancement of these activities being due to the synthesis of new molecules (*33,34*). Adrenalectomy delays or prevents the normal increases of sucrase and maltase (*31,35–37*).

In murine fetuses, alkaline phosphatase (*23*), maltase (*29*), and leucine aminopeptidase (*28*) activities all surge up during the last three days before birth. The control of these increases has received comparatively little attention, but the evidence available indicates a similar dependence on the adrenal cortex. In the rat, the cortex is actively secreting during the last few days before birth (*38,39*), and administration of adrenocortical extract to the 15-day fetus reportedly enhances alkaline phosphatase activity in the intestine (*40*). In the fetal guinea pig, which has a gestation period of almost 10 weeks, intestinal phosphatase activity increases to a maximum at the end of the seventh week, after a period of rapid adrenocortical growth and apparent secretory activity (*41*). The most direct evidence comes from the fetal rabbit, in which hypophysectomy (by decapitation) at 22 days results in severe deficiency of duodenal phosphatase at 28 days (2 days before term), unless the hypophysioprivic fetuses are given corticotropin (*42*).

At birth, the intestines of all mammals are rich in a neutral β-galactosidase (EC 3.2.1.23), lactase, which is essential for the digestion of lactose. This enzyme is also concentrated primarily in the brush border (8,43,44), and in the rat and rabbit its activity increases sharply in the last few days of prenatal life (44); high activity is maintained for about two weeks after birth, then falls to the low values characteristic of most adult mammals (26,29,44). The prenatal increase is not induced by circulating lactose synthesized by the mammary glands; activity at term is the same in fetuses of mastectomized and intact rabbit mothers (44).

The fact that neutral β-galactosidase activity declines after two weeks, at the time when activities of other enzymes begin to increase, has suggested that the decline might be an element in a corticosteroid-dependent pattern of intestinal maturation. In suckling mice afflicted with runt disease, in which the adrenals are large and apparently active, β-galactosidase activity is very low (45). Administration of cortisone in the first or second week not only fails to decrease β-galactosidase activity, however, but may even enhance it (46). Attempts to obviate the decrease by supplying lactose orally or intraperitoneally have been unsuccessful (47–49), and forcing the young to subsist only on mother's milk for a prolonged period delays the decline by no more than two or three days (50). If rat pups are hypophysectomized at 6 days, however, β-galactosidase activity at 20 days is as high as that in neonates, and even at 28 days is higher than in controls at 14 days (51). Daily injections of cortisone acetate from 19 to 22 days result in somewhat diminished β-galactosidase activity at 24 days, but thyroxine decreases this activity to the same low value found for intact animals. Thyroidectomy also inhibits the decline; again, thyroxine is much more effective than cortisone in decreasing the activity (51).

This indication that the thyroid hormone plays an important part in controlling enzyme development in the mammalian intestine has been borne out by studies on alkaline phosphatase and α-disaccharidases in hypophysectomized animals at 24 days, when these enzymes normally reach peak activities (52,53). Sucrase, which is absent at six days, does appear in hypophysioprivic rats, but the activity is less than a third of the normal value; maltase increases to only about twofold the six-day level, and alkaline phosphatase does not increase at all. Thyroxine increases phosphatase to the control value, but is less effective in normalizing maltase and sucrase (Figure 2); in contrast, cortisone exerts a stronger effect on the disaccharidases (54). In rats adrenalectomized on the 14th postnatal day, daily injections of thyroxine evoke a limited increase in sucrase and maltase after 4 days (55).

The increases in enzyme activities that occur in the intestinal surfaces of mice and rats in the transition period from nursling to self-dependent status cannot be ascribed to increase in amount of surface. Whereas the villi are longest in the duodenum and shortest in the ileum (56), sucrase, maltase, and aminopeptidase activities are highest in the jejunum; only alkaline phosphatase has its maximal activity in the duodenum (22,25–29). Although microvilli are said to lengthen in the mouse duodenum concomitantly with the upsurge of phosphatase activity (57), this does not appear to be the case in the rat (53). Rather, the alterations in enzyme activity must reflect qualitative changes in the brush-border membrane. The brush border of the neonatal rat is poor not only in enzymes that are glycoproteins (12,13), but also in periodic acid-Schiff stainable carbohydrate; maturation brings about enhancement of both enzyme activities and PAS stainability (54).

After hypophysectomy at six days, neither surface enzymes nor surface carbohydrates undergo the normal maturational increase. These deficiencies are probably related to the small size and abnormal configuration of the Golgi complexes in hypophysioprivic

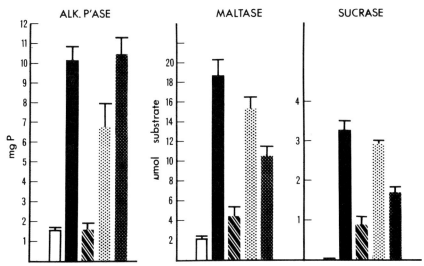

Figure 2. Alkaline phosphatase activity in the duodenum and maltase and sucrase activities in the jejunum of normal and hypophysectomized rats. In each group the first column (*open*) represents the normal 6-day activity and the second (*black*) the normal 24-day activity. The next three represent 24-day-old rats that were hypophysectomized at 6 days: third column (*diagonal stripes*), untreated; fourth (*dotted*), given cortisone acetate daily from 19–22 days; fifth (*cross-hatched*), given thyroxine daily from 19–22 days. Activities are mg P/mg protein/30 min; or μmol of substrate/mg of protein/h. (Adapted from ref. 54).

animals (54), because the Golgi membranes are the site of glycosylation of surface components, no doubt including enzymes (58,59). Administration of thyroxine from the 19th through the 22nd postnatal day restores the normal appearance of the Golgi complex at 24 days, but cortisone stimulates vacuolization in the Golgi zone without restoration of the usual configuration of elongated stacks of membranes (Figure 3) that ordinarily characterize the supranuclear zone of the mature rat (54). Taking into account the previously cited fact that thyroxine and cortisone exert positive but unequal effects on phosphatase and α-disaccharidases, these results suggest that variations in endocrine functioning might be reflected in the composition of the microvillous membrane, and hence of its functional integrity.

In addition to its enzymatic composition, the neonatal intestine also differs from that of older animals in its capacity for pinocytosis. In the suckling rat, the surface is interrupted by tubular infoldings that communicate with vacuoles in which ingested milk is apparently digested (60–62). This activity is concurrent with passive immunization, although the absorption of homologous antibodies actually depends on selective binding at the cell surface (63,64). Pinocytosis ceases abruptly after 18 days, concomitantly with a fourfold increase in plasma corticosterone concentration (65). Adrenalectomy at 18 days delays closure (65), but it can be elicited a week or more prematurely by cortisone (24,60,66) or thyroxine (67). In rats hypophysectomized at 6 days, closure is virtually complete by 24 days, at least in the proximal region of the intestine (53), despite the fact that the enzymes characteristic of the mature intestine do not increase normally. The failure of these animals to continue their steady though subnormal growth much beyond 24 days (53) may reflect the incapacity of the small intestine to deal adequately with either the nursling or the adult diet.

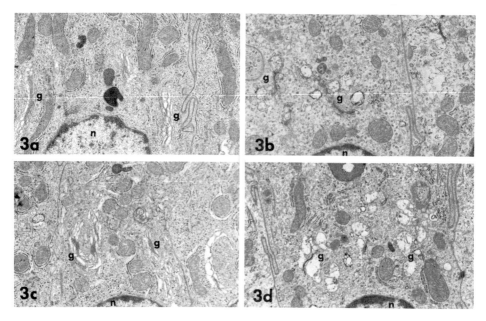

Figure 3. Supranuclear zone in villus epithelial cells of 24-day-old rats. *n*, nucleus, *g*, Golgi complex. 7200×. *3a*, intact control showing several active Golgi complexes. *3b*, hypophysectomized at 6 days, showing short, compact Golgi membranes with abnormal vesiculation. *3c*, hypophysectomized at 6 days, given thyroxine 19–22 days; Golgi complexes are large, numerous, and active. *3d*, hypophysectomized at 6 days, given cortisone acetate 19–22 days; Golgi complexes are excessively vesiculated, but lack typical stacks of membranes.

THE INTESTINAL SURFACE IN THE HUMAN FETUS AND NEONATE

In keeping with the usual pattern of a long gestation period, the human intestine passes through the basic steps of structural and biochemical differentiation early, attaining an approximation of its mature configuration by the end of the third month (*21*). As in other animals, differentiation proceeds in a proximo-distal direction. Although the villi do not attain their adult dimensions even as late as the seventh gestational month, pre-villous ridges are present by eight or nine weeks (*68,69*). The epithelial cells assume a tall columnar form that seems superficially mature by the end of the 12th week; the cytoplasm is, however, laden with glycogen (*70,71*), and the microvilli vary in size and density (*69,71*), probably depending on the intestinal region from which the sample was derived. (The regions usually cannot be determined in specimens from embryos obtained by suction curettage.) By the 14th week, infoldings of the plasma membrane appear between the microvilli, apparently communicating with vesicles that crowd the cytoplasm (*72*). The vesicles are believed to contain meconial material taken in by pinocytosis (*72*) and subsequently degraded by acid hydrolases (*73*). Such activity, which has been experimentally demonstrated in the fetal stages of several species (*74*), reaches its peak in the sixth month, but has virtually ceased at birth (*21,72*). There is no evidence that endocytosis resumes after birth, its absence being probably related to the presence of quantities of gastric and pancreatic proteases adequate to permit breakdown of proteins to proceed extracellularly (*22*).

Alkaline phosphatase is histochemically detectable in the human fetal jejunum at seven weeks, and four weeks later gives a uniform reaction confined to the luminal surface of the epithelial cells (68); as early as ten weeks it is limited to the outer surface of the microvillus membrane (69). Activity increases steadily from the 11th to the 23rd week (68,75,76) and may subsequently increase further (77). It is not possible to decide from the data at hand whether specific activities attained in utero are equal to (77) or less than (75) adult activities. The histochemical reaction for leucine aminopeptidase is positive at 10 weeks and increases in intensity to 22 weeks, but is not sharply localized in the brush border (68). Measured quantitatively, the increase between 10 and 16 weeks is twofold in the jejunum, fivefold in the ileum (78). The activity and distribution of this enzyme beyond 22 weeks have not been reported.

By contrast, total maltase activity is high at 10 weeks and does not change in the ensuing 14 weeks (75,79,80). There may be a further increase to term (77,79), but after birth the same level of activity is maintained from the second through the eleventh month (80). Surprisingly—because no other mammal is known to have significant sucrase activity at birth—sucrase and isomaltase (EC 3.2.1.10) show the same developmental pattern as does total maltase (77,79). Formula-fed infants can utilize sucrose immediately after birth; conversely, congenital sucrase–isomaltase deficiency may lead to serious osmotic diarrhea at a very early stage (81). However, maltase-1, a sucrase-free component of the human maltase complex, is weak during fetal life, apparently attaining its adult activity at some unspecified time after birth (79). Neutral β-galactosidase, the surface enzyme whose function is most clearly established in the nursing infant, is barely detectable as late as five months in utero (75,79). It increases moderately in later fetal life, but sharply, to values greater than those found in adults of the white race, only after birth. This postnatal increase has been attributed to substrate induction (82), but the fact that it may occur before the first feeding (79) suggests that endocrine adjustments involved in the adaptation to extrauterine life may be causal.

Fetal meconium contains alkaline phosphatase, maltase, isomaltase, sucrase, and β-galactosidase activities that appear identical with those of the intestinal mucosa (77). Alkaline phosphatase is abundant in the meconium of the full-term infant, being insensitive to both trypsin (EC 3.4.21.4) and chymotrypsin (EC 3.4.21.1). Lactase and sucrase activities, however, are virtually absent from the meconium at term, and are also low in the meconium of most premature infants; maltase, which is somewhat less susceptible to proteolytic digestion, survives to a limited extent (77).

The data currently available provide a reasonably coherent account of the development of the surface enzymes of the human fetal intestine up to the age of about 20 weeks. Beyond that time, the findings are fragmentary, and suffer the additional drawback of being principally derived from nonsurviving premature or full-term infants.[1] Where biopsy specimens have been used (80), they have, of course, been obtained from infants who had been treated for ailments of probable intestinal origin. Nevertheless, the outline that emerges traces a biphasic course: an early phase, completed by four months, in which enzymes appear as the structural features of the intestinal wall become established, and a late phase, probably beginning in the eighth month, when enzyme activities attain or somewhat exceed adult values. The second phase is clearly a part of the preparation for postnatal functioning; the first may be related to the assumption of pinocytotic activity, which begins in the fourth month (72). These phases may be roughly equated

---

[1] The papers on enzyme development cited in this article were based on 234 embryos, fetuses, and newborn infants, comprising the following groups: 32 specimens between 7–24 weeks, examined histochemically, half of them with the electron microscope (68,69); 75 examined quantitatively for several enzymes, of which 39 were between 10–14 weeks and 36 between 14–24 weeks (75-80); and 52 infants, of which about half were premature (77,79,80).

to the prenatal and postnatal periods of differentiation in rats, mice, and other small mammals, and may be controlled by similar agencies. The adrenal cortex can apparently secrete steroids by the end of the third month (83), when the fetal thyroid is also functionally competent (84). A parallel study of phosphatase activity in the duodenum and of lipid accumulation in the definitive cortex of human fetuses between 18 and 21 weeks has, in fact, suggested a causal relationship between the two (85). The paucity of information about the secretory activity of the adrenal and thyroid in the third trimester offers no basis for inferences about the endocrine control of the final phases of functional differentiation of the intestinal epithelium. The cessation of pinocytosis, and the modest increases in enzyme activity that occur during the period, however, are events affected by glucocorticoids and thyroxine in other animals, and it is likely that they are similarly regulated in the human fetus and neonate. Hence, endocrine deficiencies in late fetal life might be reflected in subnormal functioning of the intestine at birth.

SUMMARY

Numerous enzymes involved in digestion and absorption are components of the plasma membrane covering the apical surface of intestinal epithelial cells. In rats and mice such enzymes (alkaline phosphatase, lactase, maltase, sucrase, aminopeptidase) accumulate during a short critical period before birth; lactase activity subsequently declines, but the others increase again in a second critical period before weaning. Glucocorticoids and thyroxine appear to regulate these patterns of enzyme development, possibly by acting on the glycosylation of these enzymes, which are glycoproteins. In the intestine of the human fetus, there is a period of structural differentiation and enzyme accumulation at the end of the first and the beginning of the second trimester, when the intestinal epithelium begins to degrade meconium taken in by pinocytosis. Fragmentary evidence suggests that there may be a second stage of enzyme increase in the third trimester, or at the time of birth. Normal adrenocortical and thyroid function may be required for maturation of the intestinal surface in the perinatal period.

ACKNOWLEDGEMENT

Original work reported in this paper was supported by grant HD-03490 from the NIH. I am indebted to Kwo-yih Yeh for permitting me to use the unpublished material shown in Figure 3.

REFERENCES

1. Crane, R. K., Digestive-absorptive surface of the small bowel mucosa, *Annu. Rev. Med.* **19,** 57 (1968).
2. Ugolev, A. M., Membrane digestion, *Gut* **13,** 735 (1972).
3. Trier, J. S., Morphology of the epithelium of the small intestine. In *Handbook of Physiology*, section 6, **III.** Amer. Physiol. Soc., Washington, D.C., 1968, pp 1125–1175.
4. Ito, S., Structure and function of the glycocalyx, *Fed. Proc.* **28,** 12 (1969).
5. Parsons, D. S. and Boyd, C. A. R., Transport across the intestinal mucosal cell: Hierarchies of function. *Int. Rev. Cytol.* **32,** 209 (1972).

6. Rao, S. N., Mukherjee, T. M., and Williams, A. W., Quantitative variation in the disposition of the enteric surface coat in mouse jejunum, *Gut* 13, 33 (1972).

7. Miller, D. and Crane, R. K., The digestive function of the epithelium of the small intestine. II. Localization of disaccharide hydrolysis in the isolated brush border portion of intestinal epithelial cells, *Biochim. Biophys. Acta* 52, 293 (1961).

8. Eichholz, A., Fractions of the brush border. *Fed. Proc.* 28, 30 (1969).

9. Hugon, J. and Borgers, M., Ultrastructural localization of alkaline phosphatatase activity in the absorbing cells of the duodenum of the mouse, *J. Histochem. Cytochem* 14, 629 (1966).

10. Overton, J., Eichholz, A., and Crane, R. K., Studies on the organization of the brush border in intestinal epithelial cells. II. Fine structure of fractions of tris-disrupted hamster brush borders. *J. Cell Biol.* 26, 693 (1965).

11. Oda, T., Seki, S. and Watanabe, S., Molecular basis of structure and function of the microvillus membrane of intestinal epithelial cells, *Acta Med. Okayama* 23, 357 (1969).

12. Forstner, G. G., Release of intestinal surface membrane glycoproteins associated with enzyme activity by brief digestion with papain. *Biochem. J.* 121, 781 (1971).

13. Kelly, J. J. and Alpers, D. H., Blood group antigenicity of purified human intestinal disaccharidases. *J. Biol. Chem.* 248, 8216 (1973).

14. Bertalanffy, F. D. Cell renewal in the gastrointestinal tract of man, *Gastroenterology* 43, 472 (1962).

15. Nelson, J. M., Influence of intestinal mucosal renewal rate on development of gastrointestinal injury and survival time in irradiated gerbils, *Radiat. Res.* 49, 367 (1972).

16. Nordstrom, C., Dahlqvist, A., and Josefsson, L., Quantitative determination of enzymes in different parts of the villi and crypts of rat small intestine, *J. Histochem. Cytochem.* 15, 713 (1967).

17. Nordstrom, C. and Dahlqvist, A., Quantitative distribution of some enzymes along the villi and crypts of human small intestine, *Scand. J. Gastroenterol.* 8, 470 (1973).

18. Das, B. C. and Gray, G. M., Protein synthesis in small intestine: Localization and correlation with DNA synthesis and sucrase activity, *Biochim. Biophys. Acta* 195, 255 (1969).

19. James, W. P. T., Alpers, D. H., Gerber, J. E. and Isselbacher, K. J., The turnover of disaccharidases and brush border proteins in rat intestine, *Biochim. Biophys. Acta* 230, 194 (1971).

20. Grand, R. J., Chong, D. A., and Isselbacher, K. J., Intracellular processing of disaccharidases: The effect of actinomycin D, *Biochim. Biophys. Acta* 261, 341 (1972).

21. Deren, J. J., Development of intestinal structure and function. In *Handbook of Physiology*, Section 6, **III**. Amer. Physiol. Soc., Washington, D. C., 1968, pp. 1099–1123.

22. Koldovsky, O., Hormonal and dietary factors in the development of digestion and absorption. In *Nutrition and Development*, M. Winick, Ed. John Wiley & Sons, New York, N.Y., 1972, pp. 135–200.

23. Moog, F., The functional differentiation of the small intestine. The differentiation of alkaline phosphomonoesterase in the duodenum of the mouse. *J. Exp. Zool.* 118, 187 (1951).

24. Halliday, R., The effect of steroid hormones on the absorption of antibody by the young rat. *J. Endocrinol.* 18, 56 (1959).

25. Moog, F. and Yeh, K.Y., Intestinal alkaline phosphatase of the rat: Development and distribution of activity with phenylphosphate and β-glycerophosphate. *Comp. Biochem. Physiol.* 44B, 657 (1973).

26. Rubino, A., Zimbalatti, F. and Auricchio, S., Intestinal disaccharidase activities in adult and suckling rats, *Biochim. Biophys. Acta.* 92, 305 (1964).

27. Noack, R. et al., Proteolytic and peptidase activities of the jejunum and ileum of the rat during postnatal development, *Biochem. J.* 100, 775 (1966).

28. Moog, F., Birkenmeier, E. H., and Glazier, H. S., Leucylnaphthylamidase activity in the small intestine of the mouse: Normal development and influence of cortisone and antibiotics, *Dev. Biol.* 25, 398 (1971).

29. Moog, F., Denes, A. E., and Powell, P. M., Disaccharidases in the small intestine of the mouse: Normal development and influence of cortisone, actinomycin D, and cycloheximide. *Dev. Biol.* 35, 143 (1973).

30. Moog, F., The functional differentiation of the small intestine. The influence of the pituitary-adrenal system on the differentiation of phosphatase in the duodenum of the suckling mouse, *J. Exp. Zool.* **124**, 329 (1953).

31. Koldovsky, O., Jirsova, V., and Heringova, A., Effect of aldosterone and corticosterone on β-galactosidase and invertase activity in the small intestine of rats, *Nature* **206**, 300 (1965).

32. Doell, R. G. and Kretchmer, N., Intestinal invertase: Precocious development of activity after injection of hydrocortisone, *Science* **143**, 42 (1964). Abstract.

33. Doell, R. G., Rosen, G., Kretchmer, N., Immunochemical studies of intestinal disaccharidases during normal and precocious development, *Proc. Natl. Acad. Sci. U.S.A.* **54**, 1268 (1965).

34. Galand, G. and Forstner, G. G. Isolation of microvillus plasma membranes from suckling rat intestine.   The influence of premature induction of digestives enzymes by injection of cortisol acetate, *Biochem. J.* **144**, 293 (1974).

35. Galand, G. and Jacquot, R., Effect of hydrocortisone and adrenalectomy on sucrase activity in rat intestine during weaning. *C. R. Acad. Sci.* (Paris), **271**, 1107 (1970).

36. Lebenthal, E., Sunshine, P., and Kretchmer, N., Effect of carbohydrate and corticosteroids on activity of α-glucosidases in intestine of infant rat. *J. Clin. Invest.* **51**, 1244 (1972).

37. Koldovsky, O., Jumawan, J., Herbst, J. J., and Palmieri, M., Corticosteroid dependent cyclo-heximide-evoked increase of sucrase and maltase in the jejunum of suckling rats, *Biochim. Biophys. Acta* **309**, 370 (1973).

38. Kitchell, R. L., and Wells, L. J., Reciprocal relation between the hypophysis and adrenals in fetal rats: Effect of unilateral adrenalectomy and of implanted cortisone, DOCA, and sex hormones, *Endocrinology* **50**, 83 (1952).

39. Josimovich, J. B., Ladman, A. J., and Deane, H. W., A histophysiological study of the developing adrenal cortex of the rat during fetal and early postnatal stages, *Endocrinology* **54**, 627 (1954).

40. Verne, J. and Hebert, S., L'apparition de l'activité phosphomonoesterasique au cours du developpement et ses rapports avec le fonctionnement cortico-surrenal, *Ann. Endocrinol.* (Paris) **10**, 456 (1949).

41. Moog, F. and Ortiz, E., The functional differentiation of the small intestine. VII. The duodenum of the foetal guinea pig, with a note on the growth of the adrenals, *J. Embryol. Exp. Morphol.* **8**, 182 (1960).

42. Bearn, J. C., The influence of the foetal pituitary-adrenal axis on the accumulation of alkaline phosphatase in the duodenal epithelium of the foetal rabbit, *J. Anat.* **100**, 449 (1966).

43. Koldovsky, O. et al., Activity of β-galactosidase in homogenates of isolated microvilli fraction of jejunal mucosa from suckling rats, *Biochem. J.* **96**, 492 (1965).

44. Doell, R. G. and Kretchmer, N., Studies of small intestine during development.   I. Distribution and activity of β-galactosidase, *Biochim. Biophys. Acta* **62**, 353 (1962).

45. Hedberg, C. A., Reiser, S., and Reilly, R. W., Intestinal phase of the runting syndrome in mice. II. Observations on nutrient absorption and certain disaccharidase abnormalities, *Transplantation* **6**, 104 (1968).

46. Koldovsky, O. and Sunshine, P., Effect of cortisone on the developmental pattern of the neutral and the acid β-galactosidase of the small intestine of the rat, *Biochem. J.* **117**, 467 (1970).

47. Goldstein, R., Klein, T., Freier, S., and Menczel, J., Alkaline phosphatase and disaccharidase activities in the rat intestine from birth to weaning. I. Effect of diet on enzyme development, *Am. J. Clin. Nutr.* **24**, 1224 (1971).

48. Schlegel-Haueter, S., Hore, P., Kerry, K. R., and Semenza, G., The preparation of lactase and glucoamylase of the rat small intestine, *Biochim. Biophys. Acta* **258**, 506 (1972).

49. Leichter, J., Effect of dietary lactose on intestinal lactase activity in young rats, *J. Nutr.* **103**, 392 (1973).

50. Lebenthal, E., Sunshine, P., and Kretchmer, N., Effect of prolonged nursing on the activity of intestinal lactase in rats. *Gastroenterology* **64**, 1136 (1973).

51. Yeh, K. Y. and Moog, F., Intestinal lactase activity in the suckling rat: Influence of hypophysectomy and thyroidectomy, *Science* **183**, 77 (1974).

52. Yeh, K. Y. and Moog, F., Effects of hypophysectomy and thyroidectomy on the maturation of the small intestine, *Amer. Zool.* **13**, 1318 (1973).

53. Yeh, K. Y. and Moog, F., Development of the small intestine in the hypophysectomized rat. I. Growth, histology, and activity of alkaline phosphatase, maltase, and sucrase, *Dev. Biol.* **47**, 156 (1975).

54. Yeh, K. Y. and Moog, F., Development of the small intestine in the hypophysectomized rat. II. Effects of cortisone, thyroxine, growth hormone, and prolactin, *Dev. Biol.* **47**, 173 (1975).

55. Koldovsky, O., Jumawan, J. and Palmieri, M., Thyroxine-evoked precocious decrease of acid hydrolases in the ileum of suckling rats, *Proc. Soc. Exp. Biol. Med.* **146**, 661 (1974).

56. Altmann, G. G. and Leblond, C. P., Factors influencing villus size in the small intestine of adult rat as revealed by transposition of intestinal segments, *Am. J. Anat.* **127**, 15 (1970).

57. Overton, J., Fine structure of the free cell surface in developing mouse intestinal mucosa, *J. Exp. Zool.* **159**, 195 (1965).

58. Bennett, G. and Leblond, C. P., Formation of cell coat material for the whole surface of columnar cells in the rat small intestine, as visualized by radioautography and L-fucose-³H, *J. Cell Biol.* **46**, 409 (1970).

59. Whaley, W. G., Dauwalder, M., and Kephart, J. E., Golgi apparatus: Influence on cell surfaces, *Science*, **175**, 596 (1972).

60. Clark, S. L., The ingestion of proteins and colloidal materials by columnar absorptive cells of the small intestine in suckling rats and mice, *J. Biophys. Biochem. Cytol.* **5**, 41 (1959).

61. Cornell, R. A. and Padykula, H. A., A cytological study of intestinal absorption in the suckling rat, *Am. J. Anat.* **125**, 291 (1969).

62. Worthington, B. B. and Graney, D. O., Uptake of adenovirus by intestinal absorptive cells of the suckling rat. I. The neonatal jejunum, *Anat. Rec.* **175**, 63 (1973).

63. Brambell, F. W. R., The passive immunity of the young mammal, *Biol. Rev.* **33**, 488 (1958).

64. Rodewald, R., Intestinal transport of antibodies in the newborn rat, *J. Cell Biol.* **58**, 189 (1973).

65. Daniels, V. G., Hardy, R. N., and Malinowsea, K. W., The effect of adrenalectomy or pharmacological inhibition of adrenocortical function on the macromolecule uptake by the newborn rat intestine, *J. Physiol.* **229**, 697 (1973).

66. Daniels, V. G., Hardy, R. N., Malinowska, K., and Nathanielez, P. W., The influence of exogenous steroids on macromolecule uptake by the small intestine of the newborn rat, *J. Physiol.* **229**, 681 (1973).

67. Chan, W. S., Daniels, V. G., and Thomas, A. L., Premature cessation of macromolecule uptake by the young rat following thyroxine administration, *J. Physiol.* **231**, 112P (1973).

68. Lev, R., Siegel, H., and Bartman, J., Histochemical studies of developing human fetal small intestine, *Histochem.* **29**, 103 (1972).

69. Kelley, R. O., An ultrastructural and cytochemical study of developing small intestine in man, *J. Embryol. Exp. Morphol.* **29**, 411 (1973).

70. Nagakawa, T., Histogenic and cytological studies of the duodenal mucosa in human foetuses, *Arch. Histol. Jap.* **16**, 495 (1959).

71. Lev, R. and Weisberg, H., Human foetal epithelial glycogen: A histochemical and electron microscopic study, *J. Anat.* **105**, 337 (1969).

72. Bierring, H. et al., On the nature of the meconium corpuscles in human foetal intestinal epithelium. 1. Electron microscope studies, *Acta Pathol. Microbiol. Scand.* **61**, 365 (1964).

73. Andersen, H. et al., On the nature of the meconium corpuscles in human foetal intestinal epithelium. 2. A cytochemical study, *Acta Pathol. Microbiol. Scand.* **61**, 377 (1964).

74. Williams, R. M. and Beck, F., A histochemical study of gut maturation, *J. Anat.* **105**, 487 (1969).

75. Dahlqvist, A. and Lindberg, T., Development of the intestinal disaccharidase and alkaline phosphatase activities in the human foetus, *Clin. Sci.* **30**, 517 (1966).

76. Pelichova, H. et al., Fetal development of non-specific esterases and alkaline phosphatase activities in the small intestine of man, *Biol. Neonat.* **10**, 281 (1966).

77. Eggermont, E., Enzymic activities in meconium from human fetuses and newborns, *Biol. Neonat.* **10,** 266 (1966).

78. Heringova, A. et al., Proteolytic and peptidase activities of the small intestine of human fetuses, *Gastroenterology.* **51,** 1023 (1966).

79. Auricchio, S., Rubino, A. and Murset, G., Intestinal glycosidase activities in the human embryo, fetus, and newborn, *Pediatrics* **35, 944** (1965).

80. Antonowicz, I., Chang, S. K., and Grand, R. J., Development and distribution of lysosomal enzymes and disaccharidases in human fetal intestine, *Gastroenterology.* **67,** 51 (1974).

81. Antonowicz, A., Lloyd-Still, J. D., Khaw, K. T. and Schwachman, D., Congenital sucrase-isomaltase deficiency, *Pediatrics* **49,** 847 (1972).

82. Boellner, S. W., Beard, A. G., and Panos, T. C., Impairment of intestinal hydrolysis of lactose in newborn infants, *Pediatrics* **36,** 542 (1965).

83. Bloch, E., Fetal adrenal cortex: Function and steroidogenesis. In *Functions of the Adrenal Cortex,* **2,** K. W. McKerns, Ed. Appleton-Century-Crofts, New York, N.Y. 1968, pp 721–772.

84. Shephard, T. H., Development of the human fetal thyroid. In *Hormones in Development,* M. Hamburgh and E. J. W. Barrington, Eds., Appleton-Century-Crofts, New York, N.Y. 1971, pp 767–780.

85. Levina, S. E., Some data on the development of the adrenal and thymus glands in human embryogenesis, *Biull. Eksp. Biol. Med.* **59** (3), 89 (1965).

Adjustment to Extrauterine Life

Circulatory and Thermal Homeostasis in the Fetus and Neonate

THOMAS BLUMENFELD, M.D.

RICHARD E. BEHRMAN, M.D.

CIRCULATORY HOMEOSTASIS

The maternal blood flowing through the placenta is, in effect, the external environment of the fetus. Under optimal conditions this environment is remarkably constant. However, changes may occur, generally for one of two reasons.

First, fetal mechanisms for homeostasis of moderate change in the external environment are not always able to prevent change—for example, in maternal hypoglycemia due to starvation. Obviously, for the newborn faced with a more varied external environment, fetal homeostatic mechanisms may be less effective or nonexistent.

Secondly, for the fetus, maternal homeostatic mechanisms may not be directed to minimize physiological changes that may adversely affect the fetus—e.g., constancy of uterine blood flow during acute moderate fetal hypoxia from cord occlusion—or the effect of maternal physiological adjustments may be in the wrong direction from the fetus's point of view, as in uterine vasoconstriction by catecholamines. In general, specific maternal adaptive mechanisms are geared to maternal survival because this is the *sine qua non* of fetal survival.

The fetal circulatory shunts are of particular importance in the circulatory homeostasis of the fetus and neonatal infant. These consist of:

1. The ductus venosus, through which a portion of the oxygenated blood returning from the placenta in the umbilical vein bypasses the liver and goes to the inferior vena cava to return to the heart

2. The foramen ovale, through which oxygenated blood returning to the right atrium is shunted, bypassing the lungs, to the left atrium and thence to the ascending aorta, brain, and coronary arteries

3. The ductus arteriosus connecting the aorta with the pulmonary artery, allowing mixed oxygenated blood to bypass the high-pressure pulmonary circulation to the collapsed lungs and return to the descending aorta

Normally, none of these shunts is functioning in the adult, but all may be relevant to tissue perfusion in the newborn.

The circulatory homeostasis of the fetus at term and the changes that occur in this system during the first few days of life are illustrated by the circulatory adjustment to moderately severe hypoxia and acidosis in rhesus monkeys (*1*). Two groups of fetal rhesus monkeys were studied and maternal hypoxia was induced in one group. When the fetuses developed a controlled moderately severe acidosis and hypoxia, differently radiolabeled microspheres were injected into the inferior vena cava, umbilical vein, and superior vena cava and their distribution was used to estimate fetal organ-blood flows. Umbilical blood flows and cardiac outputs were measured by an independent technique.

The maternal acid-base balance did not change significantly during the period of experimental maternal hypoxia in which maternal arterial saturation decreased from an average of 99% to an average of 78% and p_{O_2} from a mean of 17.2 kPa (129 mmHg) to a mean of 9.6 kPa (72 mmHg).

The fetuses of the mothers subjected to hypoxia developed a mixed metabolic and placental respiratory acidosis with elevation in p_{CO_2} from 6.1 kPa (46 mmHg) to 7.1 kPa (53 mmHg) and lactate from 2.3 mmol/litre to 5.2 mmol/litre. Oxygen consumption decreased by more than 50% from 7 ml/min per kilogram to 3 ml/min per kilogram as p_{O_2} and saturation fell from 3.1 kPa (23 mmHg) to 1.9 kPa (14 mmHg) and 55 to 19%, respectively. The lactate/pyruvate ratio increase averaged 21 to 44.

The distressed fetuses increased the amount of oxygenated umbilical-vein blood going to the inferior vena cava, bypassing the liver, from 53 to 90%, as the umbilical blood flow and cardiac output decreased markedly from 91 to 40 ml/min and 194 to 134 ml/min, respectively. The percentage of cardiac output going to the placenta also decreased from 48 to 29%. Thus, a greater portion of umbilical-vein blood was returned to the heart, although it was less well oxygenated and the overall volume of venous blood returning to the heart was significantly less. Obviously, this fetal mechanism of response to hypoxia is not available to the newborn after birth.

This adaptation to stress results in the maintenance of the percentage of the cardiac output that returns to the heart from the placenta via the ductus venosus, despite an absolute decrease in placental blood flow and cardiac output. In contrast, the return to the heart from the inferior vena cava is significantly less, decreasing from 40% of the cardiac output to 24%. The proportion of the cardiac output derived from the superior vena cava during fetal distress increases from 23 to 42%.

When viewed from the perspective of the fetal organs, the homeostatic adjustments become evident. The percentage of cardiac output supplying the lungs decreases from 10.7 to 3.2%, leading to decreased pulmonary perfusion from 2.9 ml/min/g to 0.5 ml/min/g. This further increases shunting through the ductus arteriosus, thus augmenting the cardiac output that had initially been decreased during fetal distress. However, this may adversely affect subsequent normal pulmonary function, contributing to the development of respiratory distress in the newborn period. This vasoconstrictive response of the pulmonary circulation to hypoxia and acidosis continues during the newborn period. In contrast, the perfusion of the adrenals is maintained by an increase in the percentage of the cardiac output going to this organ.

The volume of blood perfusing the heart and brain during moderate fetal distress is maintained by significant increases in the percentage of the cardiac output going to these organs. The percentage of cardiac output going to the brain increased from 16 to 31%, and that to the heart increased from 2.7 to 4.9%. However, the perfusing blood has a low p_{O_2} and saturation and an increased p_{CO_2} and lactate concentration, an adjustment accomplished by a dramatic increase in shunting through the foramen ovale.

During moderate fetal distress, the coronary blood flow derived from the superior vena cava via the foramen ovale increases from 4 to 19%. This increased shunting through the foramen ovale results in an increase from 1 to 26% in the amount of blood going to the brain that is derived from the superior vena cava. Although this is the least oxygenated blood, it does serve to maintain circulatory volume to the brain acutely. Similar shunting through the foramen ovale occurs in the infant monkey maintained on a positive pressure respirator and to the human infant subjected to severe postnatal stress, especially shock, acidosis, and hypoxia.

In the newborn, responses to stress are superimposed on a developing circulation (2). Oxygen uptake increases in the newborn. The percentages of the cardiac output going to the brain and heart increase. There is also a dramatic increase in the cardiac output provided to the liver coincident with the abrupt cessation of umbilical blood flow, about half of which supplies the fetal liver with oxygen-rich blood. These trends continue during the first week of life.

The circulatory adjustments that the fetus makes to hypoxia and acidosis persist into the newborn period. These responses tend to maintain a steady-state environment, protecting the brain and heart, but they may have untoward effects on other tissue such as the lungs and ductus arteriosus.

THERMAL HOMEOSTASIS

The newborn infant is a homeotherm capable of prompt thermal regulatory responses to maintain deep body temperature near its set point. In response to heat, the infant vasodilates—especially the hands and feet—and sweats. The infant's response to cold is cutaneous vasoconstriction and increased heat production.

A neutral thermal environment is one in which heat production is minimal, yet deep body temperature is maintained within normal range. Adult humans in a neutral thermal environment have a skin temperature range of 33–35 °C. However, term infants show an increased metabolic rate at skin temperatures below 36.2 °C and low-birth-weight infants do likewise at 36.5 °C (3). Investigation suggests that a relative humidity of 50% may be considered optimal for full-term newborn infants on the first day of life (4). The increased metabolic rate at 20% relative humidity is due to increased evaporative heat loss, and the increased metabolic rate at 80% relative humidity is at present unexplained.

Heat production can be determined by measuring oxygen consumption, and the oxygen consumption can be converted to Calories (kcal) by multiplying by 4.83, the number of Calories produced per litre of oxygen consumed. Calories are converted to the SI unit, the joule, by multiplying by 4184. The minimal rate of heat production for full-term (3500 g) infants at birth to 6 h of age, the latter half of the first day, and the second or third day, is 32, 37, and 43 Cal/kg/24 h, respectively. With increasing postnatal age, the metabolic rate of premature infants exceeds that of a full-term baby of the same weight.

Infants who are small for gestational age also have a higher rate of oxygen consumption than do normal infants of similar birth weight and postnatal age (5).

Heat is lost from the interior of the body to the skin surface (internal gradient) and from skin surface to adjacent air (external gradient). The former may be controlled by vasomotor activity; the latter is dependent on the environment. Heat loss may occur by four mechanisms: convection, radiation, evaporation, and conduction. Compared to the adult, the newborn infant is at a disadvantage in dealing with the external gradient because he has a relatively large surface area proportional to body mass and his tissue insulation is less because of thinner subcutaneous tissue. With increasing gestational age, postures tend toward increased flexion of the extremities, which decreases the exposed surface area and thus the heat loss by radiation and convection (6).

The infant's physiological response to excessive environmental temperature is vaso-dilatation and sweating. Vasodilatation decreases tissue insulation; it occurs after the rectal temperature exceeds 36.6 to 37.3 °C and requires an intact central nervous system (7). Under resting conditions in a neutral thermal environment, a quarter of the heat loss in infants is owing to evaporation (8). The infant's ability to increase evaporation is its principal defense against hyperthermia. The threshold for sweating is about 37.2 °C (rectal) and tends to be higher on the first day of life (8). Term infants can triple evap-orative water loss, but infants who are more than three weeks premature have a decreased— or no—ability to increase evaporative water loss (8). Thus, sweating is a function of gestational age and not of size.

The infant's physiological response to decreased environmental temperatures is periph-eral vasoconstriction and increased heat production (9). The thermoregulatory stimulus to cold may originate in the peripheral skin, because exposure to cold without a change in interior temperature can cause vasoconstriction and nonshivering thermogenesis. The face is particularly sensitive to cold; application of a cold stimulus can result in a distinct increase in metabolic rate (9,10). Abnormalities of the central nervous system can impair the metabolic response to cold, so an intact nervous system may be necessary for an ade-quate metabolic response to cold (11). Vasoconstriction has the effect of increasing the tissue insulation and increases the internal temperature gradient. The newborn's range of control of tissue insulation is similar to that of the adult (7), but because of the smaller body size the maximum tissue insulation is less.

Healthy term newborn infants, when exposed to cold, may increase their heat produc-tion by two and half times the resting rate. There is an approximately linear increase in metabolic rate with temperature decrease (12). Infants in a cool environment may appear restless and cry but do not appear to shiver unless there is rapid fall in rectal temperature (9); however, for human adults, shivering is the principal source of additional heat pro-duction on exposure to cold. The age at which nonshivering thermogenesis ceases to be a major factor in heat production in the child is not known, but from evidence in chil-dren with congenital heart disease it appears to be of substantial importance up to at least six months of age (13,14).

Even though the newborn may under some circumstances produce heat by shivering, nonshivering thermogenesis is largely responsible for increased heat production. There is very strong, although indirect, evidence that brown fat is the important site of non-shivering heat production in the human infant. In the human fetus, the primitive brown fat cells begin to differentiate from reticular cells at 26 to 30 weeks of gestation. Develop-ment of brown fat is not complete at term; the cells continue to enlarge after birth and by the third to fifth postpartum week the amount of cytoplasm per cell is almost double that at birth (*15*). Brown fat in infants is found in five principal sites: (*a*) a large diamond-shaped interscapular mass; (*b*) small deposits adjacent to muscles and blood vessels of neck, the major one following the course of the internal jugular veins and the common carotid arteries; (*c*) large axillary deposits; (*d*) deposits adjacent to the great vessels entering the thoracic inlet and from there following the intercostal arteries and internal mammary vessels; and (*e*) deposits adjacent to posterior abdominal wall structures, the largest enveloping the kidneys and adrenals (*15*). Nerve fibers, capillaries, and blood vessels are numerous in brown fat and one third or more of the surface of each cell is in contact with a capillary (*15*). Mitochondria of brown fat cells have prominent cristae and numerous adjacent fat vacuoles. This ultrastructure indicates the great metabolic potential of these cells.

When newborn infants are exposed to cool conditions, the surface temperature of the skin of the trunk falls sharply while the surface temperature of the nape of the neck falls significantly less, suggesting increased metabolic activity and increased profusion of nuchal brown fat (*16,17*). On acute cold exposure, the spinal cord, paravertebral ganglia, adrenal glands, kidneys, axilla, and aortic arch (i.e., body core) are protected by heat produced by the closely applied brown fat. In infants dying with cold syndrome, brown fat was totally depleted, indicating that these infants may not have been able to produce heat in response to cold exposure (*15*). In cold-exposed animals, the temperature of the venous blood draining the brown fat increases and heat is transferred to other sites by vascular convection (*18*). It is interesting that warming the spinal cord of newborn guinea pigs at the level of C6-T1 tends to suppress shivering (*19*).

In newborn animals and infants, norepinephrine is intensely thermogenic, and in animals its effect can be blocked by hexamethonium and reserpine, norepinephrine blocking agents (*20,21,22,23*). Increased susceptibility to cold injury has been reported in infants whose mothers received reserpine before delivery (*24*). Stimulation of the sympathetic nerves innervating the brown fat or intravenous infusion of norepinephrine increases the temperature of the brown fat, suggesting that the thermogenic response is mediated primarily through the sympathetic nervous system, with norepinephrine being the probable transmitting agent (*25*). After cold stress, newborn infants have been observed not to shiver but have elevated body temperature, increased urinary excretion of norepinephrine and dopamine, and a significant increase in free fatty acids in the plasma (*23*). Norepinephrine infusion produces a similar increase in plasma-free fatty acids and in rectal temperature. In another study, newborn infants subjected to a cooling temperature had a significant increased oxygen consumption and plasma glycerol but not a significant increase in plasma free fatty acids, blood glucose, or blood-lactate concentrations (*26*). Newborn rabbit brown fat, in vitro, has a lipolysis rate threefold that of white fat and an oxygen consumption rate twentyfold that of adult rabbit fat, which is predominantly white (*11*). Heat production in the newborn rabbit is accompanied by a fourfold increase in plasma glycerol and a slightly significant rise in plasma free fatty acids (*27*). Brown fat tissue has no glycerol kinase (EC 2.7.1.30), and the increase in plasma glycerol is an indication of lipolysis of triglycerides (*27*). The small concomitant increase in free fatty acids in the plasma suggests that fatty acids are being oxidized locally in brown fat, with the production of heat. These observations strongly suggest that nonshivering heat production in the cold-stressed infant is due to norepinephrine-stimulated metabolism of brown fat.

There is evidence (25) that norepinephrine mediates the acute cold-induced thermogenic response of brown fat by stimulating production of 3',5'-cyclic adenosine monophosphate, which activates a lipase that catalyzes hydrolysis of tryglycerides to fatty acids and glycerol. Fatty acids and glycerol can be readily oxidized in vitro by brown fat, and it appears that either or both may serve as the fuel during norepinephrine stimulation of brown fat thermogenesis. Thermogenesis may occur by the triglyceride re-esterification cycle in which triglycerides are hydrolyzed to glycerol and fatty acids and then re-esterified or by the fatty acid resynthesis cycle in which fatty acids are oxidized to acetyl CoA and then resynthesized to fatty acids, or by both mechanisms. It has also been proposed that norepinephrine may also produce a thermogenic response by uncoupling oxidative phosphorylation (adenosine diphosphate–adenosine triphosphate) in brown fat mitochondria (Figure 1).

Nonincubated infants have significantly higher values for protein-bound iodine and higher thyroid radioiodine clearance at 48 h than do incubated infants, suggesting that feedback suppression of thyrotropin (thyroid stimulating hormone) secretion is inoperative in infants in the colder environment (28). These findings are consistent with the hypothesis that the neonatal hyperthyroid state results from thermal receptor stimulation of thyrotropin secretion by the relatively cold extrauterine environment. Thyroxine evidently affects the metabolic response of brown fat to norepinephrine, because continued exposure to cold or norepinephrine injection of euthyroid mice—but not of hypothyroid mice—increases their oxygen consumption (29). These findings are consistent with the suggestion that, in adipose tissue, thyroid hormone may regulate the activity of adenyl cyclase (EC 4.6.1.1), which may mediate the thermogenic effect of norepinephrine (30).

Recently it has been proposed that thyroid thermogenesis results from thyroxine indirectly activating sodium pumps in the cell membrane, which increases active sodium transport, increasing adenosine triphosphate hydrolysis and formation of adenosine diphosphate, and paces oxidative phosphorylation in mitochondria at a new and higher

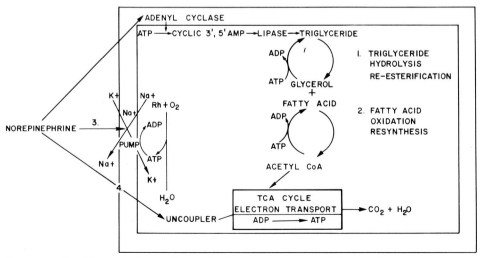

Figure 1. Possible mechanisms of brown fat thermogenesis activated by norepinephrine.

level. In mammals the sodium pump constitutes one of the principal sources of heat, as well as serving to regulate intracellular ion composition (*31*).

Studies of metabolism of brown fat have shown that the addition of ouabain, a specific inhibitor of the sodium pump, or removal of sodium from the medium decreased oxygen consumption evoked by norepinephrine by 60%, implying that more than half of the thermogenic action of norepinephrine on this system is a consequence of increased energy turnover coupled to sodium transport (*32*). Data from this study also indicated that ouabain inhibition of the norepinephrine-induced increase in brown fat thermogenesis did not reflect an inhibition of cyclic adenosine monophosphate synthesis or lipolytic activity. Thus, there is evidence that the activity of the sodium pump accounts for a significant portion of oxygen consumption and thermogenic response of the activated brown fat cell.

Nonshivering thermogenesis activated by norepinephrine may therefore be produced by any one or a combination of the following: (*a*) triglyceride re-esterification, (*b*) fatty acid resynthesis, (*c*) uncoupling adenosine diphosphate–adenosine triphosphate oxidative phosphorylation, and (*d*) augmented adenosine triphosphate turnover coupled to active sodium transport (Figure 1). These mechanisms may be augmented by thyroid hormone action. However, knowledge of the exact mechanism or mechanisms by which norepinephrine can induce a sustained increase in the rate of oxygen consumption/thermogenesis in brown fat is incomplete.

SUMMARY

In summary, the infant can respond to increased environmental temperature by sweating and vasodilatation and can respond to decreased environmental temperature by vasoconstriction and nonshivering thermogenesis, primarily from brown fat. Thus, the healthy term newborn is a homeotherm capable of thermal adaption of changing environmental temperatures; however, the range of response is different from that of the adult.

REFERENCES

1. Behrman, R. E. et al., Distribution of the circulation in the normal and asphyxiated fetal primate, *Am. J. Obstet. Gynecol.* **108**, 956 (1970).

2. Behrman, R. E. and Lees, M. H., Oxygen blood flows of the fetal, newborn and adult rhesus monkey. A comparative study, *Biol. Neonate.* **18**, 330 (1971).

3. Hey, E. N. and Katz, G., The optimum thermal environment for naked babies, *Arch. Dis. Child.* **45**, 328–334 (1970).

4. Sulyok, E., Jequier, E., and Ryser, G., Effect of relative humidity on thermal balance of the newborn infant, *Biol. Neonate.* **21**, 210–218 (1972).

5. Sinclair, J. C., Heat production and thermoregulation in the small-for-date infant, *Pediatr. Clin. North Am.* **17**, 147–158 (1970).

6. Amiel-Tison, C., Neurological evaluation of the maturity of newborn infants, *Arch. Dis. Child.* **43**, 89–93 (1968).

7. Hey, E. N. and Katz, G., The range of thermal insulation in the tissue of the newborn baby, *J. Physiol.* (London) **207**, 667–681 (1970).

8. Hey, E. N. and Katz, G., Evaporative water loss in the newborn baby, *J. Physiol.* **200**, 605–619 (1969).

9. Bruck, K., Temperature regulation in the newborn infant, *Biol. Neonate.* **3**, 65–119 (1961).

10. Mestyan, J., Jarar, I., Bata, G., and Fekete, M., Surface temperature versus deep body temperature and the metabolic response to cold of hypothermic premature infants, *Biol. Neonate.* **7**, 230–242 (1964).

11. Scopes, J. W., Metabolic rate and temperature control in the human body, *Br. Med. Bull.* **22**, 88–91 (1966).

12. Hey, E. N., The relation between environmental temperature and oxygen consumption in the newborn baby, *J. Physiol.* **200**, 589–603 (1969).

13. Baum, D. and Mullins, G. H., Core temperature in infants undergoing cardiac catheterization, *Pediatrics* **36**, 88–93 (1965).

14. Lees, M. H., Bristow, J. D., Griswold, H. E., and Olmsted, R. W., Relative hypermetabolism in infants with heart disease and undernutrition. Presented at the annual meeting of the Society for Pediatric Research, Philadelphia, Pa., May, 1965.

15. Ahern, W. and Hull, D., Brown adipose tissue and heat production in the newborn infant, *J. Pathol.* **91**, 223–234 (1966).

16. Silverman, W. A., Zamelis, A., Sinclair, J. C., and Agate, F. J., Jr., Warm nape of newborn, *Pediatrics*, **33**, 984–987 (1964).

17. Grausz, J. P., Interscapular skin temperature in the newborn infant, *J. Pediat.* **76**, 752–756 (1970).

18. Smith, R. E. and Roberts, J. C., Thermogenesis of brown adipose tissue in cold acclimated rats, *Am. J. Physiol* **206**, 143–148 (1964).

19. Bruck, K. and Wunnenberg, W., Beziehung zwischen Thermogenese im "braunen" Fettgewebe, Temperatur im cervicalin Anteil des Vertiebralkanals und Kallezittern, *Arch. Ges. Physiol.* **290**, 167–183 (1966).

20. Moore, R. E. and Underwood, M. C., The thermogenic effect of noradrenalin in newborn and infant kittens and other small mammals. A possible hormonal mechanism in the control of heat production, *J. Physiol.* **168**, 290–317 (1963).

21. Scopes, J. W. and Tizard, J. P. M., The effect of intravenous noradrenalin on the oxygen consumption of newborn mammals, *J. Physiol.* **165**, 305–326 (1963).

22. Karlberg, P., Moore, R. E., and Oliver, T. K., Jr., The thermogenic response of the newborn infant to noradrenalin, *Acta Paediata. Scand.* **51**, 284–292 (1962).

23. Schiff, D., Stern, L., and Leduc, J., Chemical thermogenesis in newborn infants: Catecholamine excretion and the plasma non-esterified fatty acid response to cold exposure, *Pediatrics*, **37**, 577–582 (1966).

24. Anagnostakis, D. and Matsaniotis, N., Neonatal cold injury and maternal reserpine administration, *Lancet* **ii**, 471 (1974).

25. Smith, R. E. and Horwitz, B. A., Brown fat thermogenesis, *Physiol. Rev.* **49**, 330–425 (1969).

26. Dawkins, M. J. R. and Scopes, J. W., Non-shivering thermogenesis and brown adipose tissue in human newborn infants, *Nature* **206**, 201–202 (1965).

27. Dawkins, M. J. R. and Hull, D., Brown adipose tissue and the response of newborn rabbits to cold, *J. Physiol.* **172**, 216–238 (1964).

28. Fisher, D. A., Oddie, T. H., and Makoski, E. D., The influence of environmental temperature on thyroid, adrenal and water metabolism in the newborn infant, *Pediatrics* **37**, 583–591 (1966).

29. Ikemoto, H., Hiroshige, T., and Itoh, S., Oxygen consumption of brown fat adipose tissue in normal and hypothyroid mice, *Jap. J. Physiol.* **17**, 516–522 (1967).

30. Krishna, G., Hynie, S., Brodie, Brodie, B. B., Effects of thyroid hormones on adenyl cyclase in adipose tissue and on free fatty acid mobilization, *Proc. Natl. Acad. Sci. U.S.A.* **59**, 884–889 (1968).

31. Edelman, I. S., Thyroid thermogenesis, *N. Engl. J. Med.* **290**, 1303–1308 (1974).

32. Horwitz, B. A., Ouabain-sensitive component of brown fat thermogenesis, *Am. J. Physiol.* **224** 352–355 (1973).

Neonatal Physiology: Basis for the Laboratory Needs of the Nursery

GORDON B. AVERY, M.D., Ph.D.

What's wrong with those neonatologists? Why can't they do things the same way as the other departments of the hospital? Why are they always in such a hurry? Why do they want everything "stat" and "micro"? When we are geared to being cordon bleu chefs for internal medicine, why must they always make us short-order cooks?

Questions of this sort must run through the minds of laboratory directors wherever neonatal intensive-care centers are located. The strident demands of this growing sub-specialty of pediatrics have upset the routine of many a clinical laboratory, for in fact the nursery that attempts to provide truly modern intensive care does have unique needs, which cannot be met without numerous special accommodations. No other field of medicine has changed faster in the past decade, and in few others is complex physiology so intimately interwoven with daily clinical practice.

It is, in fact, the unique physiology of the newborn that lies behind the special demands that neonatology places on the laboratory. All of pediatrics is marked by infant growth and development, upon which disease entities are superimposed. The pace of change in the newborn is very rapid as the adaptation from intrauterine to extrauterine existence is made. In the case of the small premature, the goal is no less than to substitute for the maternal life-support environment from which the infant has been separated too soon.

In this paper, I will attempt to explain the physiological considerations and disease states that underlie some of the more common requests for special consideration that emanate from the intensive care nursery.

BILIRUBIN, STAT, MICRO, AROUND-THE-CLOCK (AND TOTAL PROTEIN)

The adult has abundant reserve capacity for conjugating and excreting bilirubin, so clinical jaundice is noted only in liver disease and in severe hemolytic states. In contrast, the newborn has a marginal capacity to excrete bilirubin, and many term infants as well as most premature infants experience jaundice in the first week of life. The hepatic enzyme UDP-glucuronyl transferase is adaptively synthesized in response to increased substrate, and conjugating ability increases remarkably after several postnatal days, both in the premature and in the term infant. Microsomal enzyme inducers such as adrenal steroids and phenobarbital can accelerate this process. The ductus venosus carries much of the umbilical venous and portal blood around the liver in utero, and its late closure may deprive the liver of some of its perfusion. Beta-glucuronidases (EC 3.2.1.31) in the gut lumen split some previously excreted conjugated bilirubin, and the resulting unconjugated bilirubin is reabsorbed and recirculated. This "enterohepatic recirculation" is believed to be an important contributor to so-called physiological jaundice. Thus paralytic ileus or any situation that delays evacuation of the intestinal contents will enhance jaundice in the newborn. Even in the absence of isoimmunization, these circumstances are sufficient to cause significant jaundice, in conjunction with the high amount of breakdown in hemoglobin that is normal during the first weeks of life.

The newborn is uniquely vulnerable to bilirubin encephalopathy (kernicterus) because of three factors: the frequent occurrence of high concentrations of unconjugated bilirubin in the first week of life; the low availability of plasma albumin binding sites for bilirubin; and the probability that the blood-brain barrier is somewhat more permeable to bilirubin in the newborn period. The considerations listed above, plus hemolytic states associated with erythroblastosis, sepsis, enclosed hemorrhage, and the like explain the frequency of jaundice. It is only the free, diffusible unconjugated bilirubin that is fat soluble and can enter the brain. Thus as long as bilirubin is transported strongly bound to albumin it is nontoxic. Each molecule of albumin has two bilirubin binding sites, one of which is strong and one comparatively weak. Free bilirubin begins to appear in the plasma after the first binding site has been saturated—at approximately a 1:1 molar ratio of albumin to bilirubin. The only magic of the old criterion that exchange transfusion should be performed if values for indirect bilirubin exceed 340 μmol/litre (20 mg/100 ml) is that, with the protein values seen in most term infants, the first albumin-binding site is saturated at that concentration.

It is now clear that kernicterus can occur at much lower bilirubin concentrations in sick premature infants or in infants in whom competing substances displace bilirubin from plasma albumin. Prematures are particularly at risk, because their plasma proteins are typically lower than those of term infants. Competing substances that displace bilirubin include drugs such as sulfonamides and salicylates, and endogenous substances such as free fatty acids, heme pigments, and such organic anions as lactate. The acid–base status of the infant affects the dissociation of bilirubin, which is a weak organic acid. Even the history of previous birth asphyxia is associated with kernicterus at lower bilirubin concentrations.

The clinician caring for critically ill prematures must balance a risky procedure (exchange transfusion) against the danger of kernicterus at the current bilirubin concentration, in an infant whose status is rapidly changing. He would most like to know the value of the remaining binding capacity of albumin at its strong binding site, which is his margin of safety. Providing a rapid, accurate, generally available method for this determination should be a challenge for clinical chemists in the future. In the meantime, a promptly obtained value for indirect bilirubin, together with one for total protein (which is roughly twice the albumin), will provide the basis for an extrapolation that takes into account the infant's entire clinical situation. Hence the call for bilirubins, stat, micro, in the middle of the night (with total protein).

SERUM ELECTROLYTES, IN THE DARK OF NIGHT, MICRO!

The newborn is relatively less able to maintain homeostasis of fluid and electrolytes when stressed by disease or miscalculated therapy. His water turnover is much more rapid than that of the older child, and his total body water is proportionately greater (77% of body weight for premature, 70% for term newborn, 60% for adult). Glomerular filtration rate, renal plasma flow, and tubular function are all relatively subnormal in the newborn and increase rapidly during the first few weeks of life. Urine is diluted in response to a water load, but only a limited volume can be excreted, so prematures, in particular, are liable to become edematous. On the other hand, newborns can only concentrate to 500 to 600 mosmol/litre in the urine and become rapidly dehydrated when insufficient fluid is provided. Both hyponatremia and hypernatremia occur with some frequency in sick prematures, and are accompanied by such symptoms as listlessness and apnea. These considerations make it necessary to tailor fluid and electrolyte therapy to the individual infant by titration rather than mere calculation from rules of thumb, using as indicators accurate body weights, urine volume and specific gravity, serum electrolytes, clinical assessment of the state of hydration, and, occasionally, information on urine and serum osmolarity.

The premature with hyaline membrane disease typifies the precariousness of many of our patients. Most of these infants are too sick to be fed for several days, and receive intravenous fluids during that time. Initial potassium values range up to 8 mmol/litre (mEq/litre) because intracellular potassium is leaking into the extracellular compartment. With improvement in oxygenation and acidosis, an abrupt decrease in potassium to subnormal values may occur around the second or third day. Sodium-free fluids are usually given the first day or two to avoid hypernatremia from therapy with sodium bicarbonate. However, the sudden appearance of hyponatremia is not uncommon, probably associated with abnormal renal losses. Intravenous alimentation may be attempted during this time, with the attendant dangers of metabolic acidosis, hyperammonemia, hyperglycemia, and osmotic diuresis with secondary electrolyte depletion. After initial stabilization and the institution of oral feedings, the premature is vulnerable to a syndrome called "late metabolic acidosis," resulting from inability to excrete the acid products that derive from catabolism of the relatively high-calorie, high-protein feedings required for rapid growth.

The symptoms displayed by prematures suffering from these metabolic vagaries tend to be nonspecific and to overlap with those caused by sepsis, intracranial hemorrhage, birth asphyxia, or deterioration of the child's underlying disease. We must, therefore, rely on the laboratory to help unscramble the pieces of the puzzle and plan rational therapy. All too often, sudden deterioration occurs in the dead of night or on Sunday afternoon.

CALCIUM, GLUCOSE (AND SOMETIMES MAGNESIUM), QUICK!

Low serum calcium values are extremely common in sick prematures during the first two days of extrauterine life. This early-onset hypocalcemia has been attributed to temporarily reduced parathyroid function, because of high in utero serum calcium concentrations, kidney tubule unresponsiveness to parathyroid hormone, asphyxial stimulation of calcitonin, temporary lack of dietary calcium, and the adrenal steroid response to stress. Each of these explanations is supported by some evidence, and all may play a part. An additional type of hypocalcemia occurs after a week or so of life, affecting term babies more often than prematures, and associated with feeding milk that has a high phosphate content.

Certain classes of newborns are particularly vulnerable to hypoglycemia: those with intrauterine growth failure, the smaller of twins of differing weights, infants of diabetic mothers, and severely erythroblastotic babies. Physiological explanations include limited glycogen and fat stores in the former two categories and pancreatic islet-cell hyperplasia with increased insulin response to glucose loading and epinephrine depletion in the latter two categories. Limited dietary intake and increased metabolic demands often contribute to the problem in sick infants.

Hypocalcemia and hypoglycemia are linked clinically, in that both may cause the same symptoms and both occur in some of the same infants. The symptoms are nonspecific and overlap with those of many other conditions, but in general consist of apnea, brady-cardia, jitteriness, seizures, pallor, and general clinical deterioration. Symptomatic hypo-glycemia is followed by neurological sequelae in about 50% of all cases, and hypocal-cemia by sequelae in about 10%. Thus the issue of finding and treating these metabolic abnormalities is an important one.

Hypomagnesemia occasionally occurs together with hypocalcemia. Administration of calcium alone fails to correct either the hypocalcemia or the symptoms. Both improve when magnesium is given.

What controls neuromuscular excitability is ionized and not total serum calcium. The fraction bound to serum proteins varies with the amount of protein, especially albumin, and with pH. Hence, prematures with their lower serum protein concentration may have relatively lower total calcium values without symptoms. On the other hand, infants with acidosis may abruptly develop tetany when their acidosis is corrected with sodium bi-carbonate. A challenge for the clinical laboratory is to develop a simple and generally available method for determining ionized calcium that can be used around the clock, for sudden clinical deterioration of uncertain cause frequently occurs at inconvenient times of day.

BLOOD GASES (pH, p_{O_2}, p_{CO_2})—RESULTS WITHIN 15 MINUTES

The newborn period is one of cardiorespiratory instability. Even healthy, term infants make a dramatic transition between intrauterine and extrauterine circulation and between a fluid-filled and air-breathing lung. The pulmonary arteries have a thick, reactive mus-cular coat, and under conditions of hypoxia and acidosis they constrict, shunting blood away from the lungs and partly returning the infant to a fetal circulatory pattern. The premature is particularly vulnerable during this transition because of his lung instability and poorly developed respiratory centers.

A further complication in the small premature is susceptibility to oxygen toxicity. At this period of development, vascularization of the retina is in a critical phase, and exces-sive oxygen tensions in the blood can result in scarring, retinal detachment, and blind-ness owing to retrolental fibroplasia. Excessive oxygen can also damage the lungs, with so-called bronchopulmonary dysplasia.

It goes without saying that measurement of blood gases is a part of intensive care, and such information is wanted in a hurry and around the clock. However, the numbers of sets of gases and the urgency with which they are required in respiratory support of the newborn may seem excessively large. The sudden changes in pulmonary circulation and relative shunting of the blood around the lungs, the frequent adjustment of respirator settings (which must be guided by blood-gas results), and the need to titrate oxygen therapy against the oxygen tension of the blood may require a dozen or more sets of blood-gas measurements for a single infant on the respirator in a 24-h period.

The mortality of prematures from hyaline membrane disease has decreased dramatically in the better neonatal intensive care centers with the advent of modern techniques of respirator care and positive expiratory pressure. Happily, those centers with relatively long-term follow-up have reported good outcomes in terms of lung function and intelligence in most survivors, but such results are only possible when the laboratory is willing to make the major commitment of support needed for this type of intensive care.

BLOOD BANK—FRESH BLOOD, WALKING DONORS, FRACTIONAL UNITS!

Prematures require relatively small volumes of blood, but often require them repeatedly. Their blood volume is about 90 ml/kg of body weight, and, thus, a modest blood loss or the cumulative result of repeated sampling may significantly reduce the hemoglobin mass. Moreover, infants with respiratory distress tolerate anemia poorly. Apneic spells are more frequent when hemoglobin values are low. Rapid growth relative to initial body size—plus the normal breakdown of erythrocytes that occurs in the newborn period—makes declining hematocrits common. Intravenous alimentation, when oral feeding must be withheld for several weeks, fails to supply essential fatty acids and trace minerals needed for growth. All these considerations may mandate transfusion therapy.

In crossmatching blood for the nursery, the mother's plasma should also be crossmatched with the donor unit, because some gamma globulins pass the placenta, and significant antibodies to the donor erythrocytes may originate passively from the mother's blood. Infants may be deficient in certain immune globulins and clotting factors, and thus the use of relatively fresh donor blood will serve multiple purposes. Because the baby may require only 15 to 30 ml of blood, but may need subsequent transfusion, some centers have subdivided units into 100-ml packs, minimizing risk of mismatch and hepatitis.

Because of the importance of rapid availability, very fresh blood, and multiple small transfusions to the same infant, a number of centers have started "walking donor" programs, with a panel of medical and nursing staff registered and available for small, heparinized donation. To minimize the risks in this sort of arrangement, the donor panel is screened every six months in the usual way, including serology and test for hepatitis B antigen. Except in extreme emergencies, the donor is crossmatched against the recipient. Then the required amount of blood is drawn into a heparinized syringe and given by slow-push infusion. Should additional transfusions be required after three days, the donor is again crossmatched against the recipient to be certain that antibodies have not appeared.

Exchange transfusion places a particular burden upon the quality of blood used. Citrate-phosphate-dextrose blood that is not more than three days old is usually used. If older donor blood is used, the result will be release of potassium, buildup of acid products of metabolism, and decreased 2–3-diphosphoglycerate in the erythrocyte, which would be acceptable for a small transfusion but not for replacement of the infant's total blood volume. It is of interest that exchange transfusion in the newborn has been proposed for several other indications besides the treatment of jaundice: disseminated intravascular coagulation, intoxications such as salicylism, sepsis, critical anemia in the presence of shock, and the poor oxygen-releasing properties of fetal hemoglobin have all been treated in this way.

SUMMARY

In summary, neonatologists are not such a bad lot if you get to know them better. They will ask for special studies to aid in the diagnosis of intrauterine infections such as toxoplasmosis, rubella, cytomegalovirus, herpes, and syphilis; they want their blood cultures in special small tubes; they will accept certain ordinarily saprophytic organisms as pathogens; they will probably want anaerobic cultures as well; they will want to know the concentrations of countless drugs in the blood that have uncertain dose-response curves; they will want information on chromosomes and catecholamines, screens for inborn errors of metabolism, amino acids, ammonia, and heaven knows what else. And everything must be in a hurry and must be done on the smallest possible sample. But more often than you might suppose, there is a sound physiological consideration or a particular disease state behind these requests. We feel particularly grateful to have a laboratory director who comes up to the nursery and looks at infants with us.

Acid-Base Changes
in the Fetus and Infant
during the Perinatal Period

L. STANLEY JAMES, M.D.

Originally, it was believed that the fetus grew and thrived in a hypoxic and acidemic environment, a conclusion based on the analysis of data derived from samples of cord blood that indicated that the infant is severely hypoxic, acidotic, and hypercapnic at birth. The data were obtained from infants born by cesarean section, and it was assumed that they, therefore, represented the normal values in utero. However, when data on individual infants were examined, it was obvious that there was a large range of values for oxygen saturation, blood pH, and plasma p_{CO_2} (Table 1). In physiological situations such a wide range of values usually indicates an unsteady state. With this interpretation in mind, we proposed that the highest values were probably closest to the normal values in utero, and even these values might well have been influenced by the process of labor and delivery.

If oxygen saturation and acid-base status do change quite rapidly during delivery, it would be useful to know how fast such changes can occur. The preparation we chose to study was the newborn puppy (1). Animals were delivered by cesarean section; arterial catheters were inserted promptly and with an endotracheal tube in place, the animals were then asphyxiated by occluding the tube. Oxygen saturation decreased from 90% to near 0% in about 2.5 min, indicating that reserves of oxygen in the blood and lungs were small and would last for only a short time. Blood pH also decreased rapidly. In the newborn of all mammalian species, the heart will continue to beat after oxygen saturation has fallen to near zero; the newborn puppy survives for about 20 min, primarily because of anaerobic energy transformation of glycogen in the heart. We noted that the blood pH continued to decrease even after oxygen-saturation values were zero. Accordingly, we proposed that blood pH measurement might better indicate the duration of an asphyxial episode than oxygen values do. For instance, one would find a zero oxygen value after about 2.5 min of asphyxia, whereas a blood sample with a pH of 6.8 would indicate that the animal had been asphyxiated for 10 min.

95

Table 1.   Oxygenation and Acid–Base Status of Umbilical Arterial and Venous Blood of Healthy Infants at Birth[a]

	O_2 saturation			p_{CO_2}	
	Relative	%	pH	kPa	mmHg
Umbilical artery	0.20	20	7.26	7.2	54
	(0–0.45)	(0–45)	(7.32–7.15)	(6.0–8.5)	(45–64)
Umbilical vein	0.48	48	7.29	5.7	43
	(0.24–0.72)	(24–72)	(7.36–7.20)	(4.7–6.7)	(35–50)

[a] Mean and range of values are illustrated.

The decrease in blood pH is the result of both an accumulation of CO_2 and of a metabolic acidosis. During asphyxia, the rate of increase in CO_2 tension averaged about 1.1 kPa (8 mmHg) per minute, while about 2 mmol/litre (mEq/litre) of nonvolatile acid accumulated per minute. This decrease in blood pH was thus the result of the combined effect of increasing p_{CO_2} and decreasing buffering base in the blood.

When the technique of sampling blood from the fetal scalp during labor was introduced by Saling (2), it was observed that pH values gradually decreased as labor advanced. Data obtained in our own institution (3) showed that at 4-cm cervical dilatation, the pH of the fetal blood is about 7.32, which decreases to about 7.25 by the time of full dilatation. These values were averaged data from a large number of infants, all of whom were normal at delivery but included infants from both short and long labors, infants of both multiparas and primiparas, and some infants with abnormalities of the fetal heart rate. Using more carefully selected criteria, other investigators (4) have shown that the blood pH remains between 7.30 and 7.35 in a "normal" labor almost to the time of full cervical dilatation. But at the very end of labor, as the infant is being expelled through the vagina and the placental circulation is changing acutely, there is a brief period of asphyxia. However, if one considers normal labor in broader categories, there is a tendency for acidosis to develop as labor advances, because CO_2 and strong acids accumulate. Consequently, as the result of predictions based on values for cord blood and on measured changes in the pH of blood from the fetal scalp during labor, the infant under normal circumstances may be said to develop some "physiological" (i.e., normally expected) asphyxia during labor and delivery, from which he soon recovers after birth.

How valid are data obtained from these samples of scalp blood? If one obtains a blood sample from an edematous scalp during labor, does it have any physiological meaning? For several years many investigators were skeptical about this method of sampling. Our group made some efforts to ascertain whether results obtained with such samples validly represented systemic fetal blood (3). Over the pH range of about 7.15 to 7.35, there is a good correlation between the acid-base composition of blood in the umbilical artery and vein and that from scalp-blood sample. In the more acidotic infants, the fetal scalp has a somewhat lower pH than does the sample from the cord, probably because of peripheral vasoconstriction and some circulatory stasis. From a practical point of view, these differences are not important in evaluating the infant's condition.

Will the presence of an edematous scalp with caput formation interfere in any way with the accuracy of the sampling? When the hematocrit of fetal capillary blood from such infants is compared with that for blood from the umbilical artery and vein, there is no greater difference than would be found between samples of arterial or venous and capillary blood from newborn infants or adults. Capillary blood samples always show a somewhat higher hematocrit than do arterial or venous blood samples. These results indicate that even though the sample is obtained through an edematous scalp, the blood flow is adequate to give a fairly true representation.

The whole fetus is under relatively high intrauterine pressure during contractions, except at the presenting part where the pressure is atmospheric, or about 5.3 to 6.7 kPa (40 to 50 mmHg) lower than the intrauterine pressure. This is the probable explanation for the good blood flow during uterine contractions and the poor flow in between them.

Adamsons et al., (5) provided further data on the validity of data from fetal scalp-blood sampling. They implanted catheters in the carotid artery and jugular vein of fetal rhesus monkeys at hysterotomy, replaced the animals in the uterus, and induced labor. They measured the pH of serial samples obtained from the arterial and venous catheters and from the capillary bed of the scalp. There was a good correlation between the values from each site over a range of blood pH from 6.80 to 7.30. Thus, from a practical point of view, blood samples from the fetal scalp provide data that are meaningful in the evaluation of fetal acid-base status.

We have observed that a significant correlation ($P = 0.01$) exists between acid-base status of the infant at birth and his clinical condition, as evaluated by the Apgar scoring system (Table 2). This correlation applies also to the pH of fetal capillary blood. Infants with an Apgar score of 7 or more had a mean pH of 7.27, whereas in those with a score of 6 or less the mean pH was 7.22, a difference that was highly significant.

Table 2. Fetal Capillary Blood pH and Apgar Scores in 355 Newborns[a]

No. samples	Apgar score	Mean pH	SE
449	7 or greater	7.27	0.003
190	6 or less	7.22	0.007

[a] $P < 0.001$.

In our experience, information on fetal acid-base status does not accurately reflect the outcome in about 18% of infants, who can be categorized as the false normals (in whom the pH is in the normal range but the infant is depressed—i.e., function is diminished) and the false abnormals (the infant is acidotic but not depressed). There is essentially only one cause for the false abnormals, but there are about eight different causes for the false normals. In the false-abnormal group, the common cause is maternal acidosis and in the false-normal group, it is maternal medication. This probably explains why the proportion of infants in the "false" groups varies from hospital to hospital. If labor is prolonged and the mother is not supported with adequate hydration, calories, and sedation, then maternal and fetal acidosis are more prevalent. More liberal use of analgesia or anesthesia to the mother is likely to be associated with depressed, but not necessarily acidotic, infants.

Another cause of depression in the false-normal group is precipitous delivery. The infants make one or two gasps at birth but behave like a patient with concussion who has a secondary respiratory depression. Obstetrical manipulations, such as a difficult forceps delivery, tend to lead to some degree of depression without necessarily affecting the acid-base status of the infant. Premature infants also may fall into the false-normal category, particularly the very small infants weighing less than 1000 g who have soft chest walls and noncompliant lungs. Such babies may have quite a good acid-base status in utero but, being unable to establish effective ventilation, may remain in poor condition 1 or even 5 min after delivery. Aspiration syndromes can also fit into this group, particularly if the asphyxial episode has been relatively transient and early in labor. Congenital anomalies—including choanal atresia, laryngeal webs, hypoplastic lungs associated with diaphragmatic hernia, and edematous cysts of the lung—are likewise in this group. All of these anomalies prevent the normal onset of good lung function at birth; such infants are born with normal acid-base values but rapidly become depressed.

Another factor, somewhat difficult to evaluate, relates to previous episodes of asphyxia. After resuscitation of severely asphyxiated infants, the blood may be reoxygenated and acidosis corrected before the central nervous system returns to its normal reactivity. The infant remains hypotonic and poorly responsive for several hours. If no other cause can be found, this is the most likely cause of depression in infants in the false-normal group—those that are depressed and yet have a normal acid-base state. We can assume that at some time, either before or during labor, they have had an asphyxial episode from which the central nervous system has not recovered.

Finally, intrauterine infection may be a serious problem and has to be evaluated carefully. If acute amnionitis develops and placental exchange is undisturbed, the acid-base state of the fetus will be normal. The amnionitis will usually be associated with fetal tachycardia and discoloration of the amniotic fluid. Poor labor may progress to uterine inertia. An error in management can arise if these signs of fetal distress are ignored and only the fetal acid-base status receives attention. The longer the infant remains in an infected environment, the greater the danger of intrauterine pneumonia. At delivery, the infant is likely to be depressed both because of the infection and because good pulmonary function cannot be established in the presence of intrauterine pneumonia. The mortality in this group is high.

Thus, information on the fetal acid-base status during labor is a valuable reflection of fetal oxygenation or asphyxia, but must be evaluated in conjunction with other clinical signs of fetal distress.

If a sample indicates that the blood of the fetal scalp from the fetus is acidotic, the next step is to ascertain whether the mother is acidotic. Table 3 shows the difference in fetal and maternal acid-base status in normal and depressed infants whose mothers were not acidotic. In normal infants—i.e., those with a blood pH of 7.21—the difference in base deficit is 2.6 mmol/litre (mEq/litre), while in the low-score acidotic infants it is 7.0 mmol/litre (mEq/litre). On the other hand, if the mother is acidotic, one would expect the fetus would also become acidotic, in order to establish a new gradient for the continuing excretion of hydrogen ion, which will be principally of fetal origin. "Fixed" (i.e., nonvolatile) acid crosses the placenta very slowly. Indeed, the placenta appears to deal with CO_2 and with fixed acid in much the same way as the lung and kidney, respectively, do in the extrauterine organism. Recovery from metabolic acidosis by the fetus is a process that requires several hours. If the mother becomes acutely acidotic, the fetus may be transiently less acidotic than the mother. But the fetus will soon become more acidotic and will establish a new steady state that permits the excretion of hydrogen ion.

Table 3.   Maternal and Fetal Acid-Base Gradients

Group	No.	Mean pH (maternal)	Mean pH (fetal)	Δ pH	Base deficit mmol/l (mEq/l)
Normals	31	7.42	7.25	0.17	2.6
Acidotic mother, vigorous fetus	9	7.36	7.15	0.21	4.8
Normal mother, depressed fetus	10	7.40	7.13	0.27	7.0

Table 3 also summarizes data from infants born of mothers who were mildly acidotic. The values for fetal pH were less than 7.21 and the change in base deficit was about 4.8 mmol/litre (mEq/litre). All these infants were in the group with a high Apgar score, despite their acidosis. Fetal acidosis developing as a result of maternal acidosis does not have the serious implication that the acidosis occurring during fetal hypoxia has, because it is not a reflection of fetal hypoxemia.

Is maternal acidosis harmful to the fetus? There is some evidence that uterine blood flow is actually increased under circumstances of maternal acidosis. In this respect, the uterine circulation appears to have a response similar to that of cerebral circulation when an elevation of p_{CO_2} leads to an increase in blood flow. Thus, a mild maternal acidosis occurring as the result of a strenuous labor might actually be beneficial to the fetus if uterine blood flow were to be increased.

As for treatment, a mother who is mildly acidotic obviously requires an adequate fluid intake and calories in the form of glucose. We do not correct maternal acidosis with bicarbonate unless it is severe. In the usual mild case, one rarely finds evidence of fetal distress, and labor should be allowed to progress. Mild sedation, to decrease unnecessary muscular effort, and appropriate fluid, glucose, and electrolyte replacement will usually be sufficient.

Perhaps the major concern about maternal acidosis and associated fetal acidosis is that the fetus, when suddenly faced with an acute asphyxial episode, will have a smaller margin of reserve. If it starts with a pH of 7.10 instead of 7.35 and then becomes acutely asphyxiated, it will more rapidly develop a degree of acidosis that could depress activity of the cardiovascular and central nervous systems.

After birth, the infant normally recovers from the acidosis that has developed during labor and delivery, usually within a few hours and principally by pulmonary excretion of CO_2 and metabolism of nonvolatile acids. The kidneys appear to play little or no role in this initial adjustment.

In healthy infants, the first sample (taken 2 or 3 min after birth) is significantly more acidemic than is the sample from cord blood (6). At 10 min, the infant's acid-base status is similar to that found in his cord blood; thereafter, there is a further gradual recovery, so that when the healthy infant is an hour old, his blood pH is about 7.30. The more anoxic infants show a greater decrease in pH after birth and recover more slowly, probably because they have some degree of central nervous system and cardiovascular depression from the asphyxial process itself, as well as some difficulties in cardiopulmonary adjustments. The decrease in pH after birth is a reflection of the preceding period of asphyxia and occurs as blood flow is restored to areas that have previously been poorly perfused. The same phenomenon is observed in pearl divers and diving mammals upon resurfacing; it reflects circulatory readjustments during diving that favor perfusion of the coronary and cerebral vessels, the circulation to other areas being markedly decreased.

The healthy infant returns to the same acid-base status as the mother before the onset of labor (7), not to the usually accepted values for healthy males. The mean plasma p_{CO_2} of the mother before labor is 4.3 kPa (32 mmHg) rather than 5.3 kPa (40 mmHg); the infant adjusts his p_{CO_2} to this point. In such an infant, a value of 5.3 kPa (40 mmHg) for plasma p_{CO_2} at 24 h would be abnormal.

An important factor that interferes with acid-base readjustment after birth is the temperature of the environment.

A cold stress will aggravate the metabolic acidosis present at birth (8). The healthy newborn infant doubles or triples his oxygen consumption when exposed to a cold environment. The metabolic acidosis observed in infants in a cool environment is probably a reflection of their increased metabolic rate. In a warm environment, where the infant's metabolic rate is close to the basal rate for infants, no such augmented metabolism interferes with the normal acid-base adjustment.

The healthy infant exposed to cold compensates for the metabolic acidosis by hyperventilation; a normal blood pH is achieved, provided prompt adequate alveolar ventilation is established. Indeed, as noted above, the initial acid-base adjustment of the newborn infant can be achieved in the absence of kidneys, if good cardiopulmonary function is established. Although healthy infants can make the necessary compensation if exposed to cold stress, infants who have severe aspiration syndromes, central nervous system depression from maternal medication, or a soft chest wall and noncompliant lungs (premature infants) cannot. In these circumstances, cold stress is poorly tolerated, and the infant becomes more acidotic.

How valid are capillary blood samples (9) from a warmed heel for measurement of blood acid-base status in the newborn? Capillary blood samples have been compared with those obtained from the aorta during the first postnatal hour. The capillary pH is invariably lower than the simultaneously measured arterial value. Plasma p_{CO_2} also varies considerably. After the first postnatal hour, the arterial and capillary values for pH increase; there is now an improved correlation, which improves further after 3 h. The same is true of plasma p_{CO_2}. Thus, in general, a blood sample from a warmed heel of a 3-h-old infant closely represents an arterial blood sample in the descending aorta, but the heel must be warmed, by wrapping the extremity in a warm (40 °C) wet towel or by placing a small thermostatically controlled infrared lamp neat the infant's heel.

SUMMARY

During development, the acid-base state of the fetus is very close to that of the mother. His blood oxygen level is low by adult standards, but there is no evidence that he suffers from oxygen lack. There is a reduction of exchange of oxygen and CO_2 between mother and fetus during labor, resulting in an accumulation of hydrogen ion in the fetus. Thus, at birth the fetus is relatively asphyxiated. He recovers from this during the first 24 h of life through the establishment of pulmonary gaseous exchange, excretion of CO_2, and metabolism of the nonvolatile acids. The changes in acid-base state of the fetus as labor progresses can be followed through analysis of capillary blood samples obtained from the fetal scalp.

REFERENCES

1. James, L. S., Acidosis at birth and its relation to birth asphyxia, *Acta Paediatr. Scand.* **49**, [Suppl. 122], 17 (1960).

2. Saling, E., Die Blutgasverhältnisse und der Säure-Basen-Haushalt des Feten bei ungestörten Geburtsablauf, *Z. Gerburtshilfe. Gynaekol.* **161**, 262 (1964).

3. Bowe, E. T., Beard, R. W., Finster, M., Poppers, P. J., Adamsons, K. and James, L. S., Reliability of fetal blood sampling. *Am. J. Obstet. Gynecol* **107**, 279 (1970).

4. Hon, E. Unpublished data.

5. Adamsons, K., Jr., Beard, R. W., Cosmi, E. V., and Myers, R. E., The validity of capillary blood in the assessment of the acid-base state of the fetus. In *Diagnosis and Treatment of Fetal Disorders.* K. Adamsons, Jr., Ed., Springer-Verlag, New York, N.Y., 1968, pp. 175–178.

6. Daniel, S. S., Adamsons, K. Jr., and James, L. S., Lactate and pyruvate as an index of prenatal oxygen deprivation. *Pediatrics* **37**, 942 (1966).

7. Weisbrot, I. M., James, L. S., Prince, C. E., Holaday, D. A., and Apgar, V., Acid–base homeostasis of the newborn infant during the first 24 hours of life, *J. Pediatr.* **52**, 395 (1958).

8. Gandy, G. M., Adamsons, K. Jr., Cunningham, N., Silverman, W. A., and James, L. S., Thermal environment and acid–base homeostasis in human infants during the first few hours of life, *J. Clin. Invest.* **43**, 751 (1964).

9. Gandy, G., Grann, L., Cunningham, N., Adamsons, K., Jr. and James, L. S., The validity of pH and p_{CO_2} measurements in capillary samples in sick and healthy newborn infants, *Pediatrics* **34**, 192 (1964).

Effect on the Infant of Drug Therapy of the Mother

REBA MICHELS HILL, M.D.

MARJORIE G. HORNING, Ph.D.

Physical variants or biochemical disturbances appearing in the newborn period were previously assumed to be the result of primary physical disease in the mother or infant. As our clinical knowledge expanded and microchemical methods were developed, we became aware that many such changes may have resulted from administration of drugs to the mother. Drugs administered at any time during intrauterine development may affect the infant's ability to adjust to an extrauterine existence. This inability to adjust may be manifested by overt teratogenesis, transient metabolic aberration, or prolonged effect on behavior adaptation. Table 1 lists some reported effects of this kind.

The mean number of different drugs consumed by a middle to high socioeconomic population of gravid females has been reported to be 10.3 drugs, with a range of 3 to 29 drugs (1), not including vitamins, iron, anesthetic agents, intravenously administered fluids, cigarette smoking, alcohol consumption, or exposure to pesticides, paints, chemicals, or roentgen rays. Drugs are ingested fairly continuously during pregnancy, but peak drug ingestion occurs between 36 to 40 weeks of gestation and again during labor and delivery. Therefore, the human neonate has multiple, continuous exposure to pharmacological agents during vulnerable periods of development and adaptation. During labor and delivery, many factors (anoxia, acidosis, cold stress, trauma, and the like) may affect the infant's ability to excrete the drugs he has been exposed to during intrauterine life.

A prospective study of a middle-to-high socioeconomic group of gravid patients was designed to demonstrate biochemical transfer of maternal drugs to the developing infant and to determine if such drugs have any effect on him. A few of the early observations from this study, which is being done at St. Luke's Episcopal Hospital in Houston, are discussed here.

103

Table 1. Influence of Maternal Drug Therapy on the Infant[a]

Teratogenic[b]	Fetal death	Immediate adaption to extrauterine life	Withdrawal	Metabolism	Hematological changes
Alcohol (x)[b] Anticonvulsant agents Cancer chemotherapeutic agents Corticosteroid Estrogens Progestins Lead Mercury Quinine ? Ovulatory agents Psychotropic agents Radiation Radioisotopes Tetracyclines Thalidomide Hallucinogenic agents	Chloral hydrate (x) Chlorpropamide Salicylates (x) Dicumarol Ergot Lead Thyroid function Radiopaque dye Iodine Thioureas Radioactive drugs	Anesthetic agents Barbiturates Bromide Cholinesterase inhibitor Curare Diazepam Hexamethonium Lithium Mag. sulfate Narcotics Paraldehyde Phenothiazine Oxytocin Reserpine Salicylates (x) Pyridoxine Oxytocin, + diuretic +IV fluids	Alcohol (x) Anticonvulsant agents Barbiturates Psychotropic agents Glutethimide Amphetamines Drugs of abuse Propoxyphene	*Hypoglycemia* Chlorpropamide Alcohol iv & oral Insulin Tolbutamide *Electrolyte Imbalance* Corticosteroids Diuretics+ Hypotonic iv fluids, + Oxytocin	*Hemorrhage, anemia, ↓ platelets* Alcohol Barbiturate Dicumarol Dilantin Diuretic Hykinone Local anesthetic agents[c] Quinine Salicylates Sulfonamides Thiourea Promethazine *Jaundice* Hykinone ? Oxytocin Sulfa drugs (long & short acting)

Carcinogenic	Birth weight	Convulsions	Somatic growth	Mental ability	Sexual reproduction
Hormones	Cigarette smoking	Local anesthetic agents	Anticonvulsant agents	Carbon monoxide	? Cancer chemothera-
Radioactive drugs	Corticosteroids	Mag. sulfate	Alcohol (x)	Mercury	peutic agents
Radiation	Drugs of abuse	Oxytocin, + diuretic	Drugs of abuse	Radiation	
? Cancer chemothera-	Ovulatory agents	+ iv fluids		Radioisotopes	
peutic agents	Alcohol (x)	Pyridoxine		Thioureas	
				Alcohol (x)	

[a] Categories of drugs are listed when multiple drugs in that category are reported to cause a specific effect. Individual drugs are listed when a single drug is reported to produce an adverse effect.

[b] x = Excessive

[c] Methemoglobinemia

MATERIALS AND METHODS

Before delivery, 156 gravid women had detailed histories taken of the drugs ingested during pregnancy. Accuracy in reporting the number and type of drugs was confirmed by the prescribing physician. The validity of nonprescription drugs depended on the mother's memory and entry in a diary that she kept during pregnancy. Labor and delivery events were recorded. At the time of delivery, samples of the mother's plasma and urine, of umbilical venous blood, and of amniotic fluid were collected. Within the first days of life, a 24-h urine and plasma sample were collected from the infant, and colostrum and breast-milk samples from the nursing mother. Serial physical examinations were performed at birth and throughout the first 48 months of postnatal life. Psychometric testings (Gesell and Wechsler Preschool and Primary Scale of Intelligence) were completed at nine months and periodically during the first four years of postnatal life. Informed consent was obtained from both parents prior to sample collections and examination of the infant.

Drugs and drug metabolites were extracted from plasma, colostrum, breast milk, amniotic fluid, and urine samples by using ammonium carbonate and ethyl acetate as a salt-solvent pair (2). In quantitative studies, internal standards—preferably stable-isotope-labeled drugs—were added to the biological samples before extraction. The drugs and their metabolites were identified by gas chromatograph/mass spectrometer methods. A gas chromatograph/mass spectrometer/computer system, operated in the chemical ionization mode, was used for quantification (3).

RESULTS

The drug profiles obtained by gas-chromatographic analysis of extracts of plasma and urine from mother-infant pairs were similar at the time of birth. The parent drug and metabolites of the drugs administered to the mother during labor and delivery, or drugs consumed chronically, were identified in the various body fluids.

Two thirds of the mothers who ingested barbiturates did so during the last four weeks of pregnancy. A barbiturate was usually prescribed in the form of a sedative or was a constituent of a diet-control pill. We monitored the duration of excretion by the neonate of transplacentally acquired barbiturates. One infant excreted phenobarbital for eight days after delivery; the mother had received one grain (65 mg) of phenobarbital nightly for insomnia during the last two weeks of pregnancy.

Another mother received mephobarbital throughout pregnancy for control of seizures. Her firstborn infant had increased muscle tonus and severe tremors and signs of central nervous system agitation shortly after birth. The symptoms, which were interpreted as drug withdrawal, lasted for the first six months of postnatal life. Placental transfer of mephobarbital to the infant was demonstrated by our analyses. The second infant born to this mother had similar symptoms, which lasted for four months. Mephobarbital excretion was demonstrated for eight days after delivery and phenobarbital, a major metabolite of mephobarbital, was excreted for 22 days after delivery. The concentration of mephobarbital in urine on day 8 was 20 μg/litre; the concentration of phenobarbital on day 22 was 130 μg/litre. Excretion of the drug beyond this time could not be determined, because the attending physician administered phenobarbital to the infant.

Intravenous alcohol was administered to five gravid patients in an attempt to stop premature uterine contractions. The infants were alert and active when admitted to the nursery but by the end of the first postnatal hour they became lethargic and hypotonic. Blood glucose concentrations, at that time were about 1.4 mmol/litre (25 mg/100 ml). Administration of glucose solution (100 g/litre) restored the infants to normal activity and tonus.

One mother suffered respiratory and cardiac arrest 20 min after 35 ml of piperocaine was administered as a caudal anesthetic. The anesthetic agent produced total spinal anesthesia in the mother. Immediate cardiac and respiratory resuscitation of the mother was accomplished, and the infant, who was delivered by emergency cesarean section, manifested severe seizures for the first two days of life. Acidosis and methemoglobinemia could not be demonstrated in the infant. Asymmetrical neurological findings were present in the infant for the first year of life. Psychometric testing at 40 weeks of age revealed a developmental quotient (D.Q.) of 112 and at 18 months, 123.

Analgesic agents were consumed by two thirds of the patients during their gestation; 40% of these analgesic agents required a prescription for purchase. Many of the drugs contained acetylsalicylic acid. One patient had a respiratory and cardiac arrest after receiving a standard dose of secobarbital and meperidine. A live-born infant was delivered who had only mild respiratory distress after delivery. A hysterectomy was performed on the mother in the postpartum period for control of severe maternal uterine hemorrhage. The mother reported taking 25 325-mg aspirin tablets daily for headaches. The infant had a serum salicylate concentration of 2.9 mmol/litre (40 mg/100 ml) 22 h after delivery. Analysis of successive urines collected from the infant demonstrated that excretion of metabolites of acetylsalicylic acid continued through eight days after delivery.

One infant manifested an excessive bruising tendency during the first two days of postnatal life. Clotting studies revealed a deficiency of vitamin K-dependent factors, although 1 mg of phytonadione was given after birth. No bleeding into the central nervous system or other organ systems was evident; only peripheral bruising was obvious. The mother had ingested mephenytoin, methsuximide, and phenobarbital during pregnancy for treatment of seizures. Additional administration of phytonadione corrected the clotting defect.

Forty-one per cent of the mothers received antibiotic therapy during pregnancy. Antibiotics were most commonly prescribed between the 24th and 36 weeks of gestation. Four mothers in the group received tetracycline therapy after the fourth month of pregnancy. Pigmentation and carious formation in the teeth were observed in two infants who were still in the study group at the time of dental eruption. One of the children, who is now five years old, will require extensive dental work.

Twenty-eight infants born to mothers receiving anticonvulsant drugs manifested physical abnormalities that made them an identifiable group of neonates. Nine mothers received only diphenylhydantoin, one received only phenobarbital, and eighteen received a combination of diphenylhydantoin and a barbiturate and/or psychotropic drug or additional anticonvulsant agents.

Physical findings observed in infants exposed to anticonvulsant drugs were: simian line, Sydney line, inguinal hernia, pilonidal sinus, large anterior and posterior fontanelle, hypoplastic distal phalanges, broad alveolar ridge, hypoplastic nails, metopic ridging, short neck, broad nasal bridge, low hairline, digital thumb, and/or hirsutism. Disfiguring or life-threatening anomalies were present in 7 of the 28 infants (25%) and 7 of 165

(4%) cohort infants including: inguinal hernia, pyloric stenosis, dislocation of the hip, epidermal cyst connected to the dura, cleft lip and palate, tetralogy of Fallot with patent ductus, ventricular septal defect, and/or hypospadias.

Hypoplasia of the fingernails and distal phalanx, digitalization of the thumb, and abnormal palmar markings were present in four infants who had been exposed to anticonvulsant drugs. The presence of abnormalities of the extremities may serve to alert the observer to look for more life-threatening or disfiguring anomalies, because 6 disfiguring or life-threatening abnormalities of a total of 11 such abnormalities observed were present in these four infants.

Four infants born to mothers receiving anticonvulsant medication had similar facial features: large quantities of hair, large, wide-set eyes, depressed nasal bridge, and low-set ears. Four infants failed to thrive in the first months. The infant exposed to anticonvulsant agents during gestation showed a statistically significantly lower developmental quotient than infants not exposed. Indeed, lower scores were obtained for all areas tested (gross motor, fine motor, adaptive, language, personal social skills).

Forty-six per cent of the mothers had been exposed to x-ray examination during pregnancy; half of these x-ray exposures occurred during the first and second trimesters of pregnancy and included dental films, chest x-ray, intravenous pyelogram, spinal films, cinecystogram, and gallbladder series. Eighty per cent of the mothers who had had dental and/or chest x-rays had done so to meet requirements for work or as part of elective annual examinations. Three mothers were exposed during the first, second, and third trimesters of pregnancy while holding a child for x-ray study. None of the infants exposed during the first and second trimesters of pregnancy had significant physical malformations.

Transfer of many agents such as diphenylhydantoin, barbiturates, and ethosuximide from the maternal circulation into breast milk was confirmed by our analyses (Table 2). Both long-acting and intermediate-acting barbiturates were present in colostrum 18 to 19 h after administration to the mother. Diazepam was identified in colostrum 25 h after administration to the mother. Codeine, methadone, and tolbutamide also were identified in colostrum and breast milk, but could not be quantitated.

Table 2. Drugs Identified in Human Breast Milk and Colostrum by GC-MS-COM Procedures

Drug	Concentration mg/l	Hours after administration	Days after delivery
Phenobarbital	2.74	16	6
	3.3	—	3
Pentobarbital	0.17	19	4
Butabarbital	0.37	1.5	4
Secobarbital	+	24	4
Diazepam	0.10	25	2
Diphenylhydantoin	1.5–4.5	—	19, 38
Ethosuximide	+	—	36
Codeine	+	8	2
Methadone	+	1.25	3
	+	1.5	5
Tolbutamide	+	—	25
Caffeine	+	1	—

SUMMARY

By utilizing methods based on a gas chromatograph/mass spectrometer/computer system, we have demonstrated that the human infant excretes drugs and drug metabolites for days to weeks after delivery. The ability to excrete any given drug may be influenced by the other multiple drugs administered to the mother during pregnancy, by events surrounding labor and delivery, by maturity of the enzyme systems involved in drug metabolism, and by as-yet-unrecognized factors.

Brazleton (4) first called attention to the effect of barbiturate administration to the mother on the nutritive suck reflex and on weight gain in the human infant. Desmond et al. (5) more recently reported that infants born to mothers ingesting phenobarbital first show withdrawal symptoms at about two weeks of age. The two infants reported here were symptomatic at birth, and the second infant was shown to excrete phenobarbital for at least 22 days.

Symptoms of drug withdrawal are seen in the neonate after ingestion of various drugs by the gravid female. Narcotic preparations at one time were the most common cause for withdrawal symptoms in the neonate, but ingestion of amphetamines, anticonvulsant agents (6), glutethimide, psychotropic agents (7), or excessive quantities of alcohol (8) will produce symptoms of central nervous system agitation for various periods up to 18 months.

Drugs such as intravenous alcohol or chlorpropamide (9) may interfere with the infant's ability to adjust to the metabolic demands placed on him in the first hours of postnatal life and cause temporary or protracted hypoglycemia in the neonate. This effect has also been seen in infants born to alcoholic mothers. Wagner et al. (10) report that premature infants infused with a solution containing 80 g alcohol/litre of physiological saline solution had depressed glucose concentrations. It should be noted that combined drug therapy with chloramphenicol may potentiate the hypoglycemic effect of tolbutamide.

A mother's adverse reactions to drugs—caused by use of an improper site for injection, too-rapid administration, or too-rapid absorption of a drug—may effect the fetus. Administration of local anesthetic drugs into the fetal scalp (11) or rapid absorption of the drug after paracervical administration will cause bradycardia, metabolic acidosis, seizures, permanent neurological impairment, or even death in the neonate.

Other agents that interfere with the infant's ability to adjust to an extrauterine existence include diazepam. When it is administered in doses of 30 mg or more, neurological depression, prolonged hypotonia, and inability to maintain body temperature may result (12). Infants born to mothers requiring lithium for treatment of psychiatric disease may be cyanotic and hypotonic for 10 days after delivery and may be diagnosed as having cyanotic heart disease if the clinician is unaware of the history of lithium ingestion by the mother. When magnesium sulfate is administered to the mother in large quantities, the infant may manifest hypotonia and convulsions because of hypermagnesemia (13), although there is no correlation between the plasma magnesium concentration and the symptoms presented by the infant. Administration of large quantities of hypotonic fluid containing oxytocin to the mother will produce symptoms of hyponatremia, including convulsions, in the infant.

The consequences to the fetus of excessive use of analgesic agents by the gravid female are not appreciated by most individuals. Salicylates and barbiturates or narcotics act synergistically. Hemorrhage in patients with salicylate intoxication is a well-recognized complication. Death in utero caused by hemorrhage and thrombocytopenia from transplacentally acquired salicylate intoxication in infants has been previously described (*14,15*).

Ingestion of either barbiturate or diphenylhydantoin by gravid females reportedly causes hemorrhage in the neonate that can be attributed to vitamin K deficiency (*16*). These infants usually bleed into the heart, central nervous system, and/or peritoneal or thoracic cavity. Vitamin K should be administered to all infants born to mothers who are receiving barbiturates or hydantoin drugs. Other drugs that cause hemorrhage or thrombocytopenia are diuretics and promethazine. Methemoglobinemia is reported to occur in infants as a result of absorption of anesthesic agents (*17*). Both transplacentally acquired and direct administration of sulfonamides and menadione sodium bisulfate are associated with jaundice, hemolytic anemia, and in some instances kernicterus in the neonate.

More recently, delayed effects of intrauterine exposure to pharmacological active agents have been recognized. Linden and Henderson (*18*) reported the occurrence of vaginal cancer in adolescent girls exposed to diethylstilbestrol in utero. There is some concern that male infants will also have a higher incidence of malignancy of the genito-urinary tract system after intrauterine exposure to this agent. Nora and Nora (*19*) report a spectrum of abnormalities (vertebral, cardiac, tracheal, esophageal, and limb deformities) occurring in infants born to mothers who had received hormones during pregnancy.

The developing fetus is frequently exposed unnecessarily to radiation, with consequences that may not be recognized until years later. Because the prevalence of accidental exposure of the gravid patient to radiation is high, it is recommended that females requiring diagnostic radiation studies during the childbearing period be tested for pregnancy before being exposed.

Meadow and Speidel (*20,21*) were among the first to suggest the possible teratogenic effect of anticonvulsant drugs on the neonate. The effect may not be a direct effect of the drug on the fetus, but other factors such as genetic influence or secondary deficiency states that occur in patients on chronic drug therapy may play a significant role. Most commonly used anticonvulsant drugs were found to cross the placenta and also to be transferred into breast milk. Discontinuance of anticonvulsant drugs during pregnancy is not recommended. However, it is important that patients with seizure disorders be evaluated before they become pregnant, to see if therapy with a single drug will control the seizures as well as multiple-drug therapy.

Because most drugs ingested by the lactating mother appear in breast milk, exposure of the breast-fed infant to maternally administered drugs will continue for days or months after parturition. It should be appreciated that some drugs may cross into colostrum and breast milk and remain there until breast feeding is instituted. It is not known if the concentration of drugs present in breast milk can become sufficient to affect the behavior or welfare of the infant. However, an active, vigorous infant may consume from 850 to 1000 ml of breast milk daily. Although the drugs are present in nanogram-per-milliliter concentrations, the total amount ingested by the neonate over a 24-h period may be some milligrams. If codeine and methadone are present in milk, the possibility of neonatal addiction exists. The presence of ethosuximide in breast milk should alert the physician to observe for hematological abnormalities in the neonate. Breast-fed infants whose mothers require tolbutamide treatment should be observed closely for hyperbilirubinemia or hypoglycemia.

In summary, the amount and the transfer of drugs in various biological fluids (blood, urine, amniotic fluid, colostrum and breast milk) has been assessed by combined use of gas chromatograph/mass spectrometer/computers. It was demonstrated that the neonate excretes drugs not only for hours after delivery, but for days or even weeks. He may be further exposed to pharmacological agents if breast fed, because drugs ingested by the lactating female are present in the milk in nanogram-to-microgram-per-milliliter amounts. Whether or not such chronic exposure to pharmacologically active compounds alters or hinders the normal systematic maturation of a developing human infant is unknown but should be studied further.

ACKNOWLEDGMENT

This investigation was supported by Public Health Service research grant GM 16216 from the National Institute of General Medical Sciences, and by the Linda Fay Halbouty Premature Research Center, St. Luke's Episcopal Hospital, Houston, Texas.

REFERENCES

1. Hill, R. M., Drugs ingested by pregnant women, *Clin. Pharmacol. Ther.* **14,** 654 (1973).

2. Horning, M. G. et al., Isolation of drugs and drug metabolites from biological fluids by use of salt-solvent pairs, *Clin. Chem.* **20,** 282–287 (1974).

3. Horning, M. G. et al., Anticonvulsant drug monitoring by GC-MS-COM techniques, *J. Chromatogr.* **12,** 630–635 (1974).

4. Brazelton, T. B., Psychophysiologic reaction in the neonate. II. Effect of maternal medication on the neonate and his behavior, *J. Pediatr.* **58,** 513 (1961).

5. Desmond, M. M. et al., Maternal barbiturate utilization and neonatal withdrawal symptomatology, *J. Pediatr.* **80,** 190 (1972).

6. Hill, R. M. et al., Infants exposed in utero to antiepileptic drugs. A prospective study, *Am. J. Dis. Child.* **127,** 645 (1974).

7. Desmond, M. M. et al., Behavioral alterations in infants born to mothers on psychoactive medication during pregnancy. In *Congenital Mental Retardation*, Gordon Farrell, Ed., University of Texas Press, Austin and London, 1969, pp. 235–244.

8. Schaefer, O., Alcohol withdrawal syndrome in a newborn infant of a Yukon Indian mother, *Can. Med. Assoc. J.* **87,** 1333 (1962).

9. Zucker, P. and Simon, G., Prolonged symptomatic neonatal hypoglycemia associated with maternal chlorpropamide therapy, *Pediatrics* **42,** 824 (1968).

10. Wagner, L., Wagner, G., and Guerrero, J., Effect of alcohol on premature newborn infants, *Am. J. Obstet. Gynecol.* **108,** 308 (1970).

11. Sinclair, J. C. et al., Intoxication of the fetus by a local anesthetic, *N. Engl. J. Med.* **273,** 1173–1177 (1965).

12. Cree, J. E., Meyer, J., and Hailey, D. M., Diazepam in labour: Its metabolism and effect on the clinical condition and thermogenesis of the newborn, *Br. Med. J.* **4,** 251 (1973).

13. Lipsitz, P. J., The clinical and biochemical effects of excess magnesium in the newborn, *Pediatrics* **47,** 501 (1971).

14. Jackson, A. V., Toxic effects of salicylate on the foetus and mother, *J. Pathol. Bacteriol.* **60,** 587 (1948).

15. Earle, F., Congenital salicylate intoxication, *N. Engl. J. Med.* **265,** 1003 (1961).

16. Davies, P. P., Coagulation defect due to anticonvulsant drug treatment in pregnancy, *Lancet* **i,** 413 (1970).

17. Climie, C. R., et al., Methaemoglobinaemia in mother and foetus following continuous epidural analgesia with prilocaine. Clinical and experimental data, *Br. J. Anaesth.* **39,** 155 (1967).

18. Linden, G. and Henderson, B. E., Genital-tract cancers in adolescents and young adults, *N. Engl. J. Med.* **286**, 760–761 (1972).

19. Nora, J. J. and Nora, A. H., Birth defects and oral contraceptives, *Lancet* **i,** 941 (1973).

20. Meadow, S. R., Anticonvulsant drugs and congenital abnormalities, *Lancet* **ii,** 1296 (1968).

21. Speidel, B. D. and Meadow, S. R., Maternal epilepsy and abnormalities of the fetus and newborn, *Lancet* **ii,** 839–843 (1972).

Neonatal Narcotic Addiction

CARL ZELSON, M.D.

During the past 15 years the use of illicit drugs among the adult and adolescent population in this country has increased at an alarming rate. By 1970, it was estimated that there were 300 000 addicts in the United States. Three years later, in 1973, this estimate had been increased to 600 000. Although the vast majority of addicts live in metropolitan areas, more recent reports indicate that the problem is more widespread, occurring in many small communities not previously involved. With this marked increase in the number of drug addicts, one would anticipate an increased number of female addicts with a concomitant increase in the number of pregnant addicts. This was confirmed by our experience as well as by that of others.

OUR EXPERIENCE

During the five-year period (1955–1959) before we began our present study, only 22 infants were born to drug-addicted mothers at our institution. The following year, in 1960, there were 26 (1 of every 164 births), and each succeeding year the number of such births has increased at our hospital in spite of a progressive drop in the birth rate. By 1972, 1 of every 27 births was to a drug-addicted mother, a more than sixfold increase. The experience of many large municipal hospitals throughout the country, is similar (Table 1).

Over this same period, there has also been a marked drop in the age of the mothers. Through 1968 the mean age was between 26 and 29 years. During the past five years, more than half of the addicted mothers in our hospital have been 21 years old or younger, with a yearly mean between 21 and 23 years (Table 2).

During the early years of our study, heroin was the most commonly abused drug, but more recently methadone has become the drug most frequently used—obtained either in a methadone-maintenance program or bought "on the street."

Between 70 and 90% of all infants born to heroin- and to methadone-addicted mothers will manifest signs and symptoms of withdrawal (Table 3). Some infants show only mild signs, others severe. In our experience, infants born to methadone-addicted mothers manifest more—and more severe—signs of withdrawal than do heroin-exposed infants.

113

Table 1. Neonatal Drug Addiction: Maternal Data

Year	Total live births	Total no. addicted mothers	No. babies	Ratio of addicted mothers to total deliveries	No. mothers 21 years old or younger
1960	4284	26	26	1:164	2
1961	4396	36	36	1:122	4
1962	4290	43 (1 twin)	44	1:97	2
1963	4335	44	44	1:98	4
1964	3923	31	31	1:126	6
1965	3615	28	28	1:129	4
1966	3089	31	31	1:100	3
1967	2688	47 (1 twin)	48	1:56	7
1968	2283	46	46	1:49	12
1969	2367	50	50	1:47	26
1970	2586	58 (2 twins)	60	1:42	26
1971	2138	69 (1 twin)	70	1:30	47
1972	1658	60	60	1:27	31
1973	1504	51	51	1:29	26

Table 2. Neonatal Narcotic Addiction: Age of Mothers, 1960–1973[a]

	Total no. mothers	21 years of age or younger	Average age all mothers	Ratio of addicted infants to delivery rate
1960	26	2	27	1:164
1961	36	4	27	1:122
1962	43 (1 twin)	2	28	1:97
1963	44	4	26	1:98
1964	31	6	27	1:126
1965	28	4	27	1:129
1966	31	3	29	1:100
1967	47 (1 twin)	7	27	1:56
1968	46	12	26	1:49
1969	50	26	23.3	1:47
1970	58 (2 twins)	26	23.5	1:43
1971	60 (1 twin)	47	21.1	1:30.5
1972	60	31	22.4	1:27
1973	51	26	23.8	1:29

[a] Data of the Metropolitan Hospital Center.

Why some infants do not develop signs of withdrawal is not known. Even though the frequency with which withdrawal signs occur relates to maternal dose, to the time the last dose was taken before delivery, and to the duration of maternal addiction, the severity of withdrawal signs does not necessarily relate to the dosage or, in methadone addicts, to the concentration of methadone in the serum (1,2).

Table 3.   Signs of Withdrawal
Observed in 443 of a Total of 625
Infants Born to Addicted Mothers,
1960–1973[a]

Tremors	294
Irritability	237
Hypertonicity & hyperactivity	166
Vomiting	147
High-pitched cry	91
Sneezing	74
Respiratory distress	54
Fever	26
Diarrhea	24
Sweating	16
Mucus secretion	15
Tachypnea	14
Convulsions	12
Yawning	7
Poor feeding	6
Scratching face	5

[a] In order of frequency.

We have observed mothers with a history of heavy and long-term use of heroin whose infants showed no signs of withdrawal. We have also observed infants manifesting signs of withdrawal who were born to mothers who were taking only negligible amounts of heroin. On several occasions, we have seen mothers who manifested withdrawal signs, but their infants did not. We have observed infants who, in spite of the presence of morphine, quinine (a popularly used diluent for "street" drugs) or methadone in their urines, did not develop signs of withdrawal. These facts cannot be explained at the present time. It is generally accepted that chronic exposure to the addictive drugs produces physiological changes that result in altered cellular reactivity. How this relates to the clinical signs is not known. Cochin and Kornetsky (3) have demonstrated in animals that behavioral changes, drug-seeking tendencies, and tolerance persist long after detoxification.

We have demonstrated that exposure of the fetus to heroin or methadone interferes with the normal sleep processes in the neonate, suggesting some disturbance in the physiological function of the central nervous system.

The clinical picture of the abrupt withdrawal syndrome in the newborn infant is quite characteristic. This condition, once seen, is easily recognized thereafter. It is a severe generalized reaction, similar to that resulting from abrupt withdrawal in the adult, and is characterized in the infant by neurological, gastrointestinal, and homeostatic disturbances. It is thus imperative that all personnel involved with the care of the neonate should be familiar with the condition and be able to recognize it when it occurs.

Infants will usually manifest signs of withdrawal within the first 48 h of postnatal life, but a few will do so as late as 96 h of age or even later, particularly in the case of infants of methadone addicts. Although the first signs of withdrawal reportedly can occur as late as three weeks of age, we have not seen such onset in any infant beyond the age of 10 days. However, we have observed several infants born to methadone-addicted mothers who showed mild signs during the first 48 h of life, but who suddenly developed severe signs of withdrawal seven to 10 days later. If these infants had not been observed carefully after birth, one might well have concluded that they were showing late onset of withdrawal signs.

Conditions to be differentiated, because clinical findings are similar, include intracranial injury, tetany, hypoglycemia, meningitis, and sepsis, which must be ruled out in making the diagnosis.

Table 4 summarizes information on all such patients we have seen during a 14-year period.

Birth weights. Of the 625 infants observed, half weighed less than 2500 g at birth. Of these, 131 (44%) were full term by gestational age as judged by history and by clinical evaluation of gestation by the criteria of Dubowitz et al. (4). The remaining 327 infants weighed more than 2500 g.

Onset of withdrawal. The infants were observed carefully from birth. Three fourths of them developed signs of withdrawal of varying intensities. As judged by our criteria, 251 (40%) of these infants manifested clinical signs of withdrawal severe enough to require treatment. Of the total, two thirds developed their withdrawal signs within the first 24 h of life, another 97 (22%) within 48 h and the remaining 50 (11%) within the first four days of life.

Length of treatment. 52 (21%) of the infants responded quickly to treatment and were under control within 10 days after onset. In retrospect, we believe that most of these infants would probably have recovered spontaneously. Of the infants, 118 (47%) were treated for 10 to 20 days before complete control was obtained, and 81 (32%) of the infants required treatment for as long as 40 days before all visible signs of withdrawal had ceased.

Treatment. In general, paregoric, phenobarbital, chlorpromazine, and diazepam have been the drugs we have used in treating this condition, chlorpromazine being our drug of choice. This drug is given in a total dosage of 2.2 mg/kg body weight/24 h, in four daily doses, either orally or by injection. When vomiting is present, the drug is given by injection. The response is rapid; the infants relax and fall into quiet sleep, sleeping from feeding to feeding. They are easily awakened for feedings. After several days at the starting dose, the dose is gradually decreased as the infant remains under control—i.e., the decrease is related to decrease in signs present. Should signs of withdrawal recur, the dosage is increased and 24 to 48 h later again gradually decreased until it is apparent that no further treatment is necessary. No ill effects have been noted.

Deaths. The death rate has been quite low (3.2%). All deaths among infants born to drug-addicted mothers were included in this count, even though some of the deaths may not have been due to intrauterine drug exposure.

COMPARATIVE OBSERVATIONS AMONG INFANTS BORN TO HEROIN- AND TO METHADONE- ADDICTED MOTHERS

Because of the increased use of methadone in recent years, we made and reported (5) a comparative study of our observations in a group of 91 infants born to drug-addicted mothers during an 18-month period in 1971–1972. Of these, 46 were exposed to metha-

Table 4. Signs of Withdrawal and Frequency of Occurrence in 46 Infants of Methadone-Addicted Mothers and 45 Infants of Heroin-Addicted Mothers[a]

	Infants of methadone-addicted mothers				Infants of heroin-addicted mothers			
	Mild	Moderate	Severe	% of total group	Mild	Moderate	Severe	% of total group
Tremor	22	5	4	67.4	22	2	0	53.0
Hypertonicity[b]	22	7	7	78.2	16	2	0	40.0
Irritability[b]	6	13	4	50.0	10	0	0	22.0
Vomiting	10	5	1	34.7	4	0	0	8.9
Respiratory distress	7	2	1	21.7	11	1	1	29.0
High-pitched cry	8	0	0	17.4	5	0	0	11.1
Fever[b]	6	0	0	13.0	0	0	0	0
Hyperbilirubinemia[c]	3	4	5	26.0	0	5	2	15.5
Convulsions	3	2	0	10.9	1	0	1	4.4
Others	6	0	0	13.0	3	1	0	8.9

[a] From reference 5.

[b] Methadone % significantly ($P = 0.05$) higher than heroin %.

[c] Mild bilirubin < 110 mg/litre; moderate, bilirubin between 110 to 150/litre; severe, bilirubin > 150 mg/litre.

done and 45 were exposed to heroin (Table 5). We demonstrated that the infants born to methadone-addicted mothers were more severely involved and required longer periods of treatment than did those infants born to heroin-addicted mothers.

Table 5. Maternal Intake of Drugs

Regime	Methadone exposure (n = 46)		Heroin exposure (n = 45)	
	Methadone intake mg/day	No.	Maternal intake	No.
Methadone throughout pregnancy	20–60	9	1–5 bags or less than $10/day	32
Heroin 1st 3 mos., methadone last 6 mos. of pregnancy	10–100	8	6–10 bags or $11–$20/day	6
Heroin 1st 6 mos., methadone last 3 mos. of pregnancy	10–80	8	11+ bags or $21 or more/day	7
Heroin & methadone throughout pregnancy	10–120	21		

In addition, in a still-unpublished study we have demonstrated that the sleep patterns in methadone-exposed infants show more severe changes than do those of heroin-exposed infants.

Kron et al. (6) have demonstrated that methadone-exposed infants have less efficient sucking responses than do the heroin-exposed infants.

Respiratory distress after birth is frequent among drug-exposed infants. Hyaline-membrane disease is rare among heroin-exposed infants (7), but occurs with greater frequency in methadone-exposed infants.

The above data lead us to believe that one should hesitate before switching pregnant addicts from heroin to methadone, especially late in pregnancy.

SUMMARY

In conclusion, on the basis of our experience in over 625 infants born to heroin- and methadone-addicted mothers, we think that intrauterine exposure to these drugs is detrimental to the neonate and that methadone exposure more seriously affects the newborn infant than does heroin exposure. What the effects of this exposure will have on the long-term pattern of growth and development is still difficult to predict. Only a prolonged period of follow-up will give us this information.

REFERENCES

1. Zelson, C., Rubio, E., Wasserman, E., Neonatal narcotic addiction: 10 years observation, *Pediatrics* **48**, 178–189 (1971).

2. Rosen, T. S. and Pippenger, C. E., Neonatal withdrawal syndrome: Correlation with plasma methadone concentration and maternal methadone dosage, *Pediatr. Res.* **8**, 92 (1974).

3. Wikler, A. (Ed.) *Addictive States*, chap. 20. Williams & Wilkins, Baltimore, Md. (1968).

4. Dubowitz, L. M. S., Dubowitz, V., and Goldberg, C., Clinical assessment of gestational age in the newborn infant, *J. Pediatr.* **77**, 1–10 (1970).

5. Zelson, C., Lee, S. J., and Casalino, M., Neonatal narcotic addiction: Comparative effects of maternal intake of heroin and methadone, *N. Engl. J. Med.* **289**, 1216–1220 (1973).

6. Kron, R. E., Litt, M., and Finnegan, L. P., Behavior of infants born to narcotic addicted mothers, *Pediatr. Res.* **7**, 292 (1973). Abstract.

7. Glass, L., Rajegowda, B. K., and Evan, H. E., Absence of respiratory distress syndrome in premature infants of heroin addicted mothers, *Lancet* **ii**, 685–686 (1971).

The Neonate

Metabolic Problems Associated with the Newborn and High-Risk Infant

DONOUGH O'BRIEN, M.D., F.R.C.P.

This presentation has two quite separate and different objectives.

The first is to review the vulnerability of the newborn—especially of his central nervous system—to a number of metabolic disturbances, such as hyperphenylalaninemia, hypoglycemia, and malnutrition. The resulting implications underscore the need for clinical laboratories to be able to monitor common biochemical aberrations in this group—frequently, with microtechniques, and at all hours.

My other aim is to emphasize a second, rarely required, but sometimes lifesaving objective: the ability, promptly and accurately, to diagnose inborn errors of metabolism that are rapidly deleterious to the central nervous system. Early treatment of these conditions is potentially successful, in contrast to the often fatal consequences of delay. This places special responsibilities on ordinary hospital laboratories.

As an example of this group of disorders, the organic acidurias are a subgroup of special interest to clinical chemists because of the ease with which they can be diagnosed by gas-liquid chromatography/mass-spectrometry systems, relatively new tools on the clinical laboratory scene.

Figure 1 illustrates the rate of appearance of total cerebral DNA in man, in the rat, and in the guinea pig during gestation and afterward. The guinea pig has largely completed this stage of growth at the time of birth; the rat has only just begun. In comparison, man is in the middle of the most active phase of DNA replication at the time of birth and so is understandably vulnerable. Because the rat is at a similar stage of development about 20 days postpartum, it is a possible model to use in learning what influences cause damage to the neonatal human brain. Figures 2 and 3 are the same sort of curves, but show the somewhat similar relationships for myelin lipid and for total brain weight.

A series of experiments in a number of laboratories, notably in that of Chase et al. (1–4), have demonstrated that malnutrition, hypothyroidism, hypoglycemia, and hyperphenylalaninemia all affect these growth curves adversely.

TOTAL DNA

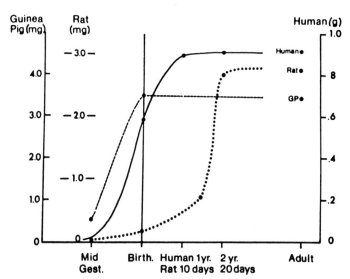

Figure 1.   Brain DNA in perinatal life.

MYELIN   LIPID

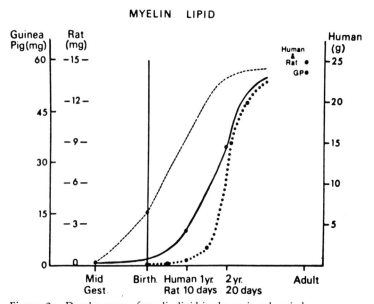

Figure 2.   Development of myelin lipid in the perinatal period.

In practice, malnutrition is probably the least important of these influences, because the brain of the human infant is resilient to perinatal malnutrition, and this is confirmed by similar figures for infants that are classified as "small for gestational age." The all-important question, of course, is whether even relatively small changes affect intellect in the long run, a question for which the answer is complicated by the many other con-current influences besides nutrition that can or may affect intellectual development in the infant.

TOTAL BRAIN WEIGHT

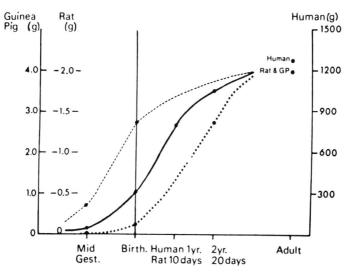

Figure 3. Perinatal changes in brain weight.

More convincing experimentally—just as the outcome is more convincing in terms of brain damage—are the effects of hypothyroidism, of hypoglycemia, and of hyperphenylalaninemia. Some effects of these homeostatic disruptions on infant rats are shown in Tables 1, 2, and 3.

Table 1. Brain Weights and Cerebral Lipids of Eight Previously Hypothyroid and Seven Control Rats, 30 Days Old[a]

	Controls	Previously hypothyroid	Reduction, %	P
Brain wt., g	1.658 ±0.048	1.459 ±0.087	12	<0.001
Lipid phosphorus[b]	2.208 ±0.068	2.093 ±0.057	—	<0.050
Cholesterol[b]	14.655 ±0.0686	12.940 ±0.0767	12	<0.001
Cerebroside[b]	5.894 ±0.675	4.288 ±0.320	28	<0.001
Sulphate[b]	1.527 ±0.099	1.181 ±0.138	23	<0.001

[a] The previously hypothyroid rats were injected daily with methimazole up to age 18 days, then allowed a 12-day period of recuperation.

[b] Lipid values are expressed as mg/g wet wt. of brain; ±values are standard deviations. From ref. 2, by permission of the publisher, Pergamon Press.

Clearly, what is true for these three conditions may in some measure also be true for aberrations of hydrogen ion concentration, of osmolality, of serum potassium, and other familiar biochemical variables. Just how well deviations from homeostasis in these are tolerated is poorly documented except in the rather gross terms of developmental follow-up studies of high-risk infants. That there is some penalty seems certain, and this surely

Table 2. Brain DNA and Protein in Control and Hypoglycemic Infant Rats[a]

| | DNA, mg | | Protein, mg | | Tissue wt. | | | |
| | | | | | Cortex–brain stem | | Cerebellum | |
	Cortex–brain stem	Cerebellum	Cortex–brain stem	Cerebellum	Weight, g	Protein, mg	Weight, g	Protein, mg
Control (18)[b]	1.24 ±0.08	1.19 ±0.12	94.6 ±7.6	12.8 ±2.0	1.01 ±0.04	76.3 ±5.6	0.15 ±0.01	10.7 ±1.0
Hypoglycemic (13)[b]	1.08 ±0.04	1.00 ±0.10	86.1 ±4.5	10.9 ±1.4	1.02 ±0.05	80.1 ±4.3	0.14 ±0.01	10.8 ±0.6
P value	<.01	<.01	<.01	<.01	>.05	<.05	<.05	<.05

[a] From ref. 3, by permission of the publisher, the American Academy of Pediatrics.
[b] No. animals.

Table 3. Effects of Phenylalanine on Brain DNA and Brain Protein in 18-Day-Old Rats[a]

| Treatment | Total DNA, mg | | Total protein, mg | | Brain wt./DNA wt., g/mg | |
	Cerebrum	Cerebellum	Cerebrum	Cerebellum	Cerebrum	Cerebellum
Phenylalanine-injected	0.846 ± 0.042[b]	1.057 ± 0.091	75.33 ± 8.64	75.33 ± 8.64	1.13	0.128
Controls	1.023 ± 0.032	1.498 ± 0.112	104.61 ± 2.54	19.18 ± .72	1.19	0.120
P value	<0.001	<0.001	<0.001	>0.5	>0.5	>0.5

[a] The control and test groups consisted of six animals each.
[b] Values represent mean ±1 SD.

justifies an alertness and competence in the clinical chemistry laboratory that will enable the clinician to do what he can to minimize these changes.

Let us next consider the clinical laboratory's responsibilities for promptly diagnosing inborn errors of metabolism. Specifically, the need is for definitive action in relation to conditions that are life threatening. Thus, screening for phenylketonuria—and perhaps also for histidinemia and homocystinuria—is an important routine duty. A delay of several days in processing the results of such screenings is of limited importance clinically. There is, however, a group of rare conditions for which immediate and accurate diagnosis may be lifesaving. These include some of the organic acidurias such as methylmalonic aciduria, galactosemia, and some of the branched-chain ketoacidurias. Screening programs are probably ineffectual in these cases. That is to say, in most systems the response time is too long-delayed for optimal therapeutic action. Rather, effective action is usually the result of a combination of the clinical acumen of the pediatrician and a prompt response from the laboratory. Laboratory diagnosis of galactosemia and maple-syrup urine disease is, of course, a relatively simple matter and the techniques are usable by the laboratory of any large hospital. For the smaller hospital, it is important to know that the American Academy of Pediatrics has established a nationwide network of centers for the diagnosis and immediate care of children with acute inborn errors of metabolism. Such centers can make available more elaborate diagnostic techniques for lysosomal disorders (e.g.) and also gas-liquid chromatography/mass-spectrometry systems for the diagnosis of organic acidurias.

A typical system is diagrammed in Figure 4, and a typical situation in which it is useful is in the diagnosis of methylmalonic aciduria. Figure 5 illustrates where a block can occur in the conversion of methylmalonyl CoA at the succinyl CoA step. Infants with this

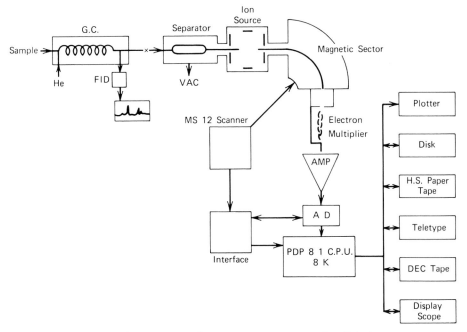

Figure 4. A typical gas chromatography/mass spectrometry system for clinical use.

metabolic defect usually show acidosis, vomiting, convulsions, and progressive neurological signs in the first few days of life. Diagnosis is especially urgent, because this rapidly deteriorating situation can be remedied either by protein restriction (when the defect is in the mutase or racemase apoenzyme) or by vitamin B_{12} (when the defect is at the cofactor site). Gas chromatography of the methyl silylated derivatives of an ether/ethyl acetate extract of urine is usually fairly typical (Fig. 6), although on one occasion we missed a case of α-methyl-β-hydroxybutyric aciduria because the peak in our systems appears at the same position as methylmalonic acid. With mass spectrometry this sort of error is eliminated. Extensive libraries of spectra of intermediary metabolites now exist, and can be used to warn of and identify unusual metabolites (5).

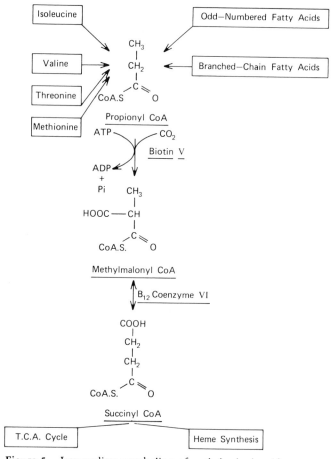

Figure 5. Intermediary metabolism of methylmalonic acid.

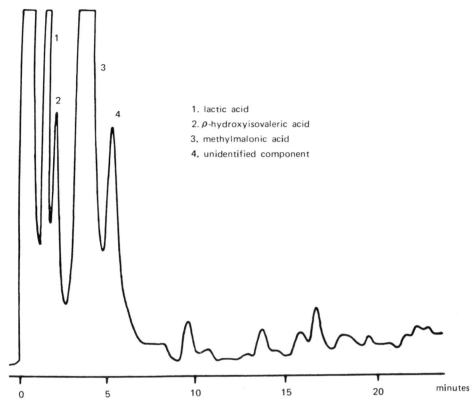

1. lactic acid
2. ρ-hydroxyisovaleric acid
3. methylmalonic acid
4. unidentified component

Figure 6. Gas-chromatographic scan of trimethylsilyl derivatives in urine from a case of methyl-malonic aciduria.

REFERENCES

1. Chase, H. P., The effects of intrauterine and postnatal undernutrition on normal brain development, *Ann. N.Y. Acad. Sci.* **205**, 231–244 (1973).

2. Walravens, P. and Chase, H. P., Influence of thyroid on formation of myelin lipids, *J. Neurochem.* **16**, 1477–1484 (1969).

3. Chase, H. P., Marlow, R. A., Dabiere, C. S., and Welch, N. N., Hypoglycemia and brain development, *Pediatrics* **52**, 513–520 (1973).

4. Chase, H. P. and O'Brien, D., The effect of excess phenylalanine and of other amino acids on brain development in the infant rat, *Pediatr. Res.*, **4**, 96–102 (1970).

5. Lawson, A. M., The scope of mass spectroscopy in clinical chemistry, *Clin. Chem.* **21**, 803–824 (1975).

Protein Metabolism in the Newborn— Some Changing Concepts

RONALD L. GUTBERLET, M.D.

The fate of protein administered to the human newborn infant is not well understood. Immaturity of digestive, enzyme, and excretory systems may result in abnormal concentrations of protein components and metabolites in blood and other tissue. These may then produce irreversible damage to developing organ systems.

Ignorance of possible toxic effects of ingested proteins is reflected in the history of infant feedings over the past two decades. It has amply been demonstrated over centuries that human milk is good for normal human babies. It contains about 12 g protein/litre and when ingested at a rate of 150 ml/kg body weight/day provides slightly less than 2 g protein/kg body weight, adequate for growth of a normal infant.

The postnatal growth of small premature babies has been of concern ever since the survival of a substantial number of such infants became possible. A major problem has been the inability to get adequate volumes of fluid and calories into and absorbed from their gastrointestinal tracts. This is especially true of infants who are sick with respiratory distress or have central nervous system immaturity manifested by recurrent apnea, and who may undergo long periods of relative starvation.

A major question is whether there exists any relationship between the observed lack of growth of the head (and therefore of the brain) and the neurological abnormalities and problems in development that are so frequent in the small premature infant. Brain growth in the human is most rapid during the last half of gestation and the first six months of extrauterine life (1). Physical head growth may be delayed for weeks, and although catch-up growth often occurs, there may be a permanent loss of brain cells, as has been noted by Winick in studies of older infants (2).

For some time, a major goal in infant nutrition has been to prevent these early failures in growth. In an effort to achieve this goal, Gordon et al. (3) showed in 1947 that more rapid weight gain could be obtained by feeding high-protein cow's milk formula instead of human milk to premature infants. The original studies were criticized on the basis that the high solute content of cow's milk led to water retention in the infant and was responsible for the weight gain. However, in 1967 Davidson et al. (4) showed that regardless of dietary mineral content, premature infants showed more rapid weight gains on 4 g than on 2 g protein/kg body weight/day, and accordingly the recommended protein intake for premature infants has been 3–4 g/kg/day, an intake achieved by giving concentrated formulas containing 3.35–3.77 MJ/litre (800–900 Cal/litre rather than the usual 2.8 MJ/litre (670 Cal/litre).

Unfortunately, aside from the fact that the babies grew faster, the other effects of giving high-protein cow's milk formulas were not appreciated. A recently recognized problem is one probably not related to the protein per se but to the high osmolarity of the formulas associated with the high protein content. In a study reported by Book et al. (5), high-osmolar formula was associated with an increased incidence of neonatal necrotizing enterocolitis, a major problem in intensive-care nurseries today. Seven of eight infants fed the high-osmolar formula (600 mosmol/litre) developed necrotizing enterocolitis as compared to only two of eight fed a 358 mosmol/litre formula. It remains to be proved whether or not the enterocolitis results from vascular stasis and intestinal ischemia secondary to distension with water being drawn into the intestine because of the high osmolarity. Human milk, aside from its low osmolarity, may protect against disease through immune mechanisms (6).

Quantitative and qualitative differences in the amino acid content of cow's milk as compared to human milk may be responsible for some problems. Table 1 shows that they differ in total protein content and in proportion of casein to lactalbumin. The proportions of the amino acids in casein may not be ideal for the premature infant. Casein is low in cystine. This amino acid is considered nonessential in the diet of mature people, being synthesized in the liver via a trans-sulfuration pathway. Gaull et al. (7) reported that the enzyme cystathionine γ-lyase [L-cystathionine cysteine-lyase (deaminating); EC 4.4.1.1], which is necessary for this to occur, is absent in the fetal and premature infant liver, and therefore cystine must be fed in the diet. Räihä (8) speculates that if cystine is then the rate-limiting amino acid in protein synthesis, high amounts of cow's-milk protein may indeed be necessary for growth. These high amounts of protein may result, however, in the observed high phenylalanine and tyrosine concentrations seen in the plasma of premature infants fed cow's-milk formula (9). Not only do the high-protein feedings result in above-normal amino acid concentrations in plasma, but also in abnormally high blood urea nitrogen concentrations (10). These increased amino acid concentrations may be associated with intellectual impairment, as are certain aminoacidurias.

Table 1.   Comparison of Protein Content of Human and Cow's Milk

	Protein g/100 ml	Casein/lactalbumin ratio (by wt.)
Human milk	1.2	40:60
Cow's milk	3.5	82:18

Goldman et al. (11) reported that more complications were observed in children five to seven years of age who had received 4 g protein/kg body weight as neonates than in those who received 2 g/kg. For example, significantly more of them developed strabismus, and 17 of 23 infants under 1.3 kg birth weight had an I.Q. of less than 90 versus only 6 of 26 on the low-protein feedings, a significant difference ($P = .01$).

Amino acid imbalance, hyperammonemia, electrolyte imbalance, dehydration, and acidosis must all be considered in the etiology of problems associated with high-protein feeding, and to date we do not know which, if any, are most important. In our present state of ignorance, we have now returned to feeding small premature infants in our nursery with formulas that contain 2.8 MJ/litre (670 Cal/litre), and provide 2 g protein/kg body weight. This is accomplished by increasing the water intake over the previously recommended 150 ml/kg and has resulted in better control of acid-base and electrolyte balance. Only after total fluid requirements are met by gastrointestinal alimentation and after continuous gastric or jejunal infusions have been discontinued are 3.35 MJ/litre (800 Cal/litre) formulas used.

Intravenous hyperalimentation is another area of protein nutrition where ignorance let us move forward more rapidly than perhaps was prudent. Not too many years ago, the supplier of intravenous fluids was the factor that determined whether fibrin hydrolysate or casein hydrolysate or synthetic amino acid mixtures were used by a particular hospital as a source of protein. Unfortunately, as reported in 1972 by several authors (*12–14*), blood ammonia sometimes increases markedly in premature infants fed these mixtures; in those infants given fibrin and casein the ammonia in the blood was thought to have originated from ammonia accumulating in the bottle on the shelf (*12,13*), but further studies of the synthetic mixtures indicated that the amino acid imbalance in the solutions caused increased ammonia production in vivo (*14*). Abnormally high blood-ammonia concentrations have been identified as a cause of intellectual and somatic retardation (*15*).

In 1973, Olney et al. added another concern (*16*). Fibrin and casein hydrolysates, injected into mice, produced acute degeneration of neurons in the developing hypothalamus. The acidic amino acids seem to be responsible. Casein hydrolysate, which produced lesions in lower concentrations than fibrin hydrolysate, is no longer given intravenously to our newborn infants.

One of the major functions of dietary protein is to provide for new tissue growth, but protein is also a source of energy and this has become an area of increasing interest in recent years. In 1970, Felig et al. described alanine as the chief gluconeogenic amino acid (*17*). Mestyan et al. (*18*) showed that the newborn's blood glucose increases after an intravenous alanine injection. The response was not seen in dysmature infants (that is, those small for gestational age). The predilection of such infants to hypoglycemia therefore appears to be related to a poor gluconeogenic capability. This concept is supported by the study of Haymond et al., who found that all potentially gluconeogenic amino acids entering the gluconeogenesis pathway at pyruvate were significantly increased above normal in these infants, in spite of the fact that their blood glucose values were lower than those for normally growing infants (*19*).

In collaboration with Pinar Ozand and Rupla Eshai, we have studied alanine utilization in full-term newborn infants who are not undergrown, but instead are large for their gestational age. Oral alanine-tolerance tests were performed at 6 h of age, before the first feeding, or at 36 h after a 4-h fast. L-Alanine (500 mg/kg body weight) was given via a nasogastric tube. We studied 12 infants. Five of these who were large for their gestational age and three who were appropriate for gestational age were studied at 6 h, and three more who were large for their gestational age and one who was appropriate for gestational age were studied at 36 h. Blood glucose, alanine, lactate, and pyruvate were measured at 0, 15, 30, 60, and 120 min.

Four of the five large infants had marked increases in blood glucose at 6 h of age (group B). These were compared to the eight infants with moderate increases in glucose (group A) and to four normal adults with regard to their blood lactate and pyruvate responses (Figure 1). The adults show no glucose response to the alanine. Group A had a slight rise in lactate with the glucose. Group B had marked but transient increases in both lactate and pyruvate, as would be expected because these metabolites represent intermediates in the conversion of alanine to glucose. The 6-h-old, large-for-gestational-age infants appear to have a much better gluconeogenic capability than do the normally growing and the older large-for-gestational-age infants.

However, the blood-alanine response to the oral load is also markedly different (Figure 2). Group A infants apparently absorb more poorly than do group B infants, but the increase in blood glucose [10 mg/100 ml (0.56 mmol/litre) during the first 30 min] about matches the increase [10–12 mg/100 ml (0.56–0.67 mmol/litre) during 40 min] reported (*18*) after an intravenous infusion of 125 mg of L-alanine/kg body weight. Therefore, the large 6-h-old infants appear to both absorb and convert more alanine to glucose, in contrast to the results reported for small-for-gestational-age infants. The mechanisms involved need to be defined, and as an understanding evolves we may be better able to provide usable calories for the sick and small premature infant. Continuing studies include measurements of hormones and other substrates involved in alanine utilization.

The results and literature cited above indicate that there needs to be continuous assessment of the fate of what is fed to newborn infants. This includes more careful biochemical monitoring of protein metabolism in the sick and premature newborn. The necessary

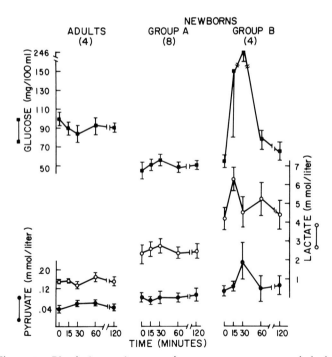

Figure 1. Blood glucose, lactate, and pyruvate responses to oral alanine.

Φ represent mean ± SE
(10 mg/100 ml glucose is 0.56 mmol/litre)

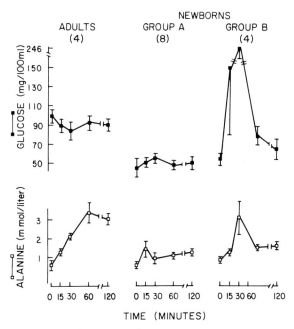

Figure 2.　Blood glucose and alanine responses to oral alanine.

Φ represent mean ± SE
(10 mg/100 ml glucose is 0.56 mmol/litre)

tests are not routinely available in hospital laboratories today. Two immediate requirements include accurate, microscale ammonia determinations in blood and measurements
of plasma amino acid concentrations (20), to allow for careful regulation of the dietary
protein based on a given infant's response. Measurements of the individual amino acids
in plasma are important, not only to prevent possible toxic concentrations of some of
them but also to indicate the availability of, or response to, amino acids in energy
metabolism.

SUMMARY

Responses to dietary protein and the role of protein in energy metabolism are influenced
by the gestational maturity and intrauterine growth of the newborn infant. Feeding premature infants high-protein cow's milk produces a more rapid weight gain, but also may
lead to necrotizing enterocolitis, amino acid imbalance, above-normal blood urea nitrogen concentration, and poor neurological outcome. Amino acid requirements differ with
maturity; e.g., cystine is essential in the premature infant's diet. Cow's milk is deficient
in cystine but rich in other amino acids.

Amino acid imbalance in solutions used for intravenous hyperalimentation may produce ammonia intoxication. Brain damage may be associated with too great an intake
of the acidic amino acids.

The role of protein in energy metabolism is still being defined. Alanine is utilized for
gluconeogenesis in normal newborns. In infants who are large for their gestational age,

absorption and metabolism may be markedly increased over that in infants appropriate for gestational age. Mechanisms and therapeutic implications need to be defined in these cases. Improved biochemical monitoring of neonatal nutrition is needed.

ACKNOWLEDGEMENT

I would like to thank Drs. Pinar Ozand, Rupla Eshai, Kulsum Merchant, Jeffrey Quartner, and Mrs. Gloria Greene, the coinvestigators in the alanine studies, for permission to present this information, and Mrs. Elaine Hanratty for help in preparing the manuscript. The alanine studies were supported in part by grants from the National Foundation and the NIH (Grant No. 03959–06).

REFERENCES

1. Dobbing, J. and Sands, J., Quantitative growth and development of human brain, *Arch. Dis. Child.* **48**, 757 (1973).

2. Winick, M., Cellular growth during early malnutrition (E. Mead Johnson Award Address), *Pediatrics* **47**, 969 (1971).

3. Gordon, H. H., Levine, S. Z., and McNamara, H., Feeding of premature infants: A comparison of human and cow's milk, *Am. J. Dis. Child.* **73**, 442 (1947).

4. Davidson, M., Levine, S. Z., Bauer, C. H., and Dunn, M., Feeding studies in low-birth-weight infants. I. Relationships of dietary protein, fat, and electrolyte to rates of weight gain, clinical courses, and serum chemical concentrations, *J. Pediatr.* **70**, 695 (1967).

5. Book, L. S., Herbst, J. J., and Jung, A. L., Necrotizing enterocolitis in infants fed an elemental formula, *Pediatr. Res.* **8**, 379 (1974). Abstract.

6. Santulli, T. V., Acute necrotizing enterocolitis: Recognition and management, *Hospital Practice* **9**(11), 129 (1974).

7. Gaull, G., Sturman, J. A., and Räihä, N. C. R., Development of mammalian sulfur metabolism: Absence of cystathionase in human fetal tissues, *Pediatr. Res.* **6**, 538 (1972).

8. Räihä, N. C. R., Biochemical basis for nutritional management of preterm infants, *Pediatrics* **53**, 147 (1974).

9. Hsia, D. Y.-Y., Berman, J. L. and Slatis, H. M., Screening newborn infants for phenylketonuria, *J. Am. Med. Ass.* **188**, 203 (1964).

10. Snyderman, S. E., Boyer, A., Kogut, M., and Holt, L. E., Jr., The protein requirement of the premature infant. I. The effect of protein intake on the retention of nitrogen, *J. Pediatr.* **74**, 872 (1969).

11. Goldman, H. I., Goldman, J. S., Kaufman, I., and Liebman, O. B., Late effects of early dietary protein intake on low-birth-weight infants, *J. Pediatr.* **85**, 764 (1974).

12. Johnson, J. D., Albritton, W. L., and Sunshine, P., Hyperammonemia accompanying parenteral nutrition in newborn infants, *J. Pediatr.* **81**, 154 (1972).

13. Ghadimi, H., Abaci, F., Kumar, S., and Rathi, M. Biochemical aspects of intravenous alimentation, *Pediatrics* **48**, 955 (1971).

14. Heird, W. C. et al., Hyperammonemia resulting from intravenous alimentation using a mixture a synthetic L-amino acids: A preliminary report, *J. Pediatr.* **81**, 162 (1972).

15. Shih, V. E., Efron, M. L., and Moser, H. W., Hyperornithinemia, hyperammonemia, and homocitullinuria. A new disorder of amino acid metabolism associated with myoclonic seizures and mental retardation, *Am. J. Dis. Child.* **117**, 83 (1969).

16. Olney, J. W., Ho, O. L., and Rhee, V., Brain-damaging potential of protein hydrolysates, *N. Engl. J. Med.* **289**, 391 (1973).

17. Felig, P., Pozefsky, T., Marliss, E., and Cahill, G. F., Jr., Alanine: Key role in gluconeogenesis, *Science* **167**, 1003 (1970).

18. Mestyan, J., Schultz, K., and Horvath, M., Comparative glycemic responses to alanine in normal term and small-for-gestational-age infants, *J. Pediatr.* **85**, 276 (1974).

19. Haymond, M. W., Karl, I. E., and Pagliara, A. S., Increased gluconeogenic substrates in the small-for-gestational-age infant, *N. Engl. J. Med.* **291**, 322 (1974).

20. Snyderman, S. E., Holt, L. E., Jr., Norton, P. M., and Phansalkar, S. V., Protein requirement of the premature infant. II. Influence of protein intake on free amino acid content of plasma and red blood cells, *Am. J. Clin. Nutr.* **23**, 890 (1970).

Carbohydrate Metabolism:
The Energy Crisis in the Newborn

JOHN F. NICHOLSON, M.D.

THE ENERGY CRISIS IN THE NEWBORN

During the last weeks of gestation, the human fetus stores large amounts of fat and carbohydrate (1). The glycogen content of liver and muscle increases to a concentration several times that present in later infancy and adulthood (2). Because only a fraction of the total energy available from the catabolism of glycogen can be mobilized anaerobically, while none of the energy available from fat can be utilized without oxygen, it seems clear that the large glycogen stores are laid down in anticipation of birth asphyxia and of the immediate needs of adaptation to extrauterine life.

Figure 1 illustrates diagrammatically the changes in respiratory quotient, blood glucose, liver glycogen, and free fatty acids that occur after birth. The arrows should be considered directional only and not indicative of magnitude, because the magnitude of change for any of these variables is a function of many other variables. In general, it can be said that liver glycogen and blood glucose concentrations decrease in the first few hours after birth and that the rate of this decrease is related to the size of the glycogen pool at birth, the thermal environment of the infant, his caloric intake, and the presence or absence of complicating energy-requiring perinatal disorders such as the respiratory distress syndrome (2). The increased concentrations of free fatty acids and glycerol that occur in the serum after birth are not as completely described as are the changes in blood glucose. However, it is clear that mobilization of free fatty acids is a normal phenomenon and that it is accompanied by the expected decrease in the respiratory quotient from a value near 1.0 at birth, indicating total dependence for energy on carbohydrate catabolism, to a value near 0.7 a few days after birth, indicating almost complete dependence on the catabolism of fat for energy (3,4). As oral intake is established in the latter part of the first week of life, the respiratory quotient increases to an intermediate value, indicating that a mixture of carbohydrate, protein, and fat is being catabolized to meet energy requirements.

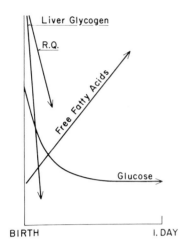

Figure 1. Changes in some variables during the first postnatal day.

The concentrations of hormones concerned with intermediary metabolism that are observed in association with the immediate postnatal metabolic adaptations of the infant seem to correlate well with the changes in substrate concentrations observed. Insulin concentrations in the serum of the normal newborn are relatively low, and remain so during the first few hours of life (5). Somatotropin (growth hormone) concentrations are relatively high and increase in the immediate postnatal period (6). Catecholamines are secreted postnatally (7), as are adrenal corticoids (8). The role of pancreatic glucagon has only recently been explored. Glucagon seems to be present at birth and to increase in the immediate postnatal period (9).

THE INFANT OF THE DIABETIC MOTHER

In order to focus on the role of hormones in the adaptation of energy metabolism to extrauterine life, it is appropriate to consider the infant of the diabetic mother. By all accounts, the basic problem of the infant of the diabetic mother is fetal hyperinsulinism, although the mechanism for islet-cell hyperplasia and for abnormally high insulin concentrations at birth is not clear. The infant of the diabetic mother is overgrown, probably as a result of the effect of excessive concentrations of insulin on the synthesis of protein and fat, and his glycogen stores are abundant. At birth, his blood sugar declines more rapidly than that of the normal infant, reaching its lowest point 1 to 2 h after birth, a change associated with higher-than-normal insulin and somatotropin concentrations. Glucocorticoid response appears to be appropriate in infants of diabetic mothers. Glucagon secretion is probably somewhat decreased (9). Two fundamental abnormalities are noted in the adaptation of the infant of the diabetic mother to extrauterine life: First, there is a failure of appropriate catecholamine excretion immediately after birth (*10*), and second, plasma free fatty acids increase only slowly in the immediate postnatal period (3). While it is difficult to generalize from an experiment of nature so complex as the infant of a diabetic mother, current general consensus would have it that the sympathetic nervous system and catecholamine release play a primary role in maintenance of blood sugar in the immediate postnatal period, through glycogenolysis and through the glucose-sparing effect of fatty acid mobilization.

OTHER DEFINED METABOLIC ABNORMALITIES

Other discrete and definable metabolic abnormalities are known to be associated with hypoglycemia in the early neonatal period. Among these are insulinoma, β-cell nesidioblastosis, hepatic glycogen-storage disease, galactosemia, hereditary fructose intolerance, and hexosediphosphatase (EC 3.1.3.11) deficiency. For reasons that are still obscure, infants with erythroblastosis have β-cell hyperplasia similar to that seen in the infant of the diabetic mother, and develop postnatal hypoglycemia with some regularity (*11*).

TRANSIENT SYMPTOMATIC NEONATAL HYPOGLYCEMIA

A relatively small proportion of full-term infants, from one to three per thousand, develop a disorder commonly known as transient symptomatic neonatal hypoglycemia (*5*). Although this entity is rather well defined, it is in the murky area surrounding it that most of the controversy concerning neonatal glucose metabolism has arisen. Given a baby who has one or more of a constellation of symptoms and signs, including "apnea, cyanosis, sudden pallor, tachypnea, jitteriness, tremors, convulsions, coma, sweating, subnormal temperature, upward rolling of the eyes, limpness, twitching, weak or high-pitched cry, refusal to feed, and irregular respirations" (*12*), whose blood sugar is less than 1.1 mmol/litre (20 mg/dl), whose clinical abnormalities appear after the first day of life and respond dramatically to intravenous glucose, all investigators would agree to the diagnosis of symptomatic hypoglycemia.

Should the clinical and chemical manifestations disappear after a few days of conservative therapy (including intravenous glucose and small doses of hydrocortisone), leaving the infant normal, all investigators would also agree to the diagnosis of transient symptomatic neonatal hypoglycemia. The etiology of this condition is unknown and may not be single, but the frequency with which such infants develop ketotic hypoglycemia in later infancy suggests that at least some of them may have intrinsic problems in adapting to glucose deprivation (*13*). Of greatest concern is the fact that transient symptomatic neonatal hypoglycemia carries a substantial risk of permanent neurological sequelae (*14*). To the physician caring for newborn infants, transient symptomatic neonatal hypoglycemia is a disorder that carries substantial risk, that is self limited, and that therefore should be prevented. Furthermore, if this well-defined clinical entity damages the brain as a result of hypoglycemia, it is reasonable to suppose that hypoglycemia that occurs during the first 24 h of life may also damage the brain. In addition, present evidence indicates that asymptomatic hypoglycemia does not carry the same risk of neurological sequelae that accompanies symptomatic hypoglycemia. Although the hypotheses and clinical considerations generated by these concepts are clear, a number of difficulties stand in the way of simple approaches to transient neonatal hypoglycemia.

Although the concentration of sugar in the blood can be expected to decrease after birth, the value to which it falls in the normal infant after normal delivery is a function of environmental temperature, as indicated by Cornblath and Schwartz (*5*). Whether the infant is fed shortly after birth or kept fasting for several hours profoundly influences blood sugar (*15,16*).

Because of these two observations, the definition of normal blood sugar in the neonatal period is in question. The values (*5*) of 1.6 to 5.6 mmol/litre (30–100 mg/dl) for the normal full-term infant and 1.1 to 5.6 mmol/litre (20–100 mg/dl) for the small infant are chemical observations made under specific nursery and feeding conditions and should not be interpreted as normal, but rather as appropriate responses to the conditions imposed on the infant.

Consider an infant whose gestation has been complicated by toxemia, premature labor, or intrauterine growth retardation; whose stores of glycogen are, therefore, less than optimal; whose fat stores may also be suboptimal; who may have a large radiant surface area requiring increased heat production; and whose glucose-metabolizing brain is relatively large with respect to his total metabolic mass. It is easy to imagine increased susceptibility to hypoglycemia, and this has indeed been shown by several investigators (17,18). However, such an infant is also at risk of cerebral anoxia, respiratory distress, and other perinatal complications associated with the underlying conditions of gestation. Since the cerebral manifestations of all disorders of the perinatal period are nonspecific, it is extremely difficult to associate low blood sugar causally with these manifestations unless intravenous glucose produces prompt and virtually complete amelioration of the manifestations.

If the clinical response to intravenous glucose is less than dramatic or does not occur at all, one is forced to conclude either that the clinical manifestations are largely not due to a low blood-sugar concentration or that the low blood-sugar concentration has so profoundly affected the infant that recovery from hypoglycemia may be prolonged or may not occur at all. In considering this group of high-risk infants, Griffiths and Bryant (19) found no evidence that low blood-sugar concentration played a part in the clinical evolution of their disorders. However, the incidence of chemical hypoglycemia in their series was several times higher than that reported in other series, raising questions about the adequacy of the chemical diagnosis. On the other hand, Pildes et al. reported a correlation between neonatal hypoglycemia and subsequent neurologic disorders (20). Unfortunately, their prospective study, which was well controlled for other perinatal conditions, was not controlled for the effects of intrauterine growth retardation on ultimate neurologic status. Therefore, the question of the direct effect of early neonatal hypoglycemia on the subsequent neurologic development of the high risk infant is not resolved

RECOMMENDATIONS

From the information generated over the past 15 years or so concerning energy metabolism in the neonate—and particularly his metabolism of glucose—it is possible to make certain recommendations:

1. Since the infant's caloric expenditure for maintenance of body temperature can be extreme at ordinary room temperature (4), it is important to maintain the neonate in a thermoneutral environment (32–34 °C). The evidence developed by Cornblath and Schwartz would suggest that this measure alone will significantly increase the mean values for blood sugar during the first day of life (5).

2. A number of investigators (15,16) have noted that the blood sugar of the neonate is maintained at concentrations much nearer fasting adult values when feedings are begun shortly after birth. In view of the known energy requirements of adaptation to extrauterine life it seems appropriate to supply a source of energy to infants soon after birth. It would appear that providing 60 ml of human milk/kg body weight during the first day of life is sufficient to ameliorate greatly the energy drain for most infants (16).

Special attention should be paid to infants born of toxemic mothers, to those born prematurely, and to infants with intrauterine growth retardation. The general recommendation (*12*) that blood glucose be monitored in these infants every few hours after birth is appropriate. Furthermore, the known stresses upon their sources of energy make it advisable that they be provided with a calorie source during adaptation to extrauterine life. Should early feeding not be feasible, intravenous glucose should be used.

The infant of the diabetic mother requires additional comment. Because catecholamine release in response to declining blood sugar is known to be impaired in the infant of the diabetic mother, it has been suggested that epinephrine be administered to these babies specifically to correct this defective response. Haworth and McRae (*14*) investigated this approach, found several deficiencies in it, and recommended as an alternative a slow infusion of dextrose (100 g/litre) from birth. While the question of the advisability of epinephrine therapy for the infant of the diabetic mother remains open, the approach of Haworth and McRae to the problem would at present appear to be a more conservative one.

SUMMARY

Summarizing current information concerning carbohydrate metabolism in the neonate, it can be said that adaptation to extrauterine life greatly stresses his energy stores. Present definitions of the lower limit of normal blood sugar in the neonate are influenced profoundly by conditions imposed in delivery-room and nursery-routine practices and cannot be considered to represent the lower limits of physiologically optimal blood-glucose values. Maintaining the neonate in a thermoneutral environment and providing an early source of calories significantly increase the mean concentration of blood glucose in all neonates. That the maintenance of higher blood sugar in high-risk infants will result in better ultimate outcome remains in question.

REFERENCES

1. Adam, P. A. J., Control of glucose metabolism in the human fetus and newborn infant, *Adv. Metab. Disord.* **5**, 184 (1971).
2. Shelly, H. J., Carbohydrate reserves in the newborn infant, *Br. Med. J.* **i**, 273 (1964).
3. Chen, C. H. et al., The plasma-free fatty acid composition and blood glucose of normal and diabetic pregnant women and of their newborns, *Pediatrics* **36**, 843 (1965).
4. Bruck, K., Temperature regulation in the newborn infant, *Biol. Neonate* **3**, 65 (1961).
5. Cornblath, M. and Schwartz, R., *Disorders of Carbohydrate Metabolism in Infancy* (Vol. 3 in the series *Major Problems in Clinical Pediatrics*), W. B. Saunders Co., Philadelphia, Pa., 1966.
6. Cornblath, M. et al., Secretion and metabolism of growth hormone in premature and full-term infants, *J. Clin. Endocrinol Metab.* **25**, 209 (1965).
7. Greenberg, R. E., Lind, J., and von Euler, U.S., Effect of posture and insulin hypoglycemia on catecholamine excretion in the newborn, *Acta Paed.* **49**, 780 (1960).
8. Kenny, F. M., Preeyasomabt, C., and Migeon, C. L., Cortisol production rate. II. Normal infants, children, and adults, *Pediatrics* **37**, 34 (1966).
9. Luyckx, A. C., Massi-Benedetti, F., Falorni, A., and Lefebvre, P. J., Presence of pancreatic glucagon in the portal plasma of human neonates. Differences in the insulin and glucagon responses to glucose between normal infants and infants from diabetic mothers, *Diabetologia* **8**, 296 (1972).

10. Stern, L., Ramos, A., and Leduc, J., Urinary catecholamine excretion in infants of diabetic mothers, *Pediatrics* **42,** 598 (1968).

11. Barrett, C. T. and Oliver, R. K., Hypoglycemia and hyperinsulinism in infants with erythroblastosis fetalis, *N. Engl. J. Med.* **278,** 1260 (1968).

12. Beard, A. et al., Neonatal hypoglycemia: A discussion, *J. Pediatr.* **79,** 314 (1971).

13. Pagliara, A. S. et al., Hypoalaninemia: A concomitant of ketotic hypoglycemia, *J. Clin. Invest.* **51,** 1440 (1972).

14. Haworth, J. C. and McRae, K. N., The neurological and developmental effects of neonatal hypoglycemia. A follow-up of 22 cases, *Can. Med. Assoc. J.* **92,** 861 (1965).

15. Ditchburn, R. K., Wilinson, R. H., Davies, P. A., and Ainsworth, P., Plasma glucose levels in infants weighing 2,500 g and less fed immediately after birth with breast milk, *Biol. Neonate* **11,** 29 (1967).

16. Bhakoo, O. N., and Scopes, J W., Minimal rates of oxygen consumption in small-for-dates babies during the first week of life, *Arch. Dis. Child.* **49,** 583 (1974).

17. Pildes, R., Forbes, A. E., O'Connor, S. M., and Cornblath, M., The incidence of neonatal hypoglycemia—A completed survey, *J. Pediatr.* **70,** 76 (1967).

18. Lubchenco, L. O. and Bard, H., Incidence of hypoglycemia in newborn infants classified by birth weight and gestational age, *Pediatrics* **47,** 831 (1971).

19. Griffiths, A. D. and Bryant, G. M., Assessment of effects of neonatal hypoglycaemia, *Arch. Dis. Child.* **46,** 819 (1971).

20. Pildes, R. S. et al., A prospective controlled study of neonatal hypoglycemia, *Pediatrics* **54,** 5 (1974).

Amino Acid Metabolism in the Newborn

CHARLES R. SCRIVER, M.D.

There are many different facets of amino acid metabolism in the newborn to be considered and it is impossible to discuss all of them, even briefly. Therefore, I will summarize three important themes only: screening, ontogeny, and catabolism. This review must exclude many of the important details concerning the metabolism of amino acids as it relates to the newborn. For consideration of this entire field in greater depth I refer you to *Amino Acid Metabolism and Its Disorders* (1).

SCREENING

Systematic screening is the essential prelude to the recognition of disordered amino acid metabolism. This must be performed early if appropriate management and treatment are to be instituted. It must differentiate the abnormal from the normal, or typical, state. The number of known disorders of amino acid metabolism and the ability to recognize these disorders have been linked to the technological developments that have become available for screening. This is illustrated in Figure 1.

Until the advent of chromatography in its various forms, only three disorders of amino acid metabolism (alcaptonuria, cystinuria, and phenylketonuria) were known. These were identified by simple chemical tests of the infant's urine. Partition chromatography on filter paper with ninhydrin as location reagent was introduced into clinical medicine in 1945. With time, additional supporting media have been used with other solvents and stains for location of the amino acids and their derivatives. Nevertheless, partition chromatography remains an invaluable technique for the qualitative analysis of amino acids. It was mainly this technique that permitted an exponential growth in the number of known amino acidopathies over the next two decades so that by 1967 some 50 "ninhydrin-positive" traits had been described.

Liquid-elution chromatography on ion-exchange resin columns became popular after 1958, when the procedure was mechanized. This remains the technique most often used

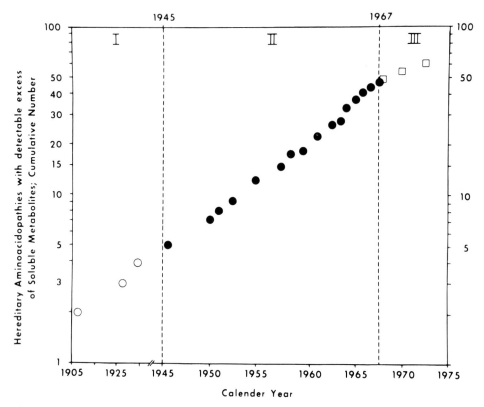

Figure 1.   Stages in the development of our knowledge about aminoacidopathies.

     I   the prechromatography era (Garrod, 1908 to Dent, 1946).
    II   the era of partition chromatography (Dent, 1946).
   III   the gas-chromatography era.

for the quantitative analysis of amino acids in body fluids. It can be modified for the rapid analysis of specific groups of amino acids.

    Gas-liquid chromatography offers theoretical advantages for the analysis of amino acids. Small volume of sample, great sensitivity, and high speed of analysis are obvious advantages, but the complexity and lack of reproducibility of the derivatization procedure have limited the application of the technique in routine practice. Gas chromatography is at present the preferred method for the identification of "ninhydrin-negative" derivatives of free amino acids. Gas chromatography is likely to have its greatest application when coupled with mass spectrometry which permits the mass numbers of compounds to be determined rapidly. Several "new" disorders of amino acid metabolism have already been discovered by the use of this technique. For example, Orval Mamer, Robert Daum, and I used gas chromatography to identify a new disorder of isoleucine metabolism in which α-methylacetoacetic acid is excreted in the urine due to a block at the β-keto-thiolase step in the metabolism of isoleucine (2). The technique also has potential application in the study of mutant traits in tissue-culture systems and for further investigation of amino acid disorders in humans following the administration of deuterated amino acids.

The difficulty in collecting urine samples from newborn infants has made screening of blood samples an attractive alternative for screening of a large population. The microbial inhibition assay of Guthrie and Susi (3) has been used to identify the high concentration of phenylalanine in the blood of infants with phenylketonuria. The assay has been adapted with different organisms and inhibitors to detect increased quantities of leucine, tyrosine, methionine, histidine, valine, and argininosuccinic acid. The Guthrie test has now been used in over 20 million infants to screen for hyperphenylalaninemia.

The collection of blood on filter paper has permitted screening tests to be applied at a few centers to large numbers of samples transported from surrounding regions. Automated colorimetric or fluorometric techniques can also be applied to the specimens collected in this manner for the quantitation of phenylalanine and tyrosine.

The various techniques of screening for disease are now being applied to over 90% of the live births in North America and are also widely used in Europe, Australia, and Japan, among other countries of the world.

RECOGNITION OF ABNORMALITY

To recognize disease or disadaptation, it is first necessary to know the normal. The concentration of any constituent in plasma reflects the balance between that added to the plasma and that removed from it. The major flux of amino acids is of their free form. It is possible to think of amino acids existing in pools in the body as indicated schematically in Figure 2. The concept of amino acid pools was elaborated by Van Slyke and Meyer (5) more than 50 years ago. They injected DL-alanine and then monitored its disappearance from plasma by the newly developed technique of formol titration for measurement of α-amino nitrogen. They discovered that the amino acid did not disappear from the blood into the urine only, but that it moved into tissues also. The major tissue pool was muscle. This observation was then "forgotten," because its importance was not recognized. It has now come into perspective, particularly as we begin to think of the metabolic interfaces between carbohydrate and amino acid metabolism.

In screening tests for blood amino acids, the extracellular pools are assayed. The plasma pool is estimated to be between 1 and 6% of the total amino acid pool. Muscle holds up to 80% of the total body pool for any of the essential amino acids and 50% for any of the

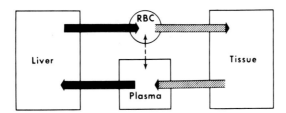

Figure 2. A hypothesis based on the studies of Elwyn (4) for the mechanism of amino acid flux between a peripheral tissue, such as muscle, and a central tissue, such as liver. Erythrocytes take up amino acids in liver sinusoids and deliver them to a peripheral capillary bed and tissue. Blood plasma extracts amino acids from peripheral tissue and delivers them to the liver. The latter tissue can clear plasma of 50 to 90% of its free amino acid load each minute. There is relatively little exchange of amino acids between the plasma and erythrocytes.

Table 1.   Amino Acid Concentration in Plasma or Serum (μmol/litre)[a]

Amino acid	"Prematures"[1]		Neonates[2]		Infants[3]		Children[4]	
	Mean	± SD	Mean	± SD	Mean	± SD	Mean	± SD
Taurine	180	75	141	40				
Hydroxyproline	40	40	32					
Aspartic acid	10	10	8	4	19	2	16	3
Threonine	215	60	217	21	177	36	145	16
Serine	270	75	163	34	131	27[c]	121	14[c]
Asp (NH$_2$) + Glu (NH$_2$)[b]	905	250	759	136				
Proline	230	75	183	32	193	52	176	33
Glutamic acid	65	35	52	25				
Glycine	460	275	343	69	213	35	219	33
Alanine	375	50	329	55	292	53	271	36
Valine	130	50	136	39	161	38	181	20
Half-cystine	65	10	62	13	42	9	44	7
Methionine	35	5	29	8	18	3	16	3
Isoleucine	40	20	39	8	39	8	44	6
Leucine	70	25	72	17	77	21	90	13
Tyrosine	120	100	69	16	54	21	45	8
Phenylalanine	90	20	78	14	55	10	47	5
Ornithine	90	20	91	25	50	11	46	8
Lysine	190	60	200	46	135	28	130	20
Histidine	50	20	77	16	78	14	80	13
Arginine	50	20	54	17	62	9	85	16
Tryptophan	30	15	32	17				
β-Alanine			14.5					

[a] All data obtained by elution chromatography on ion exchange resin columns.

[b] Asparagine and glutamine, as combined amounts.

[c] Includes asparagine.

[d] Signifies pooled glutamine and asparagine. The individual values for the mean ± SD (and range) are glu (NH$_2$) 640 ± 58, (520–742); asp (NH$_2$) 56 ± 15, (34–82).

[e] Signifies glutamine alone.

[1] Adapted from Dickinson, Rosenblum, and Hamilton, 1970. Data for the first day of life from 10 premature infants with birth weights less than 2500 grams. Some of these infants may have been small-for-gestational-age rather than prematurely born.

[2] Recalculated from Dickinson et al., 1965; 25 infants (more than 2500 grams) studied before first feeding.

nonessential amino acids. By comparison, the liver pool of any amino acid usually is less than 10% of the total pool and the kidney pool is less than 4%. The concentration of amino acids in plasma is regulated closely by the relationships between various pools. However, a single measurement of a concentration in plasma gives no indication of the flux through the pools nor of episodic variations in the pool size.

The means and standard deviations for the concentrations of individual amino acids in plasma for the human population are surprisingly constant, given the wide variation

Children[5]		Children[6]		Adults[7,8]		Adults[9]		
Mean	Range	Mean	Range	Mean[7]	Range[8]	Mean	± SD	Range
80	57–115	49	19–91	66	27–168	59	12	41–78
	25							
10	4–20	2	0–9	16	0–24			0–5
76	42–95	60	33–128	162	79–246	138	31	75–189
94	79–112	92	24–172	112	67–193	99	19	67–129
295	57–467	135	46–290	603	413–690	696[d]	73[d]	554–824[d]
106	68–148	115	51–185	233	100–442	185	48	90–270
110	23–250			58	14–192	24	12	10–67
166	117–223	170	56–308	231	120–553	284	44	162–335
234	137–305	219	99–313	344	209–659	360	74	205–496
162	128–283	127	57–262	169	116–315	225	49	151–302
60	45–77			74	48–141	49	9	34–67
14	11–16	21	3–29	21	6–39	21	4	43–32
43	28–81	44	26–94	54	35–97	60	12	38–83
85	56–178	75	45–155	100	71–175	115	23	77–162
43	34–71	45	11–122	50	21–87	54	11	40–80
42	26–61	40	23–69	57	37–115	48	7	37–61
33	27–86	40	10–107	69	29–125	58	14	32–88
111	74–151	87	45–144	173	82–236	186	36	99–249
55	24–85	64	24–112	79	31–106	88	16	65–119
53	23–86	31	11–65	81	21–137	82	17	53–115
						31	6	19–45
					25–73			

[3] Recalculated from Brodehl and Gellisen, 1968; 12 infants, 16 days to 4 months of age, studied after 6- to 8-hour fast.

[4] Recalculated from Brodehl and Gellisen, 1968; 12 children 2 to 12 years of age, studied after overnight fast.

[5] Scriver and Davies, 1965; 9 children, 3 to 10 years of age, studied after overnight fast.

[6] Soupart, 1962; 20 children, 9 months to 2 years of age, studied after overnight fast.

[7] Recalculated from Dickinson et al. 1965; 8 adults.

[8] Data on 76 adults compiled from nine sources by Dickinson et al., 1965; includes variation recorded by Soupart, 1962.

[9] Data on 10 men and 10 women (age range 33 to 56 years), from Perry and Hansen, 1969.

of environmental conditions among different races. Means and standard deviations change with time after birth, as illustrated in Table 1. It is necessary to know these data to identify abnormal values. Variations in the excretion of amino acids in the urine also occur. Urine composition is determined by certain functions such as tubular reabsorption capability. Other factors that have considerable influence include the pattern and concentration of amino acids present initially in the glomerular filtrate. Consequently, the normal pattern of aminoaciduria in man is more variable than that of plasma. Diet, age, sex, and physiological status of the individual, as well as the disease process—each accounts for some of the variability. Finally, concentrations in both plasma and urine exhibit considerable diurnal (circadian) variation.

The remarkable steady state that we maintain in our plasma concentration of amino acids in the face of many different environmental variations and diets is a reflection of the control of the many different events illustrated in Figure 3. These include ingestion of protein, hydrolysis in the gastrointestinal tract, and absorption of free amino acids and oligopeptides that are released by the hydrolysis of the protein. There is absorption across the intestinal tract, followed by entry of the amino acids into the portal circulation to the liver, where they enter the liver metabolic pool. There is flux from the liver into the peripheral circulation, which in turn delivers the amino acids to muscle. The presence of circadian variation in the concentration of amino acids in blood is indicated by the oscillating line which describes the "plasma pool." The relevance of this fact is that in order to identify carriers of some mutant genes which may affect amino acid pool size, it is important to recognize that circadian rhythmicity influences the normal mean and standard deviation for plasma amino acids.

From the plasma, the amino acids enter the metabolic pools of various tissues, eventually to flux back to plasma. The kidney receives approximately one fifth of the total circulating blood volume and has a filtration fraction of about 20%. The potentially large load of amino acids lost by filtration is reclaimed by tubular absorption with greater than 97% efficiency (Figure 4). Thus, many different events contribute to the extraordinary homeostasis of amino acid metabolism.

The fluxes between tissues are even more subtle than we had anticipated several years ago (Figure 2). For instance, we now recognize that the centrifugal flux of glutamic

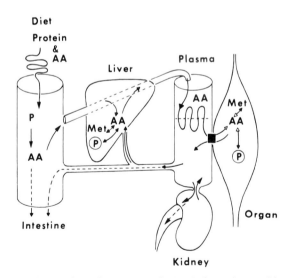

Figure 3. The flow of free (unbound) amino acids (*AA*) from the nutritional phase (intestine), through metabolic pools (*Met*) in organs such as liver and muscle, into bound pools (*P*). Plasma and erythrocytes mediate the interorgan fluxes with oscillations in the plasma steady state. Regulators such as hormones influence supply and chemical demand at various sites (viz., muscle-plasma interface).

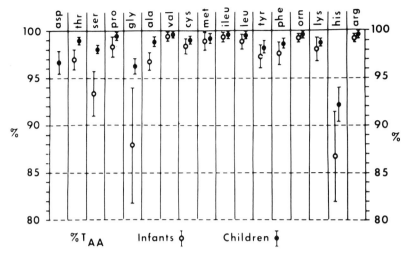

Figure 4. Net tubular absorption of amino acids, expressed as percentage of filtered load, in infants and children. Efficiency of absorption improves with age. (Redrawn from reference 6).

acid may occur predominantly in the erythrocyte. Other amino acids—for example alanine—when moving from muscle back to the splanchnic tissues, may have a significant fraction of their bulk transfer taking place in the erythrocyte as well as in the plasma. These studies, which were first undertaken in the dog, are now clearly pertinent to the interpretation of metabolism of amino acids in man. The importance of this should not be overlooked. When evaluating nutritional procedures, particularly in the newborn, it is desirable to perform studies of whole blood as well as of plasma to elucidate the compartmentation of amino acids.

REGULATION

Although the events which control amino acid pool size in man are multifactorial, the source of the regulation is genetic. An example of the major influence of heredity is shown in Figure 5, in which there is seen extraordinary similarity in the plasma amino acid patterns of monozygotic twins but much less in dizygotic twins; the differences between non-twin persons are greater still.

Regulation is important, particularly as it pertains to the interface between carbohydrate and amino acid metabolism. The alanine cycle is a good example in this context. The significance of this cycle became apparent during studies of the interface between protein and carbohydrate metabolism in healthy individuals and in those with diabetes mellitus. It is believed that glucose delivered to muscle is metabolized to pyruvate, which can undergo transamination, then take up amino groups liberated by muscle metabolism. In this way alanine is re-formed, as summarized in Figure 6. The re-formed alanine fluxes back to the splanchnic circulation, partly in erythrocytes, partly in plasma. After uptake by the liver, ammonia is released and converted to urea. The original carbon chain is once again available for conversion to glucose. The so-called alanine cycle is thus an important mechanism for recycling carbon chains and for transporting ammonia from

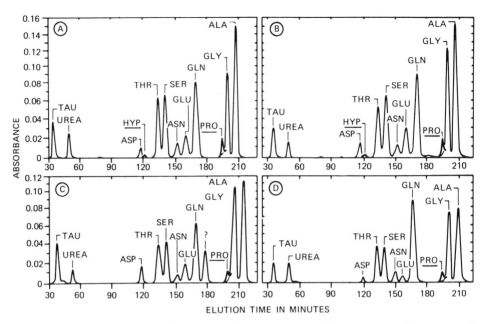

Figure 5. Comparison of serum free amino acid chromatograms of fasting 13-year-old monozygotic male twins (*A* and *B*) and 12-year-old dizygotic male twins (*C* and *D*). Both pairs were studied in identical fashion. (Data from reference 7).

peripheral to splanchnic tissues. An analogous cycle exists for glutamine (also illustrated in Figure 6). The latter is particularly important in the renal regulation of acid-base metabolism involving the synthesis and elimination of ammonium salts (*1*).

Additional significance is to be found in the alanine cycle, because alanine is the trigger for glucagon release in the same way that leucine is a trigger for insulin release. Glucagon is an important determinant of uptake by splanchnic tissues of gluconeogenic amino acids. During their first day of life, when they are most vulnerable to hypoglycemia, infants have poor ability to extract proline (another gluconeogenic amino acid which is used predominantly in the kidney) and alanine from blood. This may explain in part the vulnerability of the newborn to hypoglycemia, as he is unable to use nonglucose carbon chains stored in muscle for efficient glucogenesis. It has been suggested that the deficient critical step in the first day of life may be the transamination reaction, which allows alanine to enter into gluconeogenesis. At three days of age, after a glucagon stimulus, the infant can extract alanine and proline from plasma much more efficiently. This response coincides with less vulnerability to the occurrence of hypoglycemia.

ONTOGENY, TRANSPORT, AND CATABOLISM

The alanine cycle is an example of ontogeny involving an interface between two types of metabolic pools, and I would like to discuss two phases of amino acid metabolism which exhibit striking ontogenic processes. The first is membrane transport, whereby an amino acid enters the cell across the plasma membrane. The second concerns an intracellular catabolic process.

THE "ALANINE CYCLE"

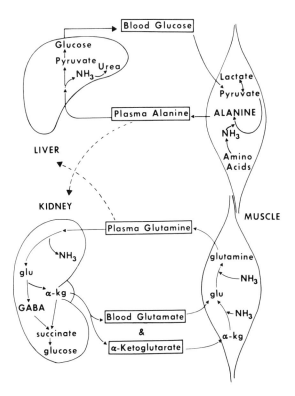

THE "GLUTAMINE CYCLE"

Figure 6. The so-called "α-alanine cycle" and "glutamine cycle," in which carbon chains and ammonia are shuttled back and forth between peripheral and central tissues. It should be noted that not all steps of either cycle have been demonstrated unequivocally, but current evidence suggests that alanine and glutamine move as shown.

With regard to transport ontogeny, classic observations have been reported by Brodehl and Gellissen's group in Germany (6). These workers have developed quantitative data for net tubular reabsorption of amino acids by the renal tubules. Their data are summarized in Figure 4. The newborn infant is less efficient in reclaiming amino acids across the tubular membrane than is the mature subject. Ontogeny of the transport process in the kidney is most clearly visible with respect to glycine, proline, some of the short-chain neutral amino acids, and histidine. Such knowledge is useful when examining urine, for example, in a mass-screening program in the newborn population. Normal ontogenic patterns should not be mistaken for disease patterns or misdiagnoses will result.

Absorptive functions for amino acids in the intestine also exhibit ontogeny. Nonetheless, protein amino acid absorption by the intestine differs from amino acid absorption by epithelium of the renal tubule, because the intestine is also exposed to large quantities of oligopeptides in addition to amino acids. It is now believed that about 80% of the amino acid load is absorbed as oligopeptides, rather than as free amino acids. This important observation tells us something about the heterogeneity of transport systems available to maintain adequate protein nutrition. It can be used to investigate how and where mutant genes affect absorptive functions which influence amino acid nutrition. Hartnup disease is an autosomal recessive condition affecting the transport function alone. The trait serves as a probe of absorption to inform us about the disposition of transport sites on the surfaces of enterocyte membranes.

There are four membrane surfaces to consider in absorptive epithelium. These are the surfaces of the luminal membrane (the brush border) and of the antiluminal membrane, each of which possesses an outer and an inner surface. An entire group of free neutral amino acids is not well absorbed in the Hartnup phenotype. On the other hand, oligo-peptides comprised of the relevant free amino acids are absorbed normally. This has been confirmed in vivo and in vitro and it implies that a separate type of transport system exists for oligopeptides. Peptidases inside the enterocyte cleave peptides into their con-stituent amino acids. Since the plasma amino acid response is normal after peptide loading in Hartnup disease, one can deduce that Hartnup disease is not a defect of efflux out of the cell at the basilar surface. One must then assume that the defect resides in the luminal membrane to affect uptake on the luminal (outer) surface of that membrane and that the defect is specific for free amino acids. Considerable specificity of absorbing sites in intestinal cells is implied.

When Christensen and Jones (8) studied uptake of an inert amino acid by rat intestine they found that the steady-state distribution between lumen and blood—that is to say, the concentration of the amino acid in the lumen relative to the blood—is the same, whether it is infused into a vein or ingested as a nutrient by mouth. Therefore, it can be assumed that amino acids at higher concentration than normal in the blood will eventually equilibrate with the intestinal lumen. Bacteria of the lower gastrointestinal tract will then produce amino acid by-products which, in turn, will be absorbed. This observation is of importance with regard to intravenous hyperalimentation. If plasma concentrations of amino acids rise out of control, there will be equilibration with the gut and undesirable metabolites may then be formed.

Ontogeny also affects catabolic processes. One of the most interesting pathways to consider is the GABA shunt (Figure 7). Gamma-aminobutyric acid is an important presynaptic inhibitory substance in brain. It is also found at high concentrations in kidney cortex. We believe that the pathway in kidney serves for disposal of the carbon chain of glutamate without the formation of a titratable dicarboxylic acid. Man's kidneys extract glutamine from the blood as a source of ammonia for maintenance of acid-base homeostasis. Thus there is a net load of glutamate for disposal in kidney after ammonia-genesis. The first enzyme that commits glutamate to the GABA shunt is glutamic acid decarboxylase. We have studied this enzyme in human kidney cortex and noted that there is an increase in its specific activity toward the end of gestation. We presume that this phenomenon permits the full-term infant to adapt more readily to the extrauterine environment and to control acid-base metabolism more readily.

Reduced specific activity can be said to characterize some phase of transadaptation in the newborn period. Alternatively, the persistence of a small but significant residual activity may make a great difference to the adaptation of the probands with a mutant enzyme regulating amino acid metabolism. Most inborn errors of metabolism are char-acterized by an almost, but not total, absence of enzyme activity. A good example is maple-syrup urine disease, in which the decarboxylation step in oxidation of the branch-chain amino acids is affected. In the "classical" form of this disease, residual activity of the α-ketoacid carboxylase (EC 4.1.1.1) is less than 2% of the normal. Probands require stringent treatment, and the disease is life threatening in the absence of early diagnosis

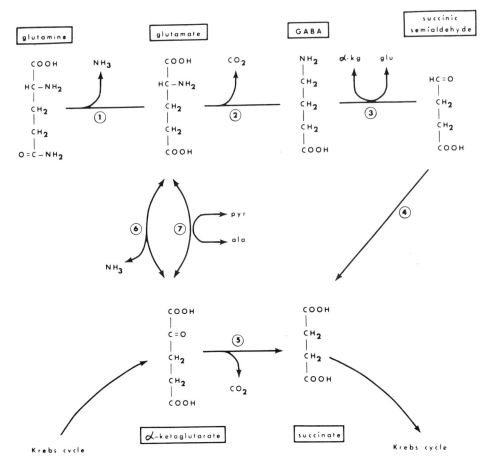

Figure 7. The GABA pathway in mammalian brain and kidney cortex, indicating the relationships of GABA to glutamate, α-ketoglutarate, and succinate metabolism.

and treatment. On the other hand, patients with a variant of maple-syrup urine disease with more than 2% of the normal enzyme activity can often tolerate a less-stringent treatment and can sometimes function well even on normal diets. Indeed, it was during the study of patients with maple-syrup urine disease that we found the need for new methods of clinical chemistry to enable us to learn more about this disease. As a result, an oximation technique was developed to measure the 2-keto branch-chain acids (9). We were then able to show that the concentration of the "toxic" keto acid in blood does not change very much relative to the concentration of amino acids in the serum when its concentration is less than 1 mmol/litre. Presumably this occurs because the keto acid is being re-aminated to the amino acid. Symptoms of maple-syrup urine disease develop only when the concentration of the keto acid rises abruptly when reamination appears to be saturated. This occurs under circumstances in which the concentration of the relevant amino acid in blood increases to greater than 1 mmol/litre. The lesson we learned is that the physician can adopt a much more relaxed attitude to the monitoring and treatment of maple-syrup urine disease because the concentration of keto acids changes very little over the amino acid range between normal and 1 mmol/litre.

SUMMARY

Application of the modern technology of clinical chemistry has made a profound difference in the management of some of the patients under our care, and advances in clinical chemistry have revealed many new facets of amino acid metabolism. It is under the control of a multifactorial spectrum of regulatory events, each of which has its own genetic component. There is a discontinuous variation, which can be detected as inborn errors of metabolism and of transport. The discontinuous variations highlight the individual steps in the various functions. The newborn exemplifies transitional disadaptation in many phases of metabolism and transport.

ACKNOWLEDGMENT

I am very grateful to the Editor for preparing this transcript of the talk given at the Conference on Clinical Biochemistry of the Neonate, Dec. 5–7, 1974. Washington, D.C.

REFERENCES

1. Scriver, C. R. and Rosenberg, L. E., *Amino Acid Metabolism and Its Disorders*. W. B. Saunders Co., Philadelphia, Pa., 1973.
2. Daum, R. S., Lamm, P. H., Mamer, O. A., and Scriver, C. R., A "new" disorder of isoleucine catabolism, *Lancet* ii, 1289 (1971).
3. Guthrie, R. and Susi, A., A simple phenylalanine method for detecting phenylketonuria in large populations of infants, *Pediatrics* 32, 338 (1963).
4. Elwyn, D. H., Launder, W. J., Parikh, H. C., and Wise, E. M., Jr., Roles of plasma and erythrocytes in interorgan transport of amino acids in dogs, *Amer. J. Physiol.* 222, 1333 (1972).
5. Van Slyke, D. D. and Meyer, G. M., The absorption of amino acids from the blood by the tissues, *J. Biol. Chem.* 16, 197 (1913).
6. Brodehl, J. and Gellissen, K., Endogenous renal transport of free amino acids in infancy and childhood, *Pediatrics* 42, 395 (1968).
7. Nance, W. E. and Nance, C., personal communication to the author, 1971.
8. Christensen, H. N. and Jones, J. C., Amino acid transport models. Renal resorption and resistance to metabolic attack, *J. Biol. Chem.* 237, 1203 (1962).
9. Lancaster, G., Mamer, O. A. and Scriver, C. R., Branched-chain alpha-ketoacids isolated as oxime derivatives: Relationship to the corresponding hydroxy acids and amino acids in maple-syrup urine disease. *Metabolism* 23, 257 (1974).

Failure to Thrive and Problems of Growth

ALLEN W. ROOT, M.D.

The infant with growth retardation is of significant concern to the family and to the physician. This presentation will include discussion of factors that influence prenatal and postnatal growth and will offer a broad perspective of neonatal failure to thrive and of retardation of growth. It will concern itself with the clinical approach to evaluation and management of such infants.

INTRAUTERINE GROWTH RETARDATION

Intrauterine growth depends on maternal, placental, and fetal factors (Table 1) (1–4). Important maternal factors that influence intrauterine growth include:

1. The socioeconomic status of the mother—the incidence of low-birth-weight infants is highest in mothers from lower socioeconomic levels because of suboptimal maternal nutrition and, perhaps, because of more frequent intercurrent maternal illness.

2. The general health of the mother—compromise of the maternal cardiovascular system owing to congenital or acquired heart disease or hypertension, poorly controlled diabetes mellitus, ulcerative colitis, and toxemia of pregnancy may impair fetal growth.

3. Maternal drug exposure—infants born of mothers addicted to narcotics or alcohol are often small for gestational age.

Malformation, infarction, or separation of the placenta from the uterine wall may impair fetal nutrition and prevent normal fetal growth. In addition to the role of the placenta in the transport of oxygen and other nutrients from the mother, it also produces a number of hormones such as choriogonadotropin (human chorionic gonadotropin), human chorionic thyrotropin, and choriomammotropin (human chorionic somatomammotropin) which are important for maintenance of pregnancy and normal fetal growth.

Choriomammotropin is a 191 amino acid polypeptide with 96% homology with somatotropin (human growth hormone). It has weak somatotropin-like biological activity but potent mammotropic and lactogenic bioactivities. It increases nitrogen retention, im-

Table 1. Causes of Intrauterine Growth Retardation

I. Maternal factors
    A. Vascular compromise
        1. Acute toxemia
        2. Hypertension
        3. Chronic renal disease
        4. Cardiac insufficiency
        5. Diabetes mellitus
        6. Ulcerative colitis
    B. Drugs
        1. Narcotics
        2. Alcohol
        3. Tobacco
    C. Malnutrition
    D. Hypoxia
        1. Altitude
        2. Sicklemia

II. Placental factors
    A. Chronic lesions
        1. Abnormal insertions of cord
        1. Hemangioma
        3. Parabiotic twinning
        4. Fibrinosis and infarctions
    B. Acute lesions
        1. Abruptio placentae
        2. Rupture of fetal vessels
        3. "Ascending chorioamnionitis"

III. Fetal factors
    A. Genetic
    B. Chromosomal
        1. Trisomic syndrome: 15,18,21
        2. Autosomal deletions: 5, 18, 21
        3. Sex chromosomes: XO, XXXXY
        4. Chromosomal breakage: Fanconi's anemia, Bloom's syndrome
    C. Infections
        1. Rubella
        2. Cytomegalic inclusion disease
    D. Twinning
    E. Congenital anomalies
        1. Single umbilical artery
        2. Dysmorphic syndromes
    F. Teratogenic agents
    G. Endocrinological causes
        1. Hypothyroidism
        2. End-organ insensitivity to somatotropin

pairs glucose tolerance, stimulates insulin release, and mobilizes free fatty acids. It may be detected in the serum of the mother by 3 to 5 weeks of gestation, increases progressively to maximum concentrations of 5.4 mg/litre at 36 weeks, and declines after the placenta is expelled (5,6). During starvation of the pregnant mother and in multiple-birth pregnancies, its concentration in plasma increases still further. Its production rate normally approaches 1 g/day, and its turnover is faster than that of any other polypeptide hormone. Determination of its concentration in the mother's blood has provided an index of placental function and of fetal distress associated with placental insufficiency. Fetal distress or abortion may be anticipated if serum values for choriomammotropin in the mother's plasma decline in the first trimester, or do not increase after 20 weeks of gestation, or are less than half the normal value after 30 weeks of gestation. In 40% of infants with intrauterine growth retardation, maternal choriomammotropin concentrations may be decreased in the mother's plasma and in the placenta (1). It is thought to provide for the "nutritional demands of the fetus" by exerting tonic metabolic effects on the mother. It may be the "growth hormone" of pregnancy, ensuring for the fetus a steady fuel supply, particularly of glucose.

Factors that influence intrauterine growth of the fetus include its genetic constitution and hormonal status, the occurrence of intrauterine infections or exposure to teratogenic agents, and the presence of more than one fetus. Intrauterine growth is impaired in fetuses with chromosomal abnormalities, particularly trisomies 13 and 18, and in association with certain sex-chromosome anomalies such as XO and XXXXY. Intrauterine growth retardation may also be associated with abnormalities of chromosome morphology, as in Fanconi's syndrome of pancytopenia and absent radius and in Bloom's syndrome of multiple telangiectases, mental retardation, broad thumbs and toes. Primordial dwarfism—i.e., growth retardation apparently due to innate "programming" of decreased rates of cell division and growth—may be observed in infants with a number of eponymic syndromes including Seckel's, Russell's, Silver's, and de Lange's. Intrauterine infections with the rubella or cytomegalic-inclusion-disease viruses result in retarded fetal and postnatal growth. Intrauterine exposure to various noxious toxins—particularly narcotics, aminopterin, and alcohol—may impair fetal growth.

Somatotropin. The role of this hormone in normal fetal growth is uncertain, because both anencephalic and hypopituitary neonates may be of normal size at birth. Somatotropin may be detected in the fetal pituitary as early as the seventh week of gestation, and its pituitary content increases progressively through the first 30 weeks of gestation (7). Its concentration in the pituitary increases between 10 to 14 and 25 to 29 weeks of pregnancy, then remains constant through the first year of postnatal life. Its concentration in fetal serum increases to peak values (119 μg/litre) at 20 to 24 weeks and then declines to term, with a mean concentration in umbilical venous blood of 33.5 μg/litre. Grumbach (7) postulates that there is sequential intrauterine development of hypothalamic control of somatotropin secretion. In early gestation, the increase in its concentrations in pituitary and serum may be independent of hypothalamic control. By midgestation, the peak concentrations of somatotropin in serum may reflect tonic stimulation by somatotropin-releasing factor while the decline in its values in late pregnancy may reflect the inhibiting activity of somatostatin.

Thyroid hormone. The absence of thyroid hormone in the fetus is associated with impaired fetal growth, and the neonate with profound hypothyroidism is often small and underweight at birth (6). The fetal pituitary-thyroid axis functions independently of the mother; there is insignificant placental transfer of either thyroxine or triiodothyronine from mother to fetus or fetus to mother (8). The fetal thyroid is histologically recognizable by the seventh week of pregnancy. Iodine is accumulated and thyroid hormone synthesized by the fetal thyroid by 10 to 12 weeks. Thyrotropin is detectable in fetal serum by 9 to 10 weeks of gestation. Concentrations of thyroxine and thyrotropin remain low until 18 to 20 weeks, then abruptly increase in serum, as does pituitary thyrotropin content; these all remain high until term. Serum triiodothyronine concentrations are low in the fetus. In the immediate postpartum period, serum thyrotropin values increase rapidly, peaking at 1 h, then declining by 48 h to adult values. Concentrations of protein-bound iodine, thyroxine, and triiodothyronine increase more slowly and peak at 24 h, slowly declining thereafter. The postpartum thyrotropin increase probably reflects a response to environmental cooling, because it may be aborted by maintaining the neonate in a warm environment.

Low-birth-weight infants—those with birth weights less than 2500 g—are of two sorts:

1. Infants born of shortened gestations whose weights are appropriate for the length of gestation—truly premature infants.
2. Infants whose weights are below those expected for infants of the stated gestational age. These neonates have sustained intrauterine growth-retarding insults, such as those discussed and are termed "small-for-gestational-age" infants (1).

The infant with intrauterine growth retardation frequently fails to "catch up" to his peer group in length, weight, or intellectual development, whereas the premature infant, depending upon the degree of prematurity, often achieves the somatic and intellectual growth of his peers. The caloric expenditure or basal metabolic rate of such infants is low in relation to chronological or height ages but normal or slightly increased when expressed per unit of body weight (9). The basal metabolic rate of infants with intrauterine growth retardation is significantly less than that of infants with postnatal onset of growth failure, in whom the basal metabolic rate is appropriate for size and greatly increased per unit of body weight. The decreased caloric expenditure of small-for-gestational-age infants probably reflects decreased rates of cell division and growth, while the normal or increased basal metabolic rate of infants with postnatal onset of growth failure indicates the reversibility of this process. The lower basal metabolic rate of small-for-gestational-age infants usually does not reflect decreased thyroid function.

In the evaluation of the infant who is small for his gestational age, thorough historical review and careful physical examination often (but not invariably) reveal the responsible factor(s). It is important to note the health and age of the mother at conception (many of the trisomic syndromes occur in older mothers), any maternal illnesses, and exposure to drugs and infectious disease during gestation. The placenta should be examined carefully in each instance. The physical findings—particularly skeletal, cranial, cardiac, or genital anomalies—should be noted. A complex of physical findings may suggest a particular syndrome (10). The presence of jaundice, petechiae, and visceromegaly suggests intrauterine infection by rubella or cytomegalic-inclusion-disease viruses. Laboratory studies that may be required include chromosome karyotyping, viral cultures, and amino acid determinations in serum and urine.

POSTNATAL GROWTH FAILURE

Postnatal growth depends on genetic, hormonal, and nutritional factors. Adult stature primarily reflects the patient's genetically endowed growth potential as modified by the hormonal, nutritional, and disease environment in which the child has existed. Thyroid and growth hormones, among others, are essential for normal postnatal growth.

The infant with "failure to thrive" is one who fails to maintain patterns of weight gain and linear growth rate appropriate for his gestational and postnatal ages. When assessing an infant's growth pattern, it is important to consider the influence of both prenatal and postnatal factors upon that individual's growth performance. Thus a premature infant may be significantly below the mean normal values for height and weight at one point in the postnatal period and yet have exhibited significant increments in height and weight since birth. The postnatal onset of growth failure may reflect structural or functional abnormalities or suboptimal caloric intake. Major causes of failure to thrive are listed in Table 2.

Malnutrition. By far the most common cause of postnatal growth failure in the infant with appropriate natal weight for gestational age is malnutrition; the infant is ingesting less food than the 540 to 630 kJ·kg^{-1} per day (130–150 Cal/kg/day) required for normal growth. Reasons for failure of the infant to receive adequate calories may be complex. Occasionally, caloric deprivation is due to socioeconomic privation, including a lack of foodstuffs. When this occurs in the non-breast-fed infant, marasmus results in less than 5 to 6 months. Infantile malnutrition occurs with dismaying frequency, even in our country, and among a broad spectrum of socioeconomic levels. However, in these instances malnutrition is usually the consequence of disturbed feeding practices. Maternal youth and inexperience may be the basis of this disturbance; if an older, more stable, mature, and experienced figure is not present in the environment, the infant may not be offered adequate calories. At the other extreme, an infant may be the youngest born of a mother with a large family, who is so busy that she lacks time to feed the newborn properly, particularly if the frequency of births burdens her with several active youngsters, all requiring supervision.

Frequently, however, the infant who fails to thrive is the second- or third-born child of a family in which older siblings are growing normally. For ill-defined reasons, the mother-infant relationship is disturbed—perhaps because the pregnancy was unplanned and the child unwanted, perhaps because of parental friction, or for some other such reason. Feeding times are periods of unrecognized combat and discontent and although the infant may be offered adequate food, the food is rejected. In this situation the mother may not recognize that the child is not ingesting adequate calories. When questioned, she recites the quantity of food offered to the infant, which she mistakenly assumes the infant has ingested. This sequence of events has been termed the "maternal deprivation syndrome" and is almost always due to decreased caloric intake by the infant.

There are many endocrinological consequences of malnutrition in infancy. Serum somatotropin values may be unduly high and not suppressible by hyperglycemia, although in prolonged states of malnutrition somatotropin concentrations may fall spontaneously. Concentrations in serum and production rates of adrenal glucocorticoids may be abnormally high, while thyroid hormone concentrations may be depressed or normal.

Table 2.   Causes of Failure to Thrive[a]

Inadequate caloric intake

A. Maternal deprivation
   1. Caloric restriction
   2. Child abuse

B. Psychosocial dwarfism
   1. Caloric restriction
   2. Emotional disorders

C. Congenital abnormalities
   1. Cleft lip or palate
   2. Tracheoesophageal fistula, esophageal webs
   3. Glossoptosis, macroglossia
   4. Chalasia, achalasia

D. Acquired abnormalities
   1. Esophageal stricture
   2. Central neural insult—subdural hematoma, hypoxia, diencephalic syndrome
   3. Diabetes insipidus
      a. Central
      b. Nephrogenic

Decreased intestinal function

A. Abnormalities of digestion
   1. Cystic fibrosis
   2. Trypsin deficiency
   3. Mono- and disaccharidase deficiencies

B. Abnormalities of absorption
   1. Celiac syndrome
   2. Gastroenteritis
   3. Biliary atresia
   4. Megacolon
   5. Giardiasis
   6. Protein-losing enteropathy

Increased utilization of calories

A. Infant of narcotic-addicted mother

B. Congenital hyperthyroidism

C. Excessive crying

D. Prolonged fever
   1. Chronic infections

E. Congenital heart disease

F. Central neural insult with spasticity

(Continued)

162

Table 2. (*Continued*)

Increased renal excretion of calories

A. Aminoaciduria

Miscellaneous

A. Chronic renal disease
   1. Renal tubular acidosis
     a. deToni–Fanconi–Debré syndrome
     b. Idiopathic
   2. Pyelonephritis
   3. Polycystic disease
   4. Congenital/acquired nephritis
   5. Congenital nephrosis
   6. Nephrogenic diabetes insipidus

B. Hypercalcemia
   1. Subcutaneous fat necrosis
   2. Hyperparathyroidism
     a. Primary, familial
     b. Secondary to maternal hypoparathyroidism
   3. Vitamin A or D intoxication
   4. Idiopathic

C. Anemia
   1. Fetal-maternal transfusion
   2. Hemoglobinopathies
   3. Iron deficiency

D. Endocrinopathy
   1. Hypothyroidism
   2. Hyposomatotropism
   3. Hypoadrenalism
     a. Congenital adrenal hyperplasia, salt losing form
     b. Congenital adrenal hypoplasia
     c. Bartter's syndrome

E. Metabolic disease
   1. Glycogen storage disease
   2. Galactosemia
   3. Hypophosphatasia
   4. Mucopolysaccharidosis
   5. Rickets
     a. Vitamin D deficient, dependent, resistant
   6. Lipidopathies

F. Central nervous system insult
   1. Subdural hematoma
   2. Intracerebral hemorrhage
   3. Tumors

[a] Adapted from Green and Richmond (*12*) and Barness (*13*).

All of these aberrations are reversible by feeding. In the syndrome of psychosocial deprivation—usually observed in children over two years of age—there may be functional hypopituitarism, with decreased secretion of somatotropin and corticotropin (adrenocorticotropic hormone). For the most part, these abnormalities reflect the long-standing consequences of malnutrition, perhaps in association with psychogenic phenomena (*11*).

Organic causes of growth failure account for only a small percentage of infants evaluated for failure to thrive. These diseases may be accompanied by decreased caloric intake, decreased intestinal absorption of foodstuffs, impaired utilization of absorbed calories, increased calorie expenditure, or abnormal excretion of nutrients. Acquired or congenital abnormalities of gastrointestinal function, diseases of the central nervous, cardiorespiratory, genitourinary, or endocrine systems, chronic infections, or drug exposure may impair postnatal growth. Growth failure was attributed to suboptimal nutrition resulting from improper feeding techniques in 87% of 200 normal-birth-weight infants and children evaluated for failure to thrive (Table 3) (*13*); the diagnoses of cystic fibrosis, hypothyroidism, or subdural hematomata were established in 8%, and in 3% no diagnosis was established.

Table 3. Causes of Failure to Thrive in a Hospital Population (*13*)

	No.	Percent
Suboptimal nutrition	174	87
Other causes		
Cystic fibrosis	6	3
Hypothyroid	5	2.5
Subdural hematoma	5	2.5
Glycogen storage disease	1	0.5
Celiac syndrome	1	0.5
Methylmalonic acidemia	1	0.5
Maple-syrup urine disease	1	0.5
Unknown	6	3
Total	200	100

Evaluation of the infant with failure to thrive is initiated by historical review of conception, gestation, labor, delivery, the early postnatal course, intercurrent illnesses, and the medical history of family members. A dietary history should be obtained, although it may well be inaccurate. Historical survey may suggest the diagnoses of feeding problems, gastrointestinal disease, genetic or familial causes for growth retardation, acute or chronic systemic diseases, or poisonings. Physical examination will disclose the child with anomalies such as congenital heart disease, dysmorphic syndromes (*10*), visceromegaly, microcephaly, macrocephaly, retinal abnormalities, genital malformations, neurological disability, etc. The typical infant who fails to thrive will be long and thin. The child's pattern of linear growth usually falls between the third and tenth percentiles, while his weight is usually below the third percentile. Thus the child presents the characteristics of nutritional deprivation—that is, he is even underweight for his height (Table 4).

Table 4. Evaluation of the Infant with Failure to Thrive

History

A. Conception—drugs, x-rays, infections
B. Gestation—drugs, infections, intercurrent illnesses (toxemia)
C. Labor and delivery—analgesia, anesthesia, fetal distress, duration and position
D. Postnatal—respiratory pattern, feeding, activity
E. Dietary
F. Systemic review
G. Family

Physical Examination

A. Measurements—length, weight, span, lower limb, head circumference
B. Somatic—congenital anomalies (neutral, skeletal, cardiac)
C. Dysmorphic syndromes—Down's, trisomy 18

Laboratory data

A. Preliminary
   Hemogram
   Urinalysis
   Bone age
   Stool for fat, occult blood, ova and parasites, pH
   Serum sodium, potassium, chloride, CO_2, creatinine, calcium

B. Intensive
   Skull roentgenogram
   Sweat chloride, sodium
   Somatotropin and thyroxine measurements
   Amino acids, serum or urine
   Electroencephalogram, brain scan, pneumoencephalogram
   Barium enema, rectal biopsy

Initially, only few laboratory tests are necessary in evaluating these infants, unless the history or physical examination suggests a specific line of inquiry. The following studies are obtained routinely:

1. Blood count—for anemia, hemoglobinopathy.
2. Urinalysis—obtained by "clean catch," for determination of pH, specific gravity, reducing substances, cellular contents, and ferric chloride reaction. Urine culture and colony count should be obtained as indicated.
3. Stool examination—for occult blood, ova and parasites, reducing substances, pH.
4. Bone age—to determine physiologic maturity and as a survey of skeletal structure.
5. Serum or plasma sodium, potassium, chloride, bicarbonate, creatinine, and calcium concentrations.
6. Tuberculin test, when appropriate.

If the reason for failure of growth should remain hidden, more intensive laboratory studies may be indicated, including:

1. Skull roentgenogram, to detect intracranial calcification and abnormalities of suture closure.

2. Sweat test, for determination of chloride and sodium concentrations.

3. Quantitative fat balance.

4. Duodenal enzyme determination.

5. Measurement of serum thyroxine and somatotropin concentrations, and other hormones as the clinical situation dictates.

6. Serum and/or urine amino acid measurements.

7. Electroencephalogram, brain scan, ventriculogram.

If, after the history and physical examination have been completed and the preliminary laboratory data reviewed, no abnormality has been defined, the infant should be permitted a period of nutritional rehabilitation before further laboratory studies are undertaken. Whitten et al. (14) have demonstrated that the syndrome of maternal deprivation is usually one of caloric starvation and that these infants will gain weight if adequate calories are available independently of the degree of attendant "mothering." Whitten and his colleagues studied several infants with failure to thrive who were provided adequate diets but were maintained in a quiet, nonstimulating environment; they gained weight rapidly. When returned to a busy ward and to a concerned nurse, their rates of weight gain did not increase further. It is usually necessary to provide a caloric intake of approximately 630 kJ/kg body weight (150 cal/kg) for optimal growth and, therefore, it is important to measure the infant's caloric intake. If a conscientious trial in which adequate calories are ingested is not followed by increase in weight, then additional investigation into other causes of growth retardation is mandatory as indicated above.

Figure 1 shows the chronicity of this problem and its natural history. This infant was first admitted to hospital at five weeks of age with a history of vomiting and diarrhea for several days. The admission weight of 3097 g was the same as the birth weight. She did not appear dehydrated, and during a five-day hospitalization she had no symptoms.

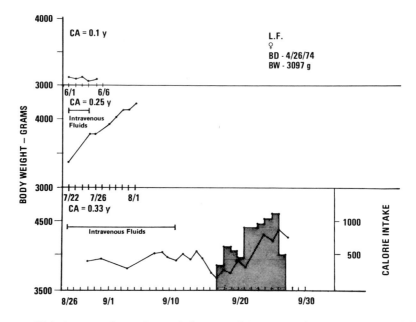

Figure 1. Clinical course of an infant with failure to thrive. *CA* is chronological age, *BD* is birth date, and *BW* is birth weight. One Calorie (kcal) is approximately 4.2 kJ.

Although she did not gain weight in this period, she was discharged to the care of the mother and father. When next seen, at three months of age, her weight had increased by only 300 g; she was admitted again, with a history of vomiting and diarrhea and with mild dehydration. In hospital, no symptoms were observed and the child gained weight rapidly, initially with intravenous hydration and then with oral feedings. At this time it became apparent that there was significant parental discord. Nevertheless, the infant was discharged to the parents' care. She was readmitted four weeks later, again with a history of vomiting and diarrhea, which did not occur in hospital. She was lethargic, dehydrated, apathetic, and ate poorly; intravenous fluids were required to maintain hydration. Spontaneous caloric intake was but 1600 kJ/24 h (380 Cal/day) or 420 kJ/kg body weight (100 Cal/kg). When a concerted effort to increase caloric intake was successful and the child ingested 3350–3770 kJ/24 h (800–900 Cal/day) or 1050 kJ/kg body weight (250 Cal/kg) her weight increased. This child had probably not received adequate calories since birth. As she aged, it became more difficult to ensure an adequate caloric supply by spontaneous oral intake alone, because she became indifferent to her surroundings. The child's course illustrates the need for persistence and calorie quantitation before assuming that failure to thrive is not due to caloric deprivation alone.

The consequences of severe malnutrition in the early neonatal period are not known with certainty. Winick (15) has demonstrated in experimental animals that starvation during critical prepartum and postpartum periods may permanently impair the rate of cell division and reduce cell number and cell size in a number of tissues, including the brain. It has been suggested that this may also occur in humans and thus be associated with impaired intellectual development. At autopsy, infants younger than six months who had succumbed to marasmus showed reduced brain-cell number and myelin content; survivors of marasmus may demonstrate retarded physical, motor, and mental development through five years of life despite adequate postmarasmus nutrition (16). However, other investigators suggest that most children subjected to nutritional deprivation in early life can be salvaged and normal growth and development restored if the normal food requirements are met and the infant is provided an adequate stimulating environment (17).

SUMMARY

Neonatal growth failure may be due to congenital or acquired abnormalities. In utero growth retardation followed by postnatal retardation of growth occurs in infants with congenital infections (rubella, cytomegalic inclusion disease, toxoplasmosis), chromosomal anomalies (trisomies D, E), chondrodystrophies and metabolic bone diseases (osteogenesis imperfecta), placental insufficiency secondary to toxemia of pregnancy or nutritional deprivation of the mother, maternal exposure to narcotics, endocrinopathies (hypothyroidism), and other insults. Postnatal growth retardation may reflect an in utero insult, but in the full-term neonate of normal size at birth, growth failure most commonly is associated with nutritional deprivation resulting from a disordered mother-child relationship. Maternal youth or inexperience, family friction, the birth order of the infant in an overly large family, or an undetected cause may lead to disorganized feeding practices and behavior and suboptimal caloric intake of the infant. In severe instances marasmus may occur, but in most such infants progressive linear growth rate with decreased weight gain is observed. Disorders of the central nervous, cardiorespiratory, gastrointestinal, genitourinary, endocrine, metabolic, and (or) musculoskeletal systems may also account for postnatal growth retardation. After careful historical review, physical examination, and appropriate laboratory studies, the infant with "failure to thrive" should be permitted a period of alimentary rehabilitation before extensive laboratory investigations are undertaken.

ACKNOWLEDGMENT

The dedicated assistance of Mrs. Eileen Morris in the preparation of this manuscript is gratefully acknowledged. This work was supported by Grant HD 08313 from the NIH, and by the National Foundation.

REFERENCES

1. Andrews, B. F., (Ed.), The small-for-dates infant, *Pediatr. Clin. North Am.* **17**, 1 (1970).

2. Cassady, G., Body composition in intrauterine growth retardation, *Pediatr. Clin. North Am.* **17**, 79 (1970).

3. Shanklin, D. R., The influence of placental lesions on the newborn infant, *Pediatr. Clin. North Am.* **17**, 25 (1970).

4. Reisman, L. E., Chromosome abnormalities and intrauterine growth retardation, *Pediatr. Clin. North Am.* **17**, 10 (1970).

5. Kaplan, S. L., Human chorionic somatomammotropin: Secretion, biologic effects, and physiologic significance. In *Third Ross Conference on Obstetric Research*, Ross Laboratories, Columbus, Ohio (1974), pp 75–80.

6. MacMillan, D. R., Endocrine influences on fetal growth, *Pediatr. Clin. North Am.* **17**, 111 (1970).

7. Grumbach, M. M., Growth hormone and prolactin secretion in the human fetus. In *Third Ross Conference on Obstetric Research*, Ross Laboratories, Columbus, Ohio (1974), pp 68–74.

8. Fisher, D. A., Development and function of the pituitary-thyroid system. In *Third Ross Conference on Obstetric Research*, Ross Laboratories, Columbus, Ohio (1974), pp 9–12.

9. Krieger, I. and Woolley, P. V., Jr., The basal metabolic rate in growth failure of prenatal onset. Comparison with growth failure of postnatal onset, *Am. J. Dis. Child.* **127**, 340 (1974).

10. Smith, D. W., *Recognizable Patterns of Human Malformation*. W. B. Saunders Co., Philadelphia, Pa., 1970, pp. 1–368.

11. Krieger, I., Endocrine and nutrition in psychosocial deprivation in the USA: Comparison with growth failure due to malnutrition on an organic basis. In *Endocrine Aspects of Malnutrition*, L. I. Gardner, and P. Amacher, Eds., Kroc Foundation, Santa Ynez, Calif. (1973), pp. 129–145.

12. Green M. and Richmond, J. B., *Pediatric Diagnosis*, 2nd ed., W. B. Saunders, Philadelphia, Pa., 1962, pp 230–235.

13. Barness, L. A., Failure to thrive, *Dallas Med. J.* **58**, 325 (1972).

14. Whitten, C. F., Pettit, M. G., and Fischoff, J., Evidence that growth failure from maternal deprivation is secondary to undereating, *J. Am. Med. Assoc.* **209**, 1675 (1969).

15. Winick, M., Cellular growth during early malnutrition, *Pediatrics* **47**, 969 (1971).

16. Winick, M. and Coombs, J., Nutrition, environment and behavioral development, *Annu. Rev. Med.* **23**, 149 (1972).

17. Cheek, D. B., Protein calorie malnutrition and intellectual competence, *Med. J. Aust.* **1**, 1119 (1973). Letter.

Medical Problems
of the Newborn

The Genetic Mucopolysaccharidoses: Clinical and Chemical Correlates in Diagnosis

IRWIN A. SCHAFER, M.D.

INTRODUCTION

Glycosaminoglycans (acid mucopolysaccharides) are a major and characteristic molecular species in connective tissues. These polymers are ubiquitous in the body and show tissue-specific patterns that may change during development and aging. Although information on their biological function remains scanty, considerable knowledge of their chemistry has arisen as a result of the study of a group of human diseases collectively termed the "genetic mucopolysaccharidoses." Recent discoveries, stemming principally from the laboratories of Elizabeth Neufeld and Albert Dorfman, have defined the enzymatic bases of specific clinical syndromes within this group. A major problem in applying this information to the prevention of these disorders is the lack of a reliable, simple screening test to detect disease in the newborn infant. Infants who later in life develop the distinctive clinical features that suggest this diagnosis to the physician appear normal at birth. It is a disturbing experience to find two or more affected children in a family simply because the disease was not identified early enough in the firstborn.

In this review, the biochemical principles underlying the genetic mucopolysaccharidoses will be related to the problems of diagnoses in the neonatal period.

BIOCHEMICAL INFORMATION

The Structure of Glycosaminoglycans

Glycosaminoglycans (GAGs) are linear polymers composed of carbohydrates linked by glycosidic bonds. In tissues, all of these compounds, with the possible exception of hyaluronic acid, are covalently linked to protein. Figure 1 depicts the structure of a tissue

171

PROTEOGLYCOSAMINOGLYCAN

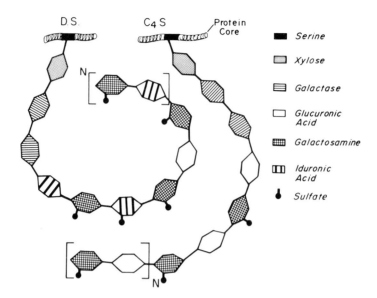

Figure 1. Schematic representation of the structure of proteoglycosaminoglycan.

proteoglycan. The linkage region differs from the remainder of the chain and consists of a serine, xylose, and two galactose residues. All sulfated GAGs—except keratan sulfate—are linked to a core protein through the hydroxyl group of serine (*1*). The remainder of the carbohydrate chain consists mainly of two saccharides, which alternate in a regular manner to form disaccharide repeating units. One component of this dimer is a hexosamine, the other either hexuronate or D-galactose.

D-Glucuronic acid, which is β-linked to an acetylated or sulfated (or both) hexosamine, is common to all GAGs except keratan sulfate. In hyaluronic acid, chondroitin-4-sulfate (chondroitin sulfate A), and chondroitin-6-sulfate (chondroitin sulfate C), glucuronic acid is the only uronic acid and is present in every disaccharide. In other GAGs, such as dermatan sulfate (chondroitin sulfate B) and heparan sulfate (heparitin sulfate), iduronic acid is the major component, but glucuronic acid may be substituted in the chain at irregular intervals (*2*). Galactose replaces uronic acid in the disaccharide unit of keratan sulfate (*3*). The hexosamine component of the disaccharide is either glucosamine or galactosamine and remains constant for a specific GAG. The amino group of the hexosamine is evidently never free; usually it is acetylated, or sulfated as in heparin and heparan sulfate (*4*). Sulfate esters are attached to the hexosamine at regularly spaced intervals in the chain and to some iduronic acid molecules (*5*).

All GAGs carry a large number of negative charges by virtue of their carboxylate and sulfate groups. In solution they behave as anionic polyelectrolytes (*6*).

This polyelectrolyte property is the basis both of the dye tests and of the turbidity tests used to screen for GAG in urine. Toluidine blue O, Alcian blue, and Azure A are cationic dyes that produce metachromatic staining when complexed with anionic polysaccharides, a saltlike compound of the dye and polysaccharide being formed. The dye cations, when concentrated on this matrix, polymerize, producing a shift in the spectrum of the dye and the metachromatic color (*7*).

The turbidity tests are also based on the polyanionic properties of the polymer. Cetyl-trimethylammonium bromide and cetylpyridinium chloride are cationic detergents containing a hydrocarbon chain with a fixed cationic group at one end. In water, they may associate to form micelles consisting of 20 to 100 cations. These complex with the anionic polysaccharides and precipitate them from solution. As might be expected, both metachromasia and precipitation with cationic detergents can be reversed or blocked by the addition of neutral salts. At acid pH, albumin becomes predominantly cationic in charge and will act like a counterion to precipitate GAG in connective tissue. This is the basis of the acid-albumin screening test (8).

Biosynthesis of GAGS

Information as to the intracellular sites where these polymers are synthesized is incomplete. As shown in Figure 2, at least seven membrane-bound enzymes add carbohydrate units in an ordered sequence to form the polymer. This multienzyme system may be arranged in a precise geometry, which is directed by specific binding sites for each enzyme on the membrane. The protein core of the polymer is synthesized first, then the trisaccharide is attached. The site of this series of reactions is thought to be the rough endoplasmic reticulum of the cell. The saccharide units are then added by specific transferases bound to the smooth endoplasmic reticulum. Sulfation may also occur in this region and in the Golgi apparatus (9).

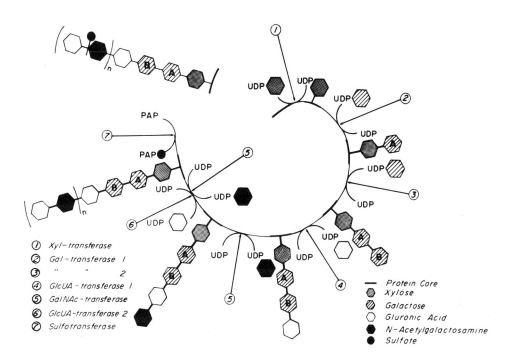

① *Xyl – transferase*
② *Gal – transferase   1*
③ *"   "   2*
④ *GlcUA – transferase 1*
⑤ *GalNAc – transferase*
⑥ *GlcUA – transferase 2*
⑦ *Sulfotransferase*

— *Protein Core*
⬡ *Xylose*
▨ *Galactose*
◯ *Gluronic Acid*
⬢ *N – Acetylgalactosamine*
● *Sulfate*

BIOSYNTHESIS OF CHONDROITIN - 4 - SO₄

Figure 2. Schematic representation of the biosynthesis of chondroitin-4-sulfate as presented in reference 9.

Human diseases attributable to defective biosynthesis of these polymers have not yet been identified. It is speculated that the etiology of certain congenital malformations may reflect aberrations of GAG biosynthesis during development.

Degradation of GAGs and the Genetic Mucopolysaccharidoses

These polymers are degraded primarily in the lysosomes of the cell by a series of hydrolytic enzymes that cleave specific linkages in the polymer chain. Questions still remain regarding the control and sequence of this process; for example, it is not clear whether proteolysis precedes or follows polysaccharide degradation. Complete degradation of a sulfated GAG results in the release of sulfate, which is excreted while the hexosamine and uronic acids are recycled through the glycolytic pathway and the hexose monophosphate shunt, respectively. If one of the enzymes in the sequence is defective, degradation is interrupted and fragments of the polymer accumulate, which may be released from the cell and excreted in the urine or retained intracellularly within lysosomes.

Such intracellular retention is progressive, producing cellular pathology that is soon reflected in clinical signs and symptoms. A block in the degradation of a specific GAG is the fundamental defect that the genetic mucopolysaccharidoses have in common (*10*).

THE CLINICAL DISEASE

The clinical effects of this process may be best illustrated by considering the most severe of the mucopolysaccharidoses, the Hurler syndrome, first reported in 1919 by the Austrian pediatrician, Gertrud Hurler. This is the prototype disease upon which the clinical classification of the mucopolysaccharidoses has been erected.

It has been clearly shown that the fetus affected with the Hurler syndrome stores dermatan sulfate and heparan sulfate in the liver, but at the time they are born these infants appear normal. During the first year, they begin to show the signs of mental and physical deterioration, which culminates in the full-blown Hurler dysmorphism. As illustrated by the patient in Figure 3, the facial features become coarsened, the tongue enlarges, the bridge of the nose is flattened, and the eyes bulge, producing the facies that characterizes all children with this disease. GAGs stored in various concentrations throughout the body produce the diffuse signs illustrated by the patient depicted in Figure 4, which include corneal clouding, impaired hearing, widespread skeletal involvement, hepatosplenomegaly, joint stiffness, cardiovascular anomalies, and mental retardation. The course of the disease is relentlessly progressive, and few such patients survive beyond the first decade.

There are at least six clinical syndromes that can be distinguished on the basis of their natural history, the clinical signs of the affected patient, and the pattern of GAG excreted in the urine. Table 1 summarizes a clinical classification of these disorders, which was adapted from McKusick (*11*). Extensive clinical descriptions of each entity are available in the reviews by Dorfman and Matalon (*12*) and in the monograph by McKusick (*11*). The clinical attribute that all of these entities share is that the affected child appears to be normal in the neonatal period. Diagnosis of the older child is not difficult if careful clinical appraisal is coupled with analytical data that identify the GAG that is being excreted in excess in urine. In children younger than two years, clinical diagnosis may prove difficult in certain syndromes. For example, Hurler's syndrome may be confused

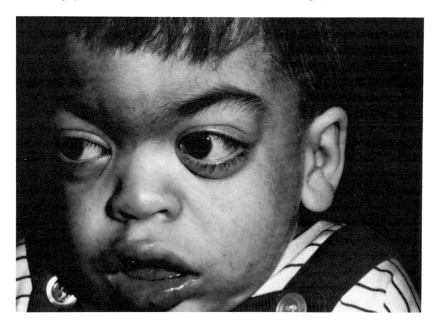

Figure 3.   Facial features of a patient with Hurler's syndrome.

with Scheie's syndrome, because the distinctive differences in these disorders depend on the assessment of intelligence and the natural history of the disease. Hunter's syndrome is distinguished from the Hurler syndrome in the older child by the absence of corneal clouding and the milder course of the disease. It should be pointed out that corneal infiltration of GAG in the Hurler patient may not be apparent on slit-lamp examination until well into the second year, and this may lead to confusion in diagnosis. Identification of the remaining syndromes is rather straightforward, in that each shows a distinctive pattern of GAG excretion in the urine.

ENZYMATIC CLASSIFICATION

Figure 5 summarizes the enzymatic defects that underlie the genetic mucopolysaccharidoses. Except for Morquio's syndrome and the chondroitin-4-sulfate mucopolysaccharidoses, the other entities are related to disturbances in the degradation of the α-linked GAGs, dermatan sulfate and heparan sulfate. The major degradative pathway for these polymers is by specific glycosidases and sulfatases that cleave the polymer from its nonreducing terminus, sequentially removing one sulfate and one sugar at a time.

Patients with the Hurler or Scheie syndromes show deficient α-L-iduronidase (EC 3.2.1.76) activity; therefore, degradation of the polymers stops when this sugar occupies the nonreducing terminus of the chain (13). As a result, heparan sulfate and dermatan sulfate accumulate in tissues and are excreted in the urine. The fact that the Hurler and Scheie patients show major clinical differences, yet have the same enzyme deficiency, has led to the speculation that the Hurler and Scheie mutations are not identical, but allelic. Patients have been described with the intermediate phenotype of the Hurler and Scheie syndromes. These individuals are presumed to represent genetic

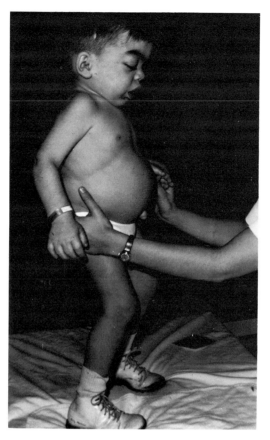

Figure 4. A patient with Hurler's syndrome who shows the characteristic skeletal deformities, growth arrest, contractures of joints, hernia, cloudy cornea and whose abdomen is distended because of enlargement of the liver and spleen.

compounds with one Hurler and one Scheie gene (*14*). Different allelic mutations may also account for the spectrum of clinical expression that has been described for the Hunter, Maroteaux-Lamy, and other clinical syndromes that comprise this group of diseases.

Some of the iduronic acid residues of dermatan sulfate and heparin are sulfated. It is presumed that heparan sulfate also contains this moiety. Before iduronic acid can be cleaved from the chain by α-L-iduronidase, this sulfate must be removed. Cultured fibroblasts and liver from patients with Hunter's syndrome have been shown to be deficient in this sulfaminidase (*15*). Degradation of both heparan sulfate and dermatan sulfate is blocked at this step, which accounts for the accumulation of these polymers in the tissues and also explains why patients with the recessively inherited Hurler's syndrome and the X-linked Hunter's syndrome excrete the same GAG in their urine.

Mutations at two different alleles have been demonstrated in the Sanfilippo syndrome. Some patients show a deficiency of α-N-acetylglucosaminidase (EC 3.2.1.50) activity (*16*); others are deficient in a specific sulfatase that cleaves the N-sulfate from glucosamine (*17*). Either mutation produces a block in the degradation of heparan sulfate. Patients with different enzyme deficiencies are phenotypically indistinguishable.

Table 1.   Clinical Classification

	Phenotype	Excess GAG in urine	Genetics
Hurler syndrome MPS IH	Mental retardation, early death, cloudy cornea, severe somatic changes, bone and viscera	Dermatan SO_4 Heparan SO_4	Homozygous H-gene
Scheie syndrome MPS IS	Normal intelligence, ? normal life-span. Otherwise similar to Hurler-MPS IH	Dermatan SO_4 Heparan SO_4	Homozygous S-gene
Hunter syndrome MPS II	Mental retardation, clear cornea milder course than Hurler MPS IH	Dermatan SO_4 Heparan SO_4	Hemizygous for X-linked gene
Sanfilippo syndrome MPS III	Mental retardation, clear cornea, minimal somatic change	Heparan SO_4	Homozygous Sanfilippo gene
Morquio syndrome MPS IV	Normal intelligence, cloudy cornea, severe bone changes	Keratan-SO_4 Chondroitin-6 SO_4	Homozygous M-gene
Maroteaux-Lamy MPS VI	Normal intelligence, corneal clouding, bone changes	Dermatan SO_4	Homozygous M-L gene
β-Glucuronidase deficiency MPS VII	Mental retardation, cloudy cornea, somatic involvement, bone and viscera	Variable Chondroitin SO_4 Dermatan SO_4	Homozygous β-glucuronidase gene
Chondroitin-4-sulfate mucopoly-saccharidoses	Mild mental retardation, "impish" face, normal life-span, cloudy cornea, somatic involvement bone and viscera	Chondroitin-4-sulfate	Homozygous ?

Patients with β-glucuronidase (EC 3.2.1.31) deficiency are of particular interest. Data are not yet available on the polysaccharides stored in their tissues; however, the clinical phenotype and pattern of GAG excretion in the urine has varied in the few patients who have been studied. One patient's urine contained excess chondroitin-4-sulfate and chondroitin-6-sulfate (*18*); another patient excreted excess dermatan sulfate (*19*). Because the chondroitin sulfates, heparan sulfate, dermatan sulfate, and hyaluronic acid all contain glucuronic acid, one would expect patients with this disorder to excrete and store all of these GAGs if the deficiency were complete. One possible explanation for the variation in phenotype may again be related to allelic mutations in which the altered enzyme retains activity for some GAGs but not for others.

Cultured fibroblasts derived from the skin of patients with the Maroteaux-Lamy syndrome are deficient in a sulfatase (EC 3.1.6.9) that removes the ester sulfate of carbon 4 from N-acetylgalactosaminine (*20*). This enzyme is uniquely related to the degradation of dermatan sulfate and accounts for the increased storage and urinary excretion of this GAG in affected individuals. Arylsulphatase B activity (EC 3.1.6.1) measured with synthetic substrates, is also deficient in cultured fibroblasts and liver of patients (*21*). This assay is not specific but may aid in diagnosis when correlated with clinical findings and the pattern of GAGs in urine.

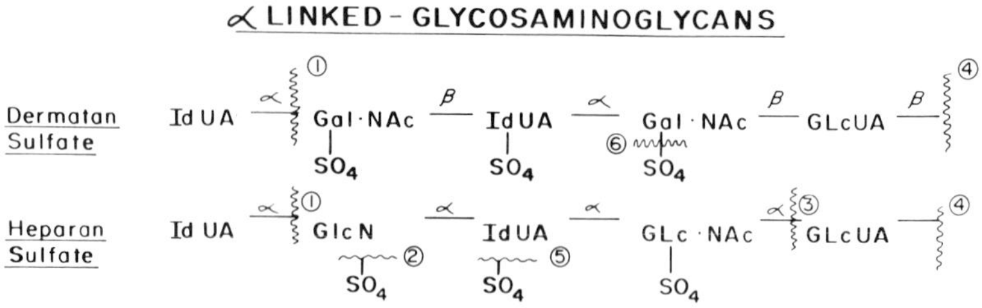

α LINKED - GLYCOSAMINOGLYCANS

Figure 5. Enzymatic defects identified in the degradation of the α-linked glycosaminoglycans. Components of the chain are abbreviated as follows: *Id Ua*, iduronic acid; *Glc Ua*, glucuronic acid; *Gal NAc*, galactosamine; *GlcN*, glucosamine. AMPS, acid mucopolysaccharide.

Turning to the β-linked GAGs—which include hyaluronic acid, keratan sulfate, chondroitin-4-sulfate, and chondroitin-6-sulfate—only two syndromes must be considered at the present time (Figure 6). The defect responsible for Morquio's disease appears to be a deficiency of the sulfatase that cleaves the ester sulfate from carbon 6 of the amino sugar. This configuration is common to both keratan sulfate and chondroitin-6-sulfate, and would account for the increased urinary excretion and storage of these polymers in patients with Morquio's disease (22).

The chondroitin-4-sulfate mucopolysaccharidoses are still ill-defined clinically and chemically, but appear to be a distinct entity. The clinical phenotypes of five affected patients, representing four unrelated families, have varied (23). One infant with the clinical picture of the Hurler syndrome was shown to store large amounts of chondroitin-4-sulfate in the liver (24). At least one patient showed normal β-glucuronidase activity. Possibly in some patients the disease will be related to a deficiency of specific glucuronidase and other patients may show a deficiency of the sulfatase necessary to cleave the sulfate ester on carbon 4 of galactosamine.

LABORATORY DIAGNOSIS

Assays for the deficient enzymes, or kinetic studies of GAG degradation in cultured fibroblasts as described by Neufeld and Crantz, provide the most direct and precise method of diagnosis (25). The complexity of these tests makes them impractical for most clinical laboratories, yet a precise diagnosis is required if the family is to have the full benefits of genetic counseling and the option of antenatal diagnosis. Increased urinary GAG excretion is the primary diagnostic sign of the genetic mucopolysaccharidoses. Initial identification of patients by screening test, coupled with the quantitative measurement of the total GAG in the urine, is not a difficult procedure and could be carried

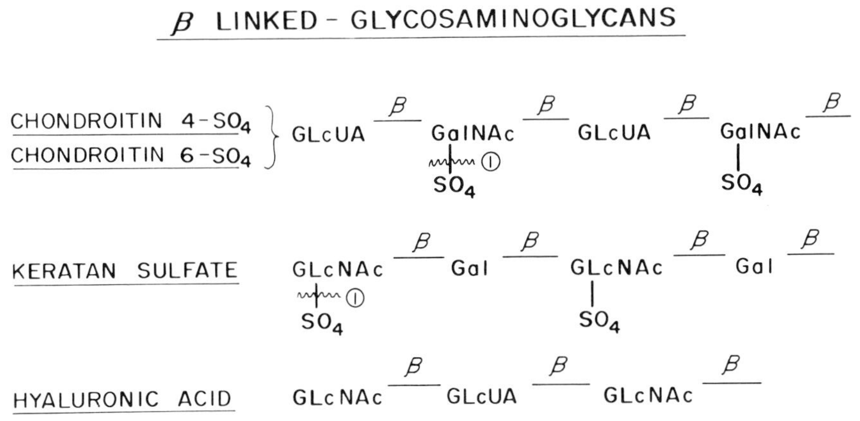

β LINKED - GLYCOSAMINOGLYCANS

Figure 6. Enzymatic defects identified in the degradation of the β-linked glycosaminoglycans. Components of the chain are abbreviated as follows: *Glc Ua*, glucuronic acid; *Gal NAc*, galactosamine; and *Gal*, galactose. AMPS, acid mucopolysaccharide.

out in most clinical laboratories. Further study of the patient to establish a precise diagnosis may require identification of the specific GAG that is being excreted in the urine and enzymatic studies of cultured fibroblasts or other tissues. These tests should be made available as a service through regional or national laboratories that are equipped and staffed to carry out these procedures.

In our clinic, we have adopted the following approach. The child with the suspected diagnosis of a genetic mucopolysaccharidosis is first screened by using the cetylpyridinium chloride turbidity test of the urine (26). This test is not specific because the cationic detergent may complex with GAG, other anionically charged polymers, or drug metabolites to produce a reaction ranging from turbidity to a flocculent precipitate. We use this particular screening test because of its sensitivity. The frequency of false-positive reaction ranges from 5 to 10%, but false-negative tests have not been recorded. If this screening test is negative, investigation of the patient is directed to other lysosomal storage disorders, which may resemble the mucopolysaccharidoses. These include the mucolipidoses and certain of the sphingoglycolipidoses. If the screening test is positive, the total GAG excreted in the urine is measured. Several simple methods for the quantitative estimation of urinary GAG have been published, in which column chromatography (27) or precipitation procedures are used to isolate the GAG (28). We used a modification of the method described by Di Ferrante and Rich (29), in which the GAGs are precipitated from 25 to 50 ml of urine with cetylpyridinium chloride. The hexuronic acid content is then measured by Bitter and Muir's modification of the Dische carbazole reaction (30). Although diurnal variations in the excretion of GAG and creatinine have been reported (31), we have encountered no problems in using casual (i.e., untimed) urine specimens collected between 10 and 16 h. The use of casual samples is a distinct advantage when dealing with small children in a clinical setting. Figure 7 shows the distribution of values for 25 patients seen in our clinic during the past five years. These values are plotted by age and compared to normal controls. The control data were generated by Dr. Wm. Van B. Robertson and are supplemented by analyses from our laboratory. They compare well with data for normals published by Teller et al. (*32*), Rich et al. (*33*), and Langunoff et al. (*34*). The excretion of GAG by patients with mucopolysaccharidoses is strikingly increased as compared to normal controls. We have encountered five patients who showed a positive turbidity screening test but had normal amounts of GAG in their urine by quantitative assay. Three of these children were shown to have other storage diseases including GM_1 gangliosidosis type I, fucosidosis, and mucolipidosis type III. The remaining two children were under one year of age when they were initially studied for a storage disorder because of unexplained hepatosplenomegaly. Subsequent follow-up showed persistently negative screening tests, normal excretion of urinary GAG, and no clinical disease.

Once we have established that the patient excretes increased quantities of GAG in the urine, the GAG is fractionated to identify it more specifically. This aids in the differential diagnosis of individual entities. For example, the X-linked Hunter's syndrome can be differentiated from the recessively inherited Sanfilippo syndrome in a male infant by the pattern of GAG in urine. Hunter's syndrome shows increased urinary concentrations of dermatan sulfate and heparan sulfate while heparan sulfate is the predominant GAG in the Sanfilippo syndrome. Finally, we attempt to confirm the diagnosis either by enzyme assay or by kinetic studies of GAG degradation in cultured fibroblasts. The latter tests are frequently done in the research laboratories of friends.

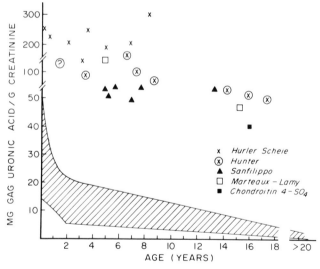

Figure 7. Urinary excretion of glycosaminoglycuronoglycans (in mg GAG glucuronic acid/mg creatinine) by normal individuals and patients with mucopolysaccharidoses. Shaded areas show the 95% confidence levels for the controls.

URINARY GAG EXCRETION BY THE NEONATE

Little data are available on the metabolism and urinary excretion of GAG by the neonate. We became aware of this problem when we were asked to exclude or confirm the diagnosis of the Hurler syndrome in a newborn infant whose parents were known to carry the mutant gene because of disease in an older child. Figure 8 presents data on the total GAG (expressed as milligrams of glucuronic acid per gram of creatinine) in the urine of newborns. These data are derived from a study published by Pennock et al. (35), supplemented with analyses from our own laboratory. The infant in question clearly showed a marked increase of uronic acid GAG as compared to normal controls. Some of our normal values exceeded the 95% confidence level in the published report. Additional data are obviously needed in this group to establish the range of reference (normal) values. The next question pertaining to diagnosis in this infant was whether the quantitative distribution of GAG in his urine differed from the normal. Again, we found few data in the literature. Table 2 summarizes some information on the pattern of GAG excretion in the newborn. The principal GAGs excreted in the urine of older children and adults are the chondroitin sulfates, chondroitin (desulfated chondroitin sulfate), and a small quantity of heparan sulfate. Only trace amounts of dermatan sulfate and keratan sulfate are present (36). In the normal neonate, the pattern apparently differs in that the proportion of nonsulfated GAG—hyaluronic acid and chondroitin—is increased. Appreciable quantities of the chondroitin sulfates are present. Like the adult, the normal neonate excretes only trace amounts of dermatan sulfate (37). Reliable information on the quantity of heparan sulfate in the urine of the normal neonate is not available. The methods used in these analyses did not clearly separate heparan sulfate from chondroitin-4-sulfate.

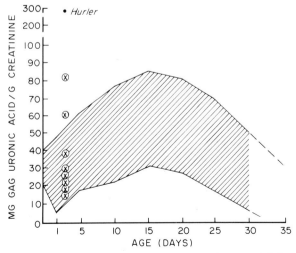

Figure 8. Urinary excretion of glycosaminoglycuronoglycans by normal infants and by an infant with Hurler's syndrome. Shaded areas show the 95% confidence levels published by Pennock (34). The symbol X indicates analyses performed in the author's laboratory.

Table 2. Composition of Urinary Glycosaminoglycans in the Neonate (% of Total of GAG Excreted)

	Older children, Adults[a]	27 Neonates[b] (10 days)	8 Neonates (3 days)	Hurler (3 days)
Keratan SO$_4$	1	9	0–15	0
Hyaluronic acid	1	35	19–25	17
Heparan SO$_4$	8	} 24	} 17–20	} 20
Chondroitin	25			
Chondroitin-4-SO$_4$	34	19	12–36	32
Chondroitin-6-SO$_4$	31	12	13–35	0
Dermatan SO$_4$	1	1	0	31

[a] See reference 36

[b] See reference 37

The suspected Hurler syndrome infant showed a distinct increase in the proportion of dermatan sulfate in his urine as compared to normal infants matched for age. Based on these data and the family history, a tentative diagnosis of the Hurler syndrome was made in this infant, who clinically appeared to be normal. The diagnosis was established by the evolution of his disease in the first year of life and by enzymatic studies which showed deficient L-iduronidase in cultured fibroblasts. This limited experience suggests that infants with the Hurler syndrome may be identified in the neonatal period by analyses of their urine. Additional data are needed on the pattern of GAG excretion in the urine of infants with the other entities, because some may show a normal pattern early in life. Analysis of the GAG composition of amniotic fluids obtained from fetuses affected with the Hurler, Hunter, or Sanfilippo syndromes suggests that abnormal excretion of GAG into the urine may begin in utero in some patients (38).

THE PROBLEM OF SCREENING

The genetic mucopolysaccharidoses collectively have a prevalence of perhaps one birth in 25 000, which puts them somewhere between that for phenylketonuria (1 in 10 000) and galactosemia (1 in 100 000).

Several screening tests for urine are available, but none readily distinguishes the affected infant from the normal neonate. The tests in common use are listed in Table 3. The urinary excretion of GAG, expressed as glucuronic acid, varies during the first seven days. Twelve infants studied by Helen K. Berry during the first day excreted 0.3 to 1.4 mg/24 h (9–65 mg/litre). Eight three-day-old infants studied in our laboratory excreted between 3–75 mg/litre. If this concentration of uronic acid is related to the lower limit of sensitivity for each test, it is clear that all will give a large number of falsely positive reactions. The range for false-positive tests given in Table 3 represents a summary of data from several studies carried out on selected populations (39–43). Pennock, who studied 800 infants, found that the urines of 5% of them gave a positive cetylpyridinium chloride turbidity test (43). Berry, using the toluidine blue O spot test, reported positive

Table 3.   Screening Tests Used to Detect Glycosaminoglycans in Urine

Dye tests	Lower limit sensitivity	Falsely positive	Falsely negative
	Uronic acid, mg/l		
		%	
Toluidine blue	10–20	0.2–30	+
Alcian blue	10–12	10–20	0
Azure A	20	0–20	0
Turbidity tests			
Cetylammonium bromide	12	2–20	0
Cetylpyridinium chloride	15	2–20	0
Acid–Albumin	28	0–8	+

results in 0.2% of 2200 infants between two and six weeks of age; however, 4 of 12 infants tested during the first day of postnatal life gave a positive test (42). Falsely negative reactions have also been reported with the toluidine blue O test and with the acid-albumin test. Comparative studies of these screening tests, carried out by several laboratories, produced widely divergent results, indicating that these tests lack specificity. Glycoproteins or anionically charged drugs, such as barbiturates, if present in the urine, may complex with the test reagent to give a false-positive reaction, or cationic compounds may combine with the GAG to produce a false-negative result. It may be possible to standardize and modify the existing screening tests to take into account the concentration of GAG in the urine of neonates. This might decrease the number of falsely positive reactions to an acceptable level. Neonates who showed a positive screening test could then be studied further to determine whether or not the positive test actually reflected an increased excretion of GAG.

A more attractive possibility would be a screening test that specifically reacted with dermatan sulfate and heparan sulfate. Except for Morquio's syndrome, patients with the other recognized mucopolysaccharidoses excrete either one or both of these polymers in excess in the urine. Both polymers contain distinctive structures that provide the basis of the color reactions now used for their quantitative measurement. Naphthoresorcinol reacts with the iduronic acid in dermatan sulfate to produce a purple color which is 40% more intense than that obtained with similar amounts of heparan sulfate or GAG containing glucuronic acid (44). The sulfated nitrogen of the amino sugar of heparan sulfate provides the unique structure that is the basis of the color reaction used for the quantitative measurement of this GAG (45).

The challenge is whether or not a screening test can be developed, based on the chemical structure and composition of these polymers, that is specific and sensitive enough to make practical the screening of all neonates. This seems a mundane problem when compared to the elegant chemical studies that have defined the principles underlying this group of storage diseases, but it is a problem of major practical importance. At our present stage of knowledge, early identification permits genetic counseling of the family. Through this process, parents who are asymptomatic carriers of the mutant gene learn the risks for recurrence in subsequent offspring. In terms of prevention, several options are open to the parents, including the monitoring of subsequent pregnancies to determine whether or not the fetus is affected. It would be a paradox if effective therapy evolved for these disorders before a reliable screening test was available for the early identification of affected infants. This scenario may become a reality if screening remains an area of investigative neglect.

SUMMARY

The enzymatic defects in most of the genetic mucopolysaccharidoses have now been elucidated. The deficient enzyme in each entity is either a glycosidase or sulfatase needed in the degradation of a specific glycosaminoglycan (GAG). As a result of the enzyme deficiency, the degradation of the polymer is blocked. The polymer fragments that result are stored in the lysosomes of the cell and excreted in the urine. Increased GAG excretion in the urine remains the primary diagnostic sign for this group of diseases. In older children in whom a storage disease is suspected, careful clinical appraisal coupled with laboratory studies to identify specific GAG excreted in excess in the urine provide sufficient data for a presumptive diagnosis in most patients. The affected neonate appears clinically normal at birth. A reliable screening test that will distinguish the affected baby from his normal counterpart is not currently available, and this is a major block in the application of existing knowledge to the prevention of this group of diseases.

REFERENCES

1. Roden, L. and Smith, R., Structure of the neutral trisaccharide of the chondroitin-4-sulfate protein linkage region, *J. Biol. Chem.* **241**, 5949 (1966).

2. Fransson, L. A. and Rodén, L., Structure of dermatan sulfate: I. Degradation by testicular hyaluronidase, *J. Biol. Chem.* **242**, 4161 (1967).

3. Meyer, K., Biochemistry and biology of mucopolysaccharides, *Am. J. Med.* **47**, 664 (1969).

4. Lindahl, U., Structure of heparin, heparan sulfate and their proteoglycans, In *NATO Advanced Study Institute on the Chemistry and Molecular Biology of the Intercellular Matrix*, **II**, E. A. Balazs, Ed., Academic Press, London, 1970, pp. 943–960.

5. Malstrom, A. and Fransson, L. A., Structure of pig skin dermatan sulfate. *Eur. J. Biochem.* **18**, 431 (1971).

6. Schubert, M. and Hamerman, D., A *Primer on Connective Tissue. Biochemistry*, Lea and Febiger, Philadelphia, Pa., 1968, p. 79.

7. Curran, R. C., The histochemistry of mucopolysaccharides, *Int. Rev. Cytol.* **17**, 149 (1964).

8. Scott, J. E., Ion binding in solutions containing acid mucopolysaccharides. In *The Chemical Physiology of Mucopolysaccharides*. G Quintarelli, Ed., Little, Brown, Boston, Mass. 1968, pp 171–197.

9. Dorfman, A., Adventures in viscous solutions, *Mol. Cell. Biochem.* **4**, 45 (1974).

10. Neufeld, E. F., The biochemical basis for mucopolysaccharidoses and mucolipidoses. *Prog. Med. Genet.* **81**, 101 (1974).

11. McKusick, V. A., *Heritable Disorders of Connective Tissue*, 4th ed., C. V. Mosby, Saint Louis, Mo. 1972, pp 521–681.

12. Dorfman, A. and Matalon R., The mucopolysaccharidoses. In *The Metabolic Basis of Inheritde Disease*, 3rd ed. J. B. Stanbury, J. B. Wyngaarden, and D. S. Fredrickson, Eds., McGraw-Hill, New York, N.Y., 1972, pp. 1233-1246.

13. Bach, G., Friedman, R., Weissman, B., and Neufeld, E. F., The defect in the Hurler and Scheie syndromes: Deficiency of α-L-iduronidase, *Proc. Natl. Acad. Sci. U.S.A.* **69**, 2048 (1972).

14. McKusick, V. A. et al., Allelism, non-allelism, and genetic compounds among the mucopolysaccharidoses, *Lancet* **i**, 933, (1972).

15. Bach, G., Eisenberg, F., Jr., Cantz, M. J., and Neufeld, E. F.: The defect in the Hunter syndrome: Deficiency of sulfoiduronate sulfatase, *Proc. Natl. Acad. Sci. U.S.A.*, **70**, 2134 (1973).

16. O'Brien, J. S., Sanfilippo syndrome: Profound deficiency of alpha-acetylglucosaminidase activity in organs and skin fibroblasts from type B patients, *Proc. Natl. Acad. Sci. U.S.A.* **69**, 1720 (1972).

17. Matalon, R. and Dorfman, A., Sanfilippo A syndrome: Sulfamidase deficiency in cultured skin fibroblasts and liver, *J. Clin. Invest.* **54**, 907 (1974).

18. Sly, W. S., Quinton, B. A., McAlister, W. H. and Rimoin, D. L., Beta glucuronidase deficiency: Report of clinical, radiologic and biochemical features of a new mucopolysaccharidosis, *J. Pediatr.* **82**, 249 (1973).

19. Beaudet, A. L. et al., Variation in the phenotypic expression of β-glucuronidase deficiency, *J. Pediatr.* **86**, 388 (1975).

20. Matalon, R. and Dorfman, A., Maroteaux-Lamy syndrome: A deficiency of N-acetyl-galactosamine 4-sulfate sulfatase, *Pediatr. Res.* **9**, 413 (1975).

21. Fluharty, A. L., Stevens, R. L., Sanders, D. L., and Kihara, H., Arylsulfatase B deficiency in Maroteaux-Lamy syndrome cultured fibroblasts, *Biochem. Biophys. Res. Commun.* **59**, 455 (1974).

22. Matalon, R., Arbogast, B., Justice, P., and Dorfman, A., Morquio's syndrome: A deficiency of chondroitin sulfate N-acetylhexosamine sulfate sulfatase, *Biochem. Biophys. Res. Comm.* **61**, 759 (1974).

23. Spranger, J. W., Schuster, W., and Freitag, F., Chondroitin-4-sulfate mucopolysaccharidosis, *Helv. Paediatr. Acta* **26**, 387 (1971).

24. Benson, P. F., Dean, M. F., and Muir, H., A form of mucopolysaccharidosis with visceral storage and excessive urinary excretion of chondroitin sulfate, *Dev. Med. Child Neurol.* **14**, 69 (1972).

25. Neufeld, E. F. and Crantz, M. J., Corrective factors for inborn errors of mucopolysaccharide metabolism, *Ann. N. Y. Acad. Sci.* **179**, 580 (1971).

26. Pennock, C. A., A modified screening test for glycosaminoglycan excretion, *J. Clin. Pathol.* **22**, 379 (1969).

27. Calatroni, A., Tests for mucopolysaccharidoses: Simple method for quantitative estimation of urinary glycosaminoglycans, *Clin. Chem.* **18**, 266 (1972).

28. Di Ferrante, N. M., The measurement of urinary mucopolysaccharides, *Anal. Biochem.* **21**, 98 (1967).

29. Di Ferrante, N. and Rich, C., The determination of acid aminopolysaccharide in urine, *J. Lab. Clin. Med.* **48**, 491 (1956).

30. Bitter, T. and Muir, H. M., A modified uronic acid carbazole reaction, *Anal. Biochem.* **4**, 330 (1962).

31. Di Ferrante, N. and Lipscomb, H., Urinary glycosaminoglycan versus creatinine excretion: A used and abused parameter, *Clin. Chim. Acta* **30**, 69 (1970).

32. Teller, W. M., Burke, E. C., Rosevear, J. W., and McKenzie, B. F., Urinary excretion of acid mucopolysaccharides in normal children and patients with gargoylism, *J. Lab. Clin. Med.* **59**, 95 (1962).

33. Rich, C., Di Ferrante, N., and Archibald, R. M., Acid mucopolysaccharide excretion in the urine of children, *J. Lab. Clin. Med.* **50**, 686 (1957).

34. Lagunoff, D., Pritzl, P., and Scott, C. R., Urinary N-sulfate glycosaminoglycan excretion in children: Normal and abnormal values, *Proc. Soc. Exp. Biol. Med.* **126**, 34 (1967).

35. Pennock, C. A., Wharton, B. A., and White, F., Urinary glycosaminoglycan excretion in the neonatal period, *Acta Paediatr. Scand.* **60**, 299 (1971).

36. Varadi, D. P., Cifonelli, J. A., and Dorfman, A., The acid mucopolysaccharides in normal urine, *Biochim. Biophys. Acta* **141**, 103 (1967).

37. Klujber, L. and Sulyok, E., Urinary glucosaminoglycan excretion in normally grown and growth retarded neonates, *Acta Paediatr. Acad. Sci. Hung.* **14**, 209 (1973).

38. Lee, T-Y. and Schafer, I. A., Glycosaminoglycan composition of human amniotic fluid, *Biochim. Biophys. Acta* **354**, 264 (1974).

39. Pennock, C. A., Mott, M. G., and Batstone, G. F., Screening for the mucopolysaccharidoses, *Clin. Chim. Acta* **27**, 93 (1970).

40. Carter, C. H., Wan, A. T., and Carpenter, D. G., Commonly used tests in the detection of Hurler's syndrome, *J. Pediatr.* **73**, 217 (1968).

41. Rezvani, I., Collipp. P. J., and Di George, A. M., Evaluation of screening tests for urinary mucopolysaccharides, *Pediatrics* **52**, 64 (1973).

42. Berry, H. K., personal communication.

43. Pennock, C. A. et al., Excess glycosaminoglycan excretion in infancy and childhood, *Acta Paediatr. Scand.* **62**, 481 (1973).

44. Pelzer, H. and Staib, W., Steroidkonjugate I. Hochspannungspapierelektrophorese von 17-Ketosteroidkonjugaten, *Clin. Chim. Acta* **2**, 407 (1957).

45. Lagunoff, O. and Warren, G., Determination of 2-deoxy-2-sulfoaminohexose content of mucopolysaccharides, *Arch. Biochem. Biophys.* **99**, 396 (1962).

Diagnosis and Understanding of Sphingolipidoses in the Newborn

ROSCOE O. BRADY, M.D.

Physicians responsible for the care of infants must be constantly alert to the possibility of an inherited metabolic disorder if there are signs of delayed or arrested development. I should like to present a brief overview of disorders of the newborn that are characterized by the accumulation of excessive quantities of lipid in various organs and tissues. I shall then describe in some detail a patient with a novel form of mental retardation that has just been discovered. The metabolic defect in this case was a failure to synthesize a particular class of lipids called gangliosides, and I shall briefly indicate the disastrous consequences attending this type of metabolic abnormality.

GAUCHER'S DISEASE AND NIEMANN-PICK DISEASE

Let me begin by presenting selected cases to illustrate how physicians may arrive at the correct diagnosis of lipid-storage diseases. Assume that an infant is presented who has not achieved well-recognized developmental milestones at 2.5 to 3 months. This fact immediately suggests central nervous system damage. One of the first clues to the nature of the disorder, in addition to the signs of mental retardation, is the presence or absence of organomegaly. If the liver and spleen are enlarged, the two principal disorders that come to mind are Gaucher's disease and Niemann-Pick disease. Bone-marrow aspiration or biopsy will almost certainly reveal large, lipid-laden cells in patients with this early onset and obvious severity. The storage cells in Gaucher's disease contain periodic acid–Schiff positive glycolipid material and those in Niemann-Pick disease show the presence of the phospholipid sphingomyelin. These cells are readily distinguishable by hematologists and pathologists. The diagnosis may be confirmed by chemical analysis of a liver biopsy specimen. An even more feasible procedure is to measure in tissue the activity of glucocerebrosidase, the enzyme deficient in Gaucher's disease (1,2) (Reaction 1).

Ceramide-glucose + H_2O $\xrightarrow{\text{glucocerebrosidase}}$ ceramide + glucose

(ceramide is N-fatty acyl sphingosine)   [1]

or sphingomyelinase (EC 3.1.4.12) which is deficient in Niemann-Pick disease (3) (Reaction 2)

Ceramide-phosphorylcholine + H_2O $\xrightarrow{\text{sphingomyelinase}}$ ceramide + phosphorylcholine   [2]

These assays are conveniently carried out with washed leukocyte preparations (4) or cultured skin fibroblasts (5,6). The latter source is preferred if the enzyme assays are to be performed by a laboratory remote from the clinic where the patient is seen, because the activity of these enzymes is much greater in cultured fibroblasts than in leukocytes, and they are more stable in frozen cultured cells when shipped. At the present time, authentic radioactive glucocerebroside is generally used to diagnose Gaucher's disease, although patients with this disorder have been detected by use of a fluorogenic substrate (5,7) (Figure 1). Currently, the diagnosis of Niemann-Pick disease absolutely depends on the use of radioactive sphingomyelin. A chromogenic substrate has been proposed for this assay (8), and it has recently been found to be an excellent reagent for the diagnosis of Niemann-Pick disease (Gal, A. E., Brady, R. O., Hibbert, S. R., and Pentchev, P. G., *New Engl. J. Med.*, **293**, 632–636 [1975]).

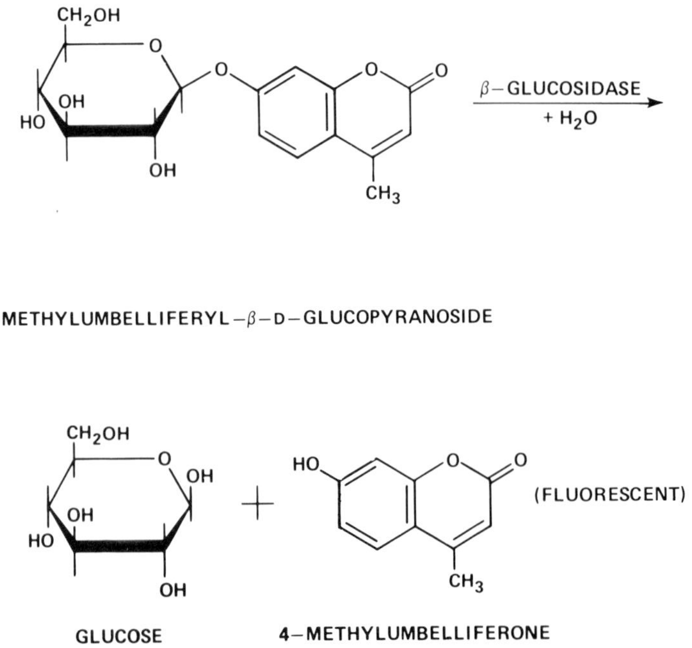

Figure 1.   Reaction involved in the fluorometric assay used in the diagnosis of Gaucher's disease.

GENERALIZED GANGLIOSIDOSIS

Consider a severely retarded infant who has skeletal deformation and joint involvement in addition to hepatomegaly and splenomegaly. This situation suggests a mucopolysaccharide storage disorder, but is also seen in the sphingolipidosis called generalized gangliosidosis. About 50% of these patients have a cherry-red spot in the retina. An acidic glycolipid called ganglioside G_{M1} [structure: ceramide–glucose–galactose–(N-acetylneuraminic acid)–N-acetylgalactosamine–galactose] accumulates because of a deficiency of the β-galactosidase (EC 3.2.1.23) that catalyzes the cleavage of the terminal molecule of galactose from this ganglioside (9). Patients with this disease may be readily diagnosed by assaying β-galactosidase activity in various tissues with artificial substrates such as 4-methylumbelliferyl-β-D-galactopyranoside or with the chromogenic nitrophenylgalactoside shown in Figure 2. Total β-galactosidase activity in these patients' organs is only about 8% of normal (10).

SANDHOFF–JATZKEWITZ DISEASE

On another occasion, a physician may be asked to see a severely retarded patient with moderate hepatomegaly and little or no splenomegaly or bone deformation, but the child is blind and has a cherry-red spot in the macular region. Here one must think of a deficiency of hexosaminidase activity and the disorder is the very severe form of Tay-Sachs disease that is often called Sandhoff-Jatzkewitz disease. Tissue hexosaminidase activity is extremely low as measured with the N-acetylglucosaminyl derivative of 4-methylumbelliferone (Figure 3) or nitrophenyl-β-D-N-acetylglucosaminide (11). Tay-Sachs ganglioside (Figure 4) accumulates primarily in neuronal cells of these individuals, and parenchymal organs have increased quantities of a neutral glycolipid called "globoside" (structure: ceramide–glucose–galactose–galactose-N-acetylgalactosamine). The latter substance is a major neutral lipid of erythrocyte stroma. Catabolism of these compounds requires a functioning hexosaminidase and it is therefore no surprise that they accumulate in the tissues of patients with this disorder (12).

TAY-SACHS DISEASE

In the more conventional form of Tay-Sachs disease, development is essentially normal until the fifth or sixth month. Thereafter, signs of increasing impairment of the central

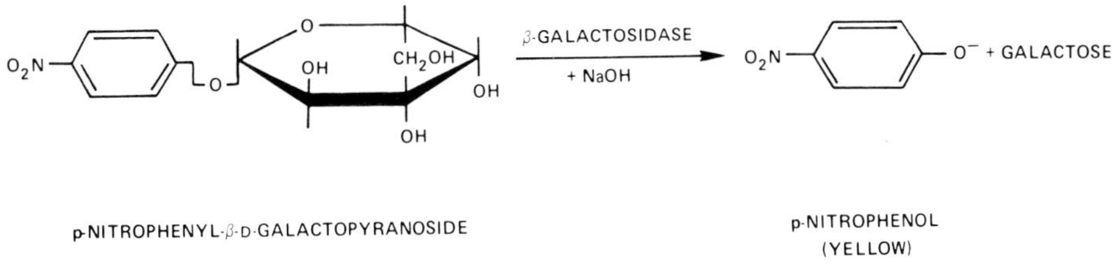

p-NITROPHENYL-β-D-GALACTOPYRANOSIDE

p-NITROPHENOL (YELLOW)

Figure 2. Reaction involved in the colorimetric assay used in the diagnosis of generalized gangliosidosis.

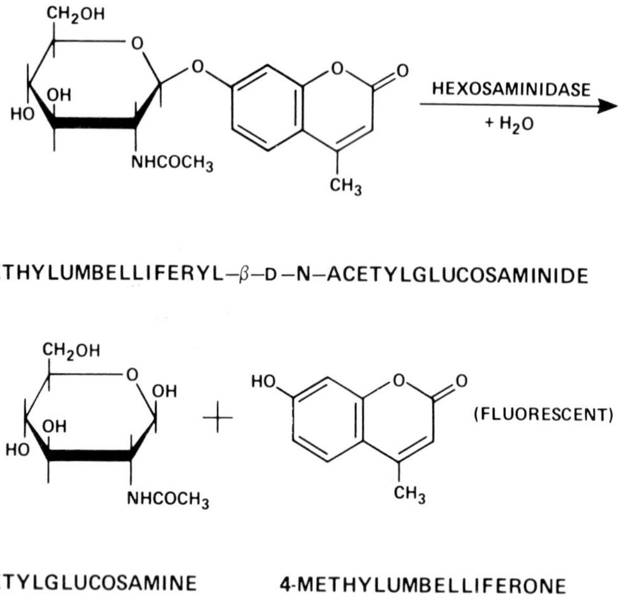

4–METHYLUMBELLIFERYL–β–D–N–ACETYLGLUCOSAMINIDE

N-ACETYLGLUCOSAMINE   **4-METHYLUMBELLIFERONE**

Figure 3.   Reaction involved in the fluorometric assay of hexosaminidase activity.

nervous system appear, as evidenced by apathy, convulsions, failure to thrive, and the onset of blindness. There is no organomegaly, but a cherry-red spot is present in the macula in virtually all of these patients. The pathological biochemistry of Tay-Sachs disease is very complicated. The fundamental defect is a deficiency of a hexosaminidase (EC 3.2.1.52) that catalyzes the cleavage of N-acetylgalactosamine from Tay-Sachs ganglioside *(13,14)* (Reaction 3).

Ceramide–glucose–galactose–(N-acetylneuraminic acid)–N-acetylgalactosamine

$$+ \ H_2O \ \xrightarrow{\text{hexosaminidase}} \ \text{Ceramide–glucose–galactose–N-acetylneuraminic acid}$$

$$+ \ N\text{-acetylgalactosamine} \quad [3]$$

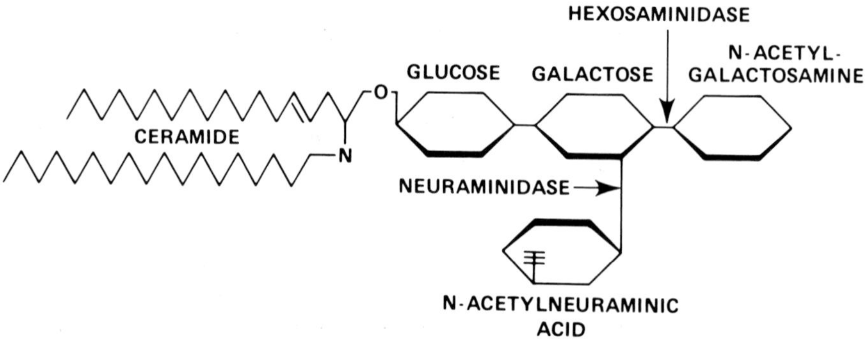

Figure 4.   Structure of Tay-Sachs ganglioside.

If one measures total hexosaminidase activity in the brain of a patient with this form of Tay-Sachs disease, one finds about a sevenfold increase over normal. There are at least two so-called hexosaminidase isoenzymes, which may be separated from each other by electrophoresis on starch gel. The isoenzyme migrating faster toward the anode is called hexosaminidase A, the slower migrating component hexosaminidase B. In these Tay-Sachs patients, hexosaminidase B is greatly increased (*15*).

Brain and other tissues also contain a neuraminidase (EC 3.2.1.18) that catalyzes the cleavage of *N*-acetylneuraminic acid from Tay-Sachs ganglioside (*16*) (Reaction 4).

Ceramide–glucose–galactose–(*N*-acetylneuraminic acid)–*N*-acetylgalactosamine

$$+ \; H_2O \xrightarrow{\text{neuraminidase}} \text{ceramide–glucose–galactose–}N\text{-acetylgalactosamine}$$

$$+ \; N\text{-acetylneuraminic acid} \quad [4]$$

The activity of this enzyme is normal in Tay-Sachs disease (*13,14,17*). An intriguing aspect of the conventional form of Tay-Sachs disease is the fact that hexosaminidase B, which is very active in these patients, can hydrolyze the asialo Tay-Sachs ganglioside produced in Reaction 4 (Reaction 5).

Ceramide–glucose–galactose–*N*-acetylgalactosamine

$$+ \; H_2O \xrightarrow{\text{hexosaminidase B}} \text{ceramide–glucose–galactose} + N\text{-acetylgalactosamine} \quad [5]$$

The question immediately arises why the whole molecule of Tay-Sachs ganglioside accumulates in Tay-Sachs disease if the alternative route for its catabolism via the neuraminidase is operating. The best estimate at present is that both the primary hexosaminidase (Reaction 3) and neuraminidase (Reaction 4) pathways must function in the neonatal period when ganglioside turnover is maximal, and catabolism via Reactions 4 and 5 cannot accommodate all of the ganglioside that is turned over at this stage of development. Some support for this line of reasoning is seen in patients with the Sandhoff-Jatzkewitz form of Tay-Sachs disease, where there is a much more rapid accumulation of Tay-Sachs ganglioside and progression of the signs and symptoms of the disease. This condition is characterized by the accumulation of a much higher percentage of asialo Tay-Sachs ganglioside in the brain than in patients with the usual form of Tay-Sachs disease.

There is some evidence that hexosaminidases A and B are different conformations (i.e., tertiary structures) of the same protein (*18*). Hexosaminidase A can be converted to hexosaminidase B simply by gentle heating, and there are indications of considerable similarities in the two forms, such as closely identical amino acid composition (*19*) and cross-reactivity to antienzyme antibodies (*20,21*). Thus, different mutations, all of which result in decreased catabolism of Tay-Sachs ganglioside, are responsible for the different clinical classes of the disorder, including patients who have normal hexosaminidase activity as measured with artificial substrates, but cannot catabolize Tay-Sachs ganglioside (*22*). This hypothesis is also compatible with the recent discovery of healthy normal individuals who have no hexosaminidase-A activity in their tissues (*23,24*). Here the mutation is such that the catabolism of Tay-Sachs ganglioside is unaffected, but only the B-configuration of the enzyme is present (*25*). In spite of the complicated biochemical phenomena that are responsible for Tay-Sachs disease, most of the patients may be diagnosed by determining hexosaminidase activity in serum, leukocytes, or cultured skin fibroblasts with fluorogenic or chromogenic derivatives of *N*-acetylglucosamine (*26*).

KRABBE'S DISEASE

Consider a patient whose postnatal course was about normal for four to five months, but who then showed hyperirritability, hyperesthesia, and episodic fever. These symptoms are gradually followed by the onset of overt mental retardation, and convulsions occur, which become severe. In addition, there may be hyperactivity, extension of arms, legs, and head, and blindness and deafness may occur. There is no organomegaly or cherry-red spot in the retina. A brain biopsy reveals involvement of the white matter in a process that is characterized by a severe lack of myelin, astrogliosis, and the presence of a large number of globoid cells. There is no net accumulation of a particular lipid in the brain because of extensive demyelination. However, once again the metabolic lesion is a deficiency of a catabolic enzyme. In this case it is the enzyme which catalyzes the hydrolysis of galactocerebroside (27) (Reaction 6).

$$\text{Ceramide–galactose} + H_2O \xrightarrow{\text{galactocerebroside-}\beta\text{-galactosidase}} \text{ceramide} + \text{galactose} \quad [6]$$

Patients with this disorder may be diagnosed by measuring the activity of galactocerebrosidase in brain biopsy specimens, washed leukocytes, or cultured skin fibroblasts. Note that this enzyme is also a β-galactosidase as in generalized gangliosidosis, but in this instance labeled galactocerebroside must be used for the diagnosis, because there is no detectable deficiency of β-galactosidase activity when the usual chromogenic or fluorogenic β-D-galactopyranosides are used as substrates.

METACHROMATIC LEUKODYSTROPHY

The most common form of metachromatic leukodystrophy is called the late-infantile type, in which flaccidity and weakness of the legs and arms appear between 12 and 18 months of age. Tendon reflexes may be diminished or even absent. The child gradually loses the ability to stand, and evidence of mental retardation appears, initially manifested by a loss of speech. Ataxia and hypertonicity occur. Some evidence of peripheral neuralgia may appear. The course of the disease progresses through blindness to complete mental deterioration.

The clinical history of the progression of the disease is indicative of white-matter pathology. Nerve-conduction time is slowed and biopsy reveals brownish-orange metachromatic droplets in the nerve fibers when the specimens are stained with cresyl violet dye.

These inclusions are the result of accumulation of sulfatide (ceramide–galactose–3-sulfate), which is also excreted in the urine in abnormally great amounts. The disorder may be diagnosed by measuring arylsulfatase (EC 3.1.6.1) activity in washed leukocyte preparations (28), with nitrocatechol sulfate as substrate (Figure 5). There are three arylsulfatases in tissues of normal individuals, designated A, B, and C. Arylsulfatase A is characteristically lacking in patients with metachromatic leukodystrophy. Some patients are deficient in all three enzymes and exhibit a number of manifestations of patients with mucopolysaccharidoses, including enlarged head, depression of the nasal bridge, hepatosplenomegaly, and bone changes. In addition to problems of gait, these infants are generally deaf. It is difficult logically to explain the mode of inheritance of this multiple sulfatase-deficiency disorder, because arylsulfatases A and B are considered to be lysosomal enzymes and arylsulfatase C and steroid sulfatases are localized in microsomes.

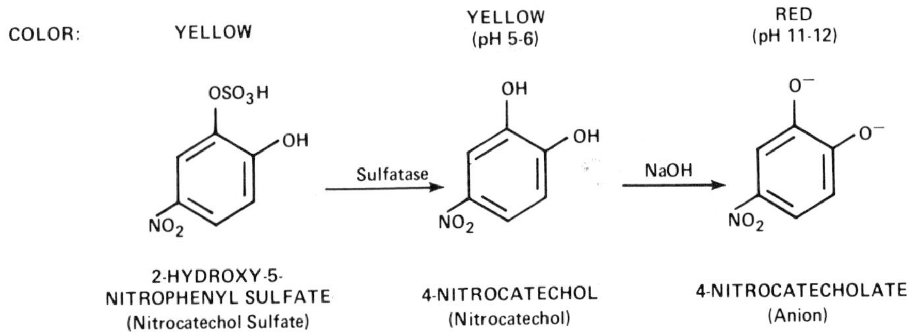

Figure 5. Chromogenic substrate used in the diagnosis of metachromatic leukodystrophy.

Furthermore, one of the missing enzymes, an iduronic acid sulfatase, is an X-linked recessive disorder (*29*).

There are at least two conceivable explanations that may account for such a total deficiency of sulfatase activity. The first is that all of the enzymes with sulfatase activity share a common subunit, which is mutated in the patients with multiple sulfatase deficiency and renders all of the enzymes inactive. The other is the possible requirement of a heat-stable "activator" substance that reportedly is necessary for sulfatide hydrolysis by arylsulfatase A (*30*). If this material is required for all sulfatase activity with natural substrates, the therapy of this type of disease will be considerably different from that for Fabry's disease (*31*) and for patients with the adult form of Gaucher's disease (*32*), in which replacing the missing enzyme appears to have striking beneficial effects.

G$_{M3}$ (HEMATOSIDE) SPHINGOLIPODYSTROPHY

I should like now to describe an infant with a novel disorder of lipid metabolism we have recently seen, which is probably illustrative of a new field of metabolic disorders. The patient was a 3.5-month-old male with severe retardation, poor motor and physical development, coarse facies, macroglossia, gingival hypertrophy, squat hands and feet, flexor contractures of the fingers, thickened, loose hirsute skin, bilateral inguinal hernias, and hepatosplenomegaly. The differential diagnosis included generalized gangliosidosis, which was ruled out by finding a normal level of β-galactosidase activity in the patient's leukocytes, and one of the mucopolysaccharidoses, which was eliminated because the urinary excretion of acid mucopolysaccharides was normal. Histologically, the brain showed large unmyelinated areas but no neuronal inclusions. A striking alteration in the pattern of brain gangliosides was observed when these substances were analyzed in a brain biopsy specimen (Figure 6). There was a 3.5-fold increase in the quantity of ganglioside G$_{M3}$ (ceramide–glucose–galactose–N-acetylneuraminic acid) [hematoside], a two-fold increase in ganglioside G$_{D3}$ (ceramide–glucose–galactose–N-acetylneuraminic acid–N-acetylneuraminic acid) [disialylhematoside], and a complete absence of all ganglioside homologs having an oligosaccharide moiety larger than that of ceramide lactoside (*33*). Ganglioside catabolism was unimpaired in homogenates of brain tissue obtained from the patient at autopsy, which eliminated the possibility of a deficiency of a catabolic enzyme as the cause of the modest accumulation of G$_{M3}$ and G$_{D3}$ in the brain. The formation of gangliosides proceeds in an orderly stepwise fashion (Figure 7), so we car-

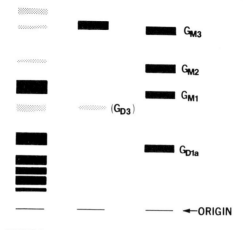

CONTROL   AFFECTED   STANDARDS

Figure 6. Tracing of a thin-layer chromatogram of brain gangliosides from a patient with G_{M3} spingolipodystrophy and from an age-matched control.

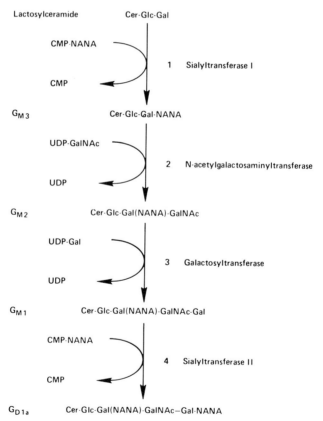

Figure 7. Pathway of synthesis of gangliosides. *Cer*, Ceramide; *Glc*, Glucose; *Gal*, galactose; *NANA*, N-acetylneuraminic acid; *GalNac*, N-acetylgalactosamine.

ried out a comprehensive series of assays to determine the activity of the transferase enzymes involved in ganglioside formation, to learn whether a deficiency of such a synthetic enzyme could account for the abnormal pattern of gangliosides. A profound deficiency of the N-acetylgalactosaminyl transferase that catalyzes the synthesis of Tay-Sachs ganglioside (G_{M2}) from G_{M3} (Figure 7, Reaction 2) was observed in a brain homogenate from this patient (Table 1). Other ganglioside-synthesizing enzymes were normal or increased in activity. Thus, the patient had a specific defect in an anabolic pathway. This observation stands in sharp contrast to all of the previously described sphingolipid disorders, which are caused by deficiencies of hydrolytic, catabolic enzymes (35). The documentation of the synthetic defect in this patient provides the first concrete evidence for the existence of a new category of metabolic disorders, caused by missing anabolic enzymes. It is difficult to speculate at this time about how frequently such defects occur, but clinicians and basic-research investigators should keep the possibility of this type of disorder in mind in patients with metabolic diseases of unknown etiology. The development of appropriate tests for detection of heterozygotes and for genetic counseling for such disorders must now be undertaken. Replacement therapy, by administration of glycosyltransferases of this type, seems now very remote because most of these enzymes are very tightly bound to microsomes (or the Golgi apparatus) and none of them has been extensively purified so far. Thus, much intensive work is required for the control and potential treatment of such patients.

Table 1. Activities of Glycosyltransferases in Brain Tissue from a Patient with G_{M3}-Sphingolipodystrophy

Reaction[a]	Activity
	Percent of age-matched controls
Sialyltransferase I	72
N-Acetylgalactosaminyltransferase	<9
Galactosyltransferase	390
Sialyltransferase II	224

[a] The reactions involved are illustrated in Fig. 7.

I think it is appropriate to conclude this presentation by citing another situation in which a deficiency of ganglioside synthesizing enzymes has been shown. If normal, contact-inhibited cultured mouse or hamster cell lines are transformed with the oncogenic DNA viruses, simian virus 40, or polyoma virus, the same N-acetylgalactosaminyl transferase is lacking in the tumorigenic-transformed cells (36). This enzymatic deficiency causes an alteration of the ganglioside pattern exactly as seen in the brain from the patient with G_{M3} sphingolipodystrophy (37). This enzymatic defect occurs only if the genome of the tumorigenic virus is inserted into the DNA of the host cell (38). These observations may be relevant to the situation in the patient, because 30 years before, a maternal uncle died at the age of two months with essentially the same symptoms as the propositus. These observations suggest an enzymatic defect that is caused by intercalation of viral DNA into one of the X-chromosomes of the infant's mother (and maternal grandmother). There are a number of important implications of this possibility that might be verified by DNA hybridization experiments. However, this investigation is very difficult in the present case because fibroblast cultures could not be established from the infant, although numerous attempts were made to do so. In addition, it should be noted that the infant did not have any obvious tumors. This may not be too surprising, because SV-40 is not tumorigenic in monkeys or other primates, and if a virus of this type is present in the genetic apparatus of the infant, it might not be expected to be tumorigenic. The major manifestation of the disorder in the central nervous system was extensive hypomyelination (39). Other work in this laboratory suggests that the pattern and metabolism of gangliosides play important roles in the formation of the myelin sheath (40). It was therefore not surprising that defective myelination is a primary manifestation of the inability to synthesize the higher ganglioside homologs. Certainly, careful consideration should be given to the possibility of this type of metabolic defect in other cases in which dysmyelination is a major pathological finding.

SUMMARY

A synopsis of the current status of the understanding of hereditary lipid-storage diseases is presented from the point of view of neonatologists and pediatricians who may be confronted with infants with such disorders. I have described the logic that can be applied in order to arrive at the correct diagnosis of these diseases and the type of laboratory determinations that may be used to confirm the nature of such disorders, as well as the signs and symptoms of a patient in whom it was recently discovered that the metabolic defect was a specific impairment of the synthesis of gangliosides. This lipodystrophy appears to be the prototype of a novel class of disorders caused by deficiencies of anabolic enzymes, and stands in sharp contrast to the abnormalities of catabolic enzymes in patients with previously described disorders of lipid metabolism.

REFERENCES

1. Brady, R. O., Kanfer, J. N., and Shapiro, D., Metabolism of glucocerebrosides II. Evidence of an enzymatic deficiency in Gaucher's disease, *Biochem. Biophys. Res. Commun.* **18**, 221 (1968).

2. Brady, R. O., Kanfer, J. N., Bradley, R. M., and Shapiro, D., Demonstration of a deficiency of glucocerebroside cleaving enzyme in Gaucher's disease, *J. Clin. Invest.* **45**, 1112 (1966).

3. Brady, R. O., Kanfer, J. N., Mock, M. B., and Fredrickson, D. S., The metabolism of sphingomyelin II. Evidence of an enzymatic deficiency in Niemann–Pick disease, *Proc. Nat. Acad. Sci. U.S.A.* **55**, 366 (1966).

4. Kampine, J. R. et al., Diagnosis of Gaucher's disease and Niemann-Pick disease with small samples of venous blood. *Science* **155**, 86 (1967).

5. Ho, M. W., et al., Adult Gaucher's disease: Kindred studies and demonstration of a deficiency of acid β-glucosidase in cultured fibroblasts, *Amer. J. Hum. Genet.* **24**, 37 (1972).

6. Sloan, H. R. et al., Deficiency of sphingomyelin-cleaving enzyme activity in tissue cultures derived from patients with Niemann-Pick disease, *Biochem. Biophys. Res. Commun.* **34**, 582 (1969).

7. Beutler, E. and Kuhl, W., Diagnosis of the adult type of Gaucher's disease and its carrier state by demonstration of a deficiency of β-glucosidase activity in peripheral blood leukocytes, *J. Lab. Clin. Med.* **76**, 747 (1970).

8. Brady, R. O., Johnson, W. G., and Uhlendorf, B. W., Identification of heterozygous carriers of lipid storage diseases, *Am. J. Med.* **51**, 423 (1971).

9. Okada, S. and O'Brien, J. S., Generalized gangliosidosis: Beta-galactosidase deficiency, *Science* **160**, 1002 (1968).

10. Brady, R. O., O'Brien, J. S., Bradley, E. M., and Gal, A. E., Sphingolipid hydrolases in brain tissue of patients with generalized gangliosidosis, *Biochim. Biophys. Acta.* **210**, 194 (1970).

11. Sandhoff, K., Andreae, U., and Jatzkewitz, H., Deficient hexosaminidase activity in an exceptional case of Tay-Sachs disease with additional storage of kidney globoside in visceral organs, *Life Sci.* **7**, 283 (1968).

12. Brady, R. O., The sphingolipidoses, *N. Engl. J. Med.* **275**, 312 (1966).

13. Kolodny, E. H., Brady, R. O., and Volk, B. W., Demonstration of an alteration of ganglioside metabolism in Tay-Sachs disease, *Biochem. Biophys. Res. Commun.* **37**, 526 (1969).

14. Tallman, J. F., Johnson, W. G., and Brady, R. O., The metabolism of Tay-Sachs ganglioside: Catabolic studies with lysosomal enzyme from normal and Tay-Sachs brain tissue, *J. Clin. Invest.* **51**, 2339 (1972).

15. Okada, S. and O'Brien, J. S., Tay-Sachs disease: Generalized absence of a beta-D-N-acetylhexosaminidase component, *Science* **165**, 698 (1969).

16. Tallman, J. F. and Brady, R. O., The catabolism of Tay-Sachs ganglioside in rat brain lysosomes, *J. Biol. Chem.* **247**, 7570 (1972).

17. Brady, R. O., Tallman, J. F., Johnson, W. G., and Quirk, J. M., An investigation of the metabolism of Tay-Sachs ganglioside specifically labeled in critical portions of the molecule, *Adv. Exp. Med. Biol.* **19**, 277 (1972).

18. Tallman, J. F. et al., Isolation and relationship of human hexosaminidases, *J. Biol. Chem.* **249**, 3489 (1974).

19. Verpoorte, J. A., Purification of two β-N-acetyl-D-glucosaminidases from beef spleen, *J. Biol. Chem.* **247**, 4787 (1972).

20. Carroll, M. and Robinson, D., Immunological properties of N-acetyl-β-D-glucosaminidase of normal human liver and of G_{M2}-gangliosidosis liver, *Biochem. J.* **131**, 91 (1973).

21. Srivastava, S. K. and Beutler, E., Hexosaminidase A and hexosamidase B. Tay-Sachs and Sandhoffs disease, *Nature* **241**, 483 (1973).

22. Sandhoff, K., Harger, K., Wassle, W., and Jatzkewitz, H., Enzyme alterations and lipid storage in three variants of Tay-Sachs disease, *J. Neurochem.* **18**, 2469 (1971).

23. Navon, R., Padeh, B., and Adam, A., Apparent deficiency of hexosaminidase A in healthy members of a family with Tay-Sachs disease, *Am. J. Hum. Genet.* **25**, 287 (1973).

24. Viogoff, J., Buist, N. R. M., and O'Brien, J. S., Absence of β-N-acetyl-D-hexosaminidase A activity in a healthy woman, *Am. J. Hum. Genet.* **25**, 372 (1973).

25. Tallman, J. F., Navon, R., Brady, R. O., and Padeh, B., Ganglioside catabolism in hexosaminidase A deficient adults. *Nature* **252**, 254 (1974).

26. O'Brien, J. S. et al., Ganglioside storage diseases, *Fed. Proc.* **30**, 956 (1971).

27. Suzuki, Y. and Suzuki, K., Krabbe's globoid leukodystrophy: Deficiency of galactocerebrosidase in serum, leukocytes, and fibroblasts, *Science* **171**, 73 (1971).

28. Percy, A. K. and Brady, R. O., Metachromatic leukodystrophy: Diagnosis with samples of venous blood, *Science* **161**, 594 (1968).

29. Bach, G., Eisenberg, F. Jr., Cantz, M., and Neufeld, E. F., The defect in Hunter's syndrome: Deficiency of sulfoiduronate sulfatase, *Prod. Nat. Acad. Sci. U.S.A.* **70**, 2134 (1973).

30. Mehl, E. and Jatzkewitz, H., Cerebroside-3-sulfate as a physiological substrate of arylsulfatase A, *Biochim. Biophys. Acta* **151**, 619 (1968).

31. Brady, R. O. et al., Replacement therapy for inherited enzyme deficiency: Use of purified ceramidetrihexosidase in Fabry's disease, *N. Engl. J. Med.* **289**, 9 (1973).

32. Brady, R. O. et al., Replacement therapy for inherited enzyme deficiency: Use of purified glucocerebrosidase in Gaucher's disease, *N. Engl. J. Med.* **291**, 989 (1974).

33. Max, S. R. et al., G_{M3} (hematoside) sphingolipodystrophy, *N. Engl. J. Med.* **291**, 929 (1974).

34. Fishman, P. H. et al., Deficient ganglioside biosynthesis: A novel human sphingolipidosis, *Science* **187**, 68 (1975).

35. Brady, R. O., The abnormal biochemistry of inherited disorders of lipid metabolism, *Fed. Proc.* **32**, 1660 (1973).

36. Cumar, F. A. et al., Enzymatic block in the synthesis of gangliosides in DNA virus-transformed tumorigenic mouse cell lines, *Proc. Nat. Acad. Aci. U.S.A.* **67**, 757 (1970).

37. Mora, P. T., Brady, R. O., Bradley, R. M., and McFarland, V. W., Gangliosides in DNA virus-transformed and spontaneously transformed tumorigenic mouse cell lines. *Proc. Nat. Acad. Sci. U.S.A.* **63**, 1290 (1969).

38. Mora, P. T., Cumar, F. A., and Brady, R. O., A common biochemical change in SV40 and polyoma virus transformed mouse cells coupled to control of cell growth in culture, *Virology* **46**, 60 (1971).

39. Tanaka, J. et al., Cerebral sponginess and G_{M3} gangliosidosis, *J. Neuropathol. Exp. Neurol.* **34**, 249 (1975).

40. Brady, R. O. and Quarles, R. H., The enzymology of myelination, *Mol. Cell. Biochem.* **2**, 23 (1973).

Neonatal and General Aspects
of Cystic Fibrosis

PAUL A. DI SANT'AGNESE, M.D., Sc.D. (Med.)

PHILIP M. FARRELL, M.D., Ph.D.

Cystic fibrosis of the pancreas (mucoviscidosis) (1,2) has been recognized as a separate entity for less than 40 years. Before this, most patients with this disease died of broncho-pneumonia in infancy, but the basic disorder was unrecognized. It is the most recently described of the major chronic diseases of man and the most common semilethal heredi-tary disease in the United States. Cystic fibrosis is transmitted as a mendelian recessive trait and the homozygotes, who have all or most manifestations of the disease, are esti-mated to be not less than 1 in 2000 live births. Five per cent of the overall population in this country—that is to say, 10 million persons—carry the cystic fibrosis gene but have no clinically recognizable symptoms. Cystic fibrosis is primarily a disease of all groups of the Caucasian race; it is rare in people of Mongolian descent and in native African Negroes. In American Negroes the incidence is probably only 1 in 10 000 to 12 000 live births, although almost 2% of the American Negro population may carry the gene.

The disease received its misnomer because of the lesions seen at autopsy in the pan-creas, which attracted the attention of the early investigators. Cystic fibrosis, however, is a generalized disorder in which the pancreas is frequently, but not necessarily, involved.

Clinically, it is characterized by the triad: chronic pulmonary disease, pancreatic de-ficiency, and increased sweat electrolytes. A family history of cystic fibrosis is common; some patients develop a distinctive type of cirrhosis of the liver, glycosuria, and other protean clinical manifestations. Cystic fibrosis is also responsible for a significant pro-portion of intestinal obstruction in newborn infants. Some of the manifestations are present at birth or develop within the first few weeks of life (Table 1); others are manifested later.

PATHOLOGICAL CHARACTERISTICS

Changes are found throughout the body wherever mucus-secreting glands are present (3). Pathologically, the basic lesion consists of obstruction and dilatation of the secretory

Table 1. Timetable for Development of Clinical Manifestations in Cystic Fibrosis

Onset	Complication	Prevalence in CF pts., %	Frequency in pediatric patient population
Birth	Meconium ileus	5–10	15–25% of intestinal obstr. of newborn
Birth	Atresia (small intest.)	occasional	∼25%
Birth	Meconium peritonitis	occasional	frequent cause
Birth	Abnormal sweat	100	almost only cause
Birth	Abnormal mesonephric derivatives in males[a]	>90	one of the causes
Usually birth	Pancreatic deficiency	85–90	almost only cause
Infancy	Obstructive jaundice	rare	one of the causes
	Hypoalbuminemia	rare	one of the causes
	Hypoprothrombinemia	occasional	one of the causes
Usually infancy	Severe malabsorption	∼75–80	most common cause
Early childhood	Chronic lung disease	eventually 100	most common cause
Early childhood	Rectal prolapse	20–25	most common cause
Early childhood	Heat prostration	occasional	most common cause

Later childhood or adolescence: Various complications of pulmonary disease, sinusitis, nasal polyps, hepatic cirrhosis with portal hypertension, glucose intolerance and glycosuria, intestinal obstructive complications (intussusception, fecal masses, meconium ileus equivalent)

[a] Epididymis, seminal vesicles, vas deferens.

gland by abnormal secretions (Figure 1). The most striking manifestations are in the pancreas (Figure 2) and consist of fibrosis or fatty replacement of the exocrine parenchyma, dilatation of the acini, and obstruction of the ducts. Usually the islets of Langerhans are normally preserved. At birth the lesions are minimal, but obstruction of pancreatic ductules and of the acini may be seen, and these lesions are usually rapidly progressive within the first few months of life.

Localized foci of biliary obstruction and fibrosis are frequently found at autopsy and have been seen as early as three days after birth. In some patients, changes become progressively more extensive and cause a distinctive type of multilobular biliary cirrhosis with large, irregular nodules.

The lungs appear normal in most infants who have died of complications other than chronic lung disease in the first few days of life. However, rarely some initial bronchial obstruction and increased mucus secretion may be present. Later bronchial obstruction by abnormally behaving secretions is the rule, with consequent progressive chronic pulmonary disease, which leads to death in 90 to 95% of cases in periods of time varying from a few months or a few years to two or three decades. Other pathological changes that are present at birth include abnormalities of mesonephric derivatives in males; absence of the vas deferens is observed in about 95% of males with cystic fibrosis, presumably due to obstruction occurring during the early part of gestation.

Other pathological evidence of antenatal obstruction may be present: meconium ileus, atresia of the small intestine, or evidence of meconium peritonitis.

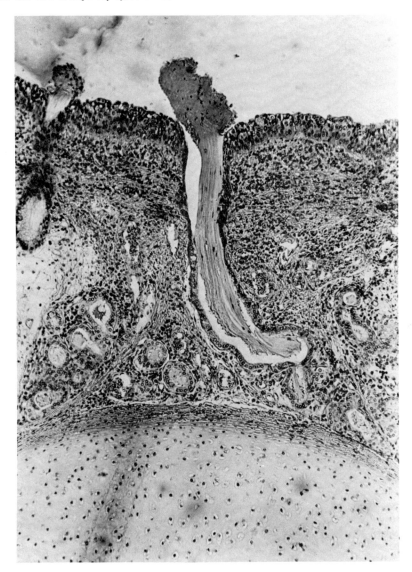

Figure 1. Microscopic section from trachea of a cystic fibrosis patient who died at six months of age. Dense eosinophilic concretion obstructs a duct of the tracheal gland. From *Nelson Textbook of Pediatrics*, 10th ed., V. C. Vaughan, III, and R. J. McKay, Eds., W. B. Saunders Co., Philadelphia, Pa., 1975, by permission.

The non-mucus-producing glands, such as the sweat glands and others, show no pathological changes, even though the chemical compositions of secretions may be markedly abnormal.

PATHOGENESIS

The unknown basic defect of cystic fibrosis leads primarily to two separate and distinct consequences: the sweat-electrolyte defect and the abnormality of "mucous secretions" (2).

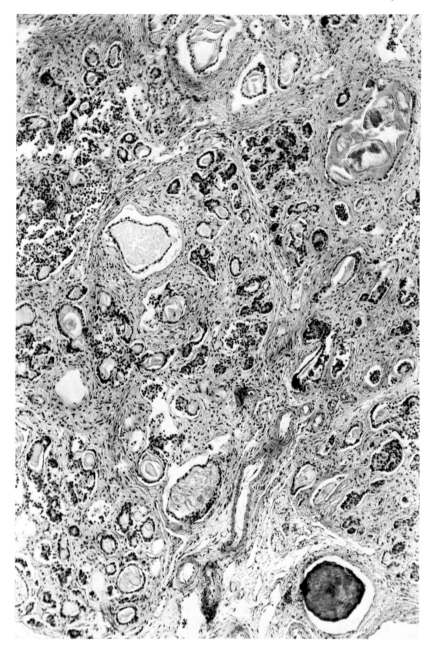

Figure 2. Microscopic section from pancreas of a cystic fibrosis patient who died at 14 months of age. Fibrosis, dilatation of ducts by eosinophilic inspissated secretion, calcified concretions, and almost complete disappearance of acini are evident. From *Nelson Textbook of Pediatrics*, 10th ed., V. C. Vaughan, III, and R. J. McKay, Eds., W. B. Saunders Co., Philadelphia, Pa., 1975, by permission.

The physicochemical abnormality of mucous secretions results in precipitation and obstruction of organ passages, causing virtually all of the clinical manifestations of cystic fibrosis. However, despite their abnormal physicochemical behavior, detailed chemical and immunological studies have thus far failed to reveal abnormalities of glycoproteins to account for this phenomenon.

The sweat-electrolyte defect is present at birth and throughout life. It is unrelated to either severity of the underlying disease or involvement of various organs. Patients with cystic fibrosis have sweat-chloride and sodium concentrations that are threefold to six-fold the hypotonic concentrations in normal individuals and in patients with almost any other disease. Mean sweat-potassium concentrations are statistically abnormal, but the overlap is too great to use this as a diagnostic test.

Except for Na, Cl, and K, the concentrations of most other solutes in sweat are normal, and the sweat glands in cystic fibrosis are morphologically and physiologically normal. This includes rate of sweating as well as the precursor solution in the sweat gland coil, as determined by micropuncture studies. Recent studies have indicated that there may be a factor present in biological fluids of patients with cystic fibrosis that inhibits sodium reabsorption in the sweat glands, thus giving reasonable explanation for the sweat-electrolyte defect. In contrast to untreated Addison's anemia, in which sweat electrolytes may also be abnormally increased, patients with cystic fibrosis have normal adrenal function, and renal conservation of electrolytes is unimpaired.

Studies have failed as yet to elucidate the basic defect (4,5). However, in tissue-culture fibroblasts obtained from skin biopsies of cystic fibrosis, homozygotes (and at times heterozygotes as well) show a number of abnormalities. These differ from laboratory to laboratory according to culture conditions, but include metachromasia, increase in acid mucopolysaccharides (glycosaminoglycuronoglycans) and high glycogen concentrations.

In both homozygotes and heterozygotes for the cystic fibrosis gene, a "cilio-toxic factor" is present in the serum that affects the symmetrical ciliary beat of epithelium obtained from oyster gills and from the trachea of mammals (e.g., rabbits). As previously mentioned, another substance is apparently found in sweat and saliva from cystic fibrosis homozygotes that inhibits sodium reabsorption. However, the experimental methods for demonstrating both of these "circulating CF factors" are difficult to perform and reproduce and have at present no practical application.

Recently the polyamine levels—and in particular the spermidine/spermine ratios in whole blood of both homozygote and heterozygote males—have been shown to be abnormal (6). Females show greater variability, probably related to hormonal changes during the menstrual cycle. These studies are being pursued at the present time and perhaps may help elucidate the basic defect and the possible relation of these abnormalities to the circulating factors.

It is important to realize that as yet none of these findings can be applied to either genetic counseling or antenatal diagnosis. In addition, these observations do suggest that cystic fibrosis is a truly generalized disease, with the gene probably expressed in every cell of the body. By analogy with the known heterogeneity of other inborn errors of metabolism (e.g., glycogen-storage disease, mucopolysaccharidoses, and others), as well as the very different clinical course of some patients, it appears possible that the cystic fibrosis syndrome in reality is a symptom complex that reflects more than one genetic error.

CLINICAL CHARACTERISTIC'S

Cystic fibrosis is not strictly a disease of neonates, but manifests itself often at the time of birth or during the first few weeks of life. Table 1 gives a timetable for the development of the clinical manifestations of cystic fibrosis. Several of the abnormalities, including the sweat defect, are present at birth.

Meconium ileus. This is the best known and most common of the perinatal obstructive complications and occurs in 5 to 10% of newborn infants with cystic fibrosis. Intestinal obstruction is present at birth; inspissated, grayish, rubbery meconium plugs the lumen of the small intestine, usually near the ileocecal valve. Proximal to it, a large amount of tenacious, viscid, abnormal meconium accumulates and leads to distention of the intestinal loop, which in a third of cases rotates upon itself, giving rise to volvulus. If the surgeon is unaware of the possibility of the occurrence of this combination, he may reduce the volvulus but disregard the obstruction. Distal to the obstructed segment, the colon is very small and apparently underdeveloped (microcolon) owing to disuse, but it returns to normal size within a few days after corrective surgery. Surgery is frequently necessary to relieve the obstruction. However, increasing success has been reported with the use of meglumine diatrizoate (Gastrografin®, Squibb) or sodium diatrizoate (Hypaque®, Winthrop) enemas to eliminate the obstructing meconium core. The patients who survive have the same course of the disease and outlook as all other fibrocystics. From Table 1 it can also be seen that meconium ileus is a complication in 15 to 25% of all patients with neonatal intestinal obstruction. Meconium ileus is always the result of cystic fibrosis, but it has been suggested that perhaps as many as 25% of patients with this complication may not have pancreatic involvement (3,7). The major factor in the pathogenesis of meconium ileus is undoubtedly the abnormal physicochemical character of intestinal secretions.

Small-intestinal atresia. This condition, resulting from antenatal volvulus (usually high in the small intestine) occurring early in fetal life, is probably due to a mechanism similar to the one in meconium ileus. There then is interference with the mesenteric blood supply and consequent perforation of the intestine, resulting in aseptic healing and the production of atresia or stenosis and frequently of meconium peritonitis. Cystic fibrosis is the cause of a significant proportion of the intestinal atresia seen in this country.

Pancreatic achylia. In 85 to 90% of patients with cystic fibrosis, pancreatic achylia is present. In the great majority, it is present at birth or in the first few weeks of life, but in some children involvement of this gland may not manifest itself until later. Untreated pancreatic insufficiency, especially among infants, leads to malnutrition despite a ravenous appetite, abdominal distention, and abnormal stools that are increased in number, bulky, greasy, and foul. On chemical examination of a three- to four-day pooled fecal specimen, marked and at times massive steatorrhea and azotorrhea are seen to be present. In contrast to fats, proteins are well tolerated, making it possible to obtain positive nitrogen balance through increased dietary intake. It has been clearly shown that soybean protein is not utilized as effectively by infants with cystic fibrosis as the protein of cow's milk and that hypoproteinemia and edema may result. Liposoluble vitamins are lost through the stools, and vitamin K deficiency and hypoprothrombinemia occasionally are the presenting symptoms. Deficiency of vitamins A and E is also found after a few weeks, but rarely gives rise to clinical symptoms. Vitamin-D-deficiency rickets apparently rarely occurs in cystic fibrosis. Lactosuria and sucrosuria are unexplained occurrences in a proportion of cystic fibrosis patients, at times even in infancy. Glucose intolerance and glycosuria usually do not develop until later in life.

   In countries with adequate diets and good public-health facilities, cystic fibrosis is at present the commonest cause of severe malabsorption in the pediatric age group. Cystic fibrosis in this country is also by far the commonest cause of prolapse of the rectum in infancy and childhood, although usually it is not seen until after a few months of life.

This complication occurs in as many as 15 to 20% of patients with cystic fibrosis and its mechanism is obscure, although symptomatic relief follows pancreatic-replacement therapy, and surgery is almost never needed.

Chronic pulmonary disease. Eventually, this disease is present in all patients and is frequently severe and progressive. However, the time of onset is variable; clinical manifestations may appear days, weeks, months, or years after birth.

When the onset is in the first few days or weeks after birth, after a variable period of coughing, generalized bronchial obstruction and obstructive emphysema appear. Alternatively, the pulmonary sequence is started at times by a sudden onset of bronchial obstruction and lobar atelectasis of one or more lobes (usually right upper lobe, or right middle lobe, or both). Generalized bronchial infection follows shortly after the obstruction and is apt to be distressingly severe. Bacterial flora from the nasopharynx, sputum, and lungs at autopsy consists primarily of *Staphylococcus aureus*. If repeated courses of antibiotic treatment are given, *Pseudomonas aeruginosa* (frequently mucoid), as the predominant or only organism, is eventually found. *Hemophilus influenzae*, *Escherichia coli*, proteus, and other bacterial species are isolated less frequently. Immunologically, patients with cystic fibrosis have been shown to develop good concentrations of circulating antibodies to pathogenic bacteria and in response to immunization and are thus competent with respect to humoral immunity. The concentrations of IgG and IgA in the serum are either normal or increased in relation to the presence of respiratory infection and severity, while IgM and IgE values are within normal limits. Cell-mediated immunity has not been adequately studied, but also appears to be normal. It is therefore difficult to explain the unusual susceptibility of patients with cystic fibrosis to respiratory infections. Bronchial obstruction preceding the pulmonary infection does not appear to be the whole answer.

Numerous complications arise in the course of severe pulmonary disease. These vary from the previously mentioned lobar atelectasis to the ones that develop later in the course of the illness: lung abscesses, recurrent pneumothorax, minor or massive hemoptysis, and eventually cor pulmonale. In older children, involvement of the paranasal sinuses is usually demonstrable roentgenographically. In the older age group, nasal polyps are a common manifestation.

Other complications. Many other complications occur after the neonatal period and at variable times during the course of the disease, such as (*a*) obstructive complications caused by inspissated or impacted feces owing to the abnormality of the fecal content (fecal masses, intussusception, volvulus, obduration); (*b*) clinically manifested cirrhosis of the liver with portal hypertension; (*c*) glucose intolerance with glycosuria; (*d*) acute pancreatitis and pancreatic lithiasis; (*e*) ocular lesions; (*f*) pulmonary hypertrophic osteoarthropathy; (*g*) massive salt loss and hypoelectrolytemia during sweating in hot weather; and (*h*) infertility because of aspermia in more than 95% of adult males (*1,8*).

DIAGNOSIS

The criteria for the diagnosis of cystic fibrosis are well established: elevated sweat electrolytes, chronic pulmonary disease, and pancreatic deficiency. At times not all three criteria are present, but in addition to an elevated sweat test, either chronic pulmonary disease or pancreatic insufficiency must be present. A family history of cystic fibrosis may be of diagnostic assistance in uncertain cases.

Pathological diagnosis in the newborn. The diagnostic situation one is faced with in a newborn may be quite different as the clinical manifestations of the disease may not have developed as yet. If death occurs in the neonatal period, firm diagnosis may rest upon autopsy findings. If, at postmortem examination, pancreatic lesions consisting of eosinophilic plugging of pancreatic ductules, dilatation of acini, and initial fibrosis are present, the diagnosis can easily be established, if it fits the clinical picture. In the absence of family history of the disease or of the characteristic lesions in the pancreas (10–15% of all patients and possibly a higher percentage in the neonatal period), it is frequently possible to make a probable or presumed diagnosis of cystic fibrosis based on the findings of ancillary pathologic lesions (3,7) as well as the preceding clinical (Table 2 and Figures 3 and 4) events.

Table 2. Perinatal Findings Compatible with Cystic Fibrosis in the Absence of Pathognomonic Lesions in the Pancreas

I. *Clinical findings:*

Meconium ileus
Small intestinal atresia
Meconium peritonitis
Pulmonary infection (usually after a few days or weeks of life)

II. *Pathological findings:*

Mucous gland hyperplasia (respiratory tract, duodenum, other GI, submaxillary)
Gallbladder mucoele or mucous metaplasia
Various intestinal "malformations" or volvulus
Abnormal male mesonephric derivatives (epididymis, seminal vesicles,
     obliteration of vas deferens)
Focal biliary cirrhosis

The "sweat test." After three weeks of age, the sweat test is the cornerstone of the laboratory diagnosis of cystic fibrosis (1,2). It is difficult to obtain a reliable test in the first three to four weeks of life, because the sweat glands do not appear to function adequately. The sweat test is the simplest and most reliable laboratory investigation for the diagnosis of cystic fibrosis. In view of the many factors that influence sweat composition (e.g., sweat rate, method of stimulation, salt intake), it is indeed surprising that this test has proved so reliable in diagnosis. This is mainly because of the wide separation of values between patients with cystic fibrosis and virtually all other normal or diseased subjects. For reliable results, it is essential that the test subject be in a stable clinical condition, because the effect of dehydration, severe malnutrition, and edema on sweat electrolytes has never been clearly established.

Quantitative tests of sweat induced by thermal stimulation in a constant-temperature room are used primarily for research. The preferred method at present for diagnostic purposes is pilocarpine iontophoresis, in which a small electric current is used to carry this cholinergic drug into the skin and stimulate sweat glands locally (Addendum I). It is safe, painless, and reliable for diagnostic purposes.

Qualitative sweat tests have been used for screening purposes. The reaction of chloride in palmar sweat with an appropriately treated agar plate or filter paper has been used for such testing. Conductivity of sweat, which is increased, has also been measured, using

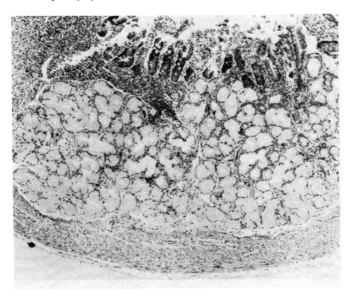

Figure 3. Duodenum showing hyperplasia of Brunner's glands, with at least seven areas of early cystic change. Baby died after partial ileectomy for ileal gangrene associated with meconium ileus (H & E, ×75) (7). From Oppenheimer, E. H., and Esterly, J. D., *Arch. Path.* 96, 149–154 (1973), by permission.

modifications of the conventional Wheatstone conductivity bridge. None of these procedures should be relied upon for a definitive diagnosis. If cystic fibrosis is suspected, a quantitative sweat test by pilocarpine iontophoresis should be obtained. With this method, from infancy to the age of 18 or 20 years, a concentration of more than 60 mmol (60 mEq) sweat chloride/litre is diagnostic of cystic fibrosis (Figure 5A), if it agrees with the clinical picture; values between 50–60 mmol/litre (50–60 mEq/litre) are highly

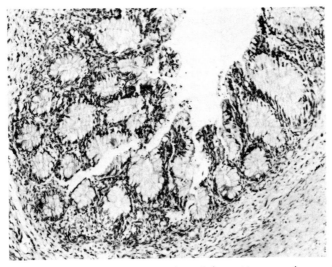

Figure 4. Goblet-cell hyperplasia in colon. Newborn infant with ruptured meconium ileus, who died 2 h after birth. Pancreas histologically normal (H & E, ×150) (7). From Oppenheimer, E. H., and Esterly, J. D., *Arch. Path.* 96, 149–154 (1973), by permission.

suggestive. Values for sweat sodium average about 10 mmol/litre higher than those for chloride (Figure 5B). Potassium concentration in sweat is significantly different on a statistical basis between patients and controls; however, because of the overlap in results, potassium determination has no diagnostic value in the single individual. It is generally agreed that for diagnostic purposes analysis for chloride in sweat is slightly more reliable than analysis for sweat sodium, probably for technical reasons. However, both should be routinely determined. Greater caution is needed to interpret results in an older age group (after 20 years of age), for sweat electrolyte concentrations may be somewhat higher and more variable in adults. In mixed saliva there is also a significant difference in the mean chloride and sodium values between patients with cystic fibrosis and others; however, the overlap is so great that this observation has no practical application. There are few conditions other than cystic fibrosis in which sweat electrolytes may be abnormally high. Untreated adrenal insufficiency and some cases of renal diabetes insipidus are the most

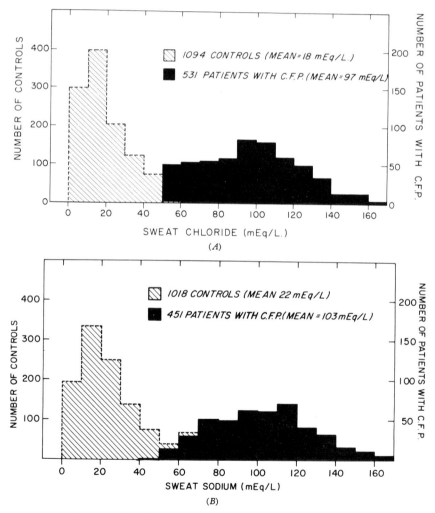

Figure 5. Sweat chloride (*A*) and sodium (*B*) values in patients with cystic fibrosis and control subjects. Pediatric age group, up to age 20 years. From di Sant'Agnese, P. A., and Powell, G. F., *Ann. N. Y. Acad. Sci.* **93**, 555–599 (1962), by permission.

important. However, neither of these is a problem in the neonatal period. It has been repeatedly stressed that all infants, children, adolescents, and young adults with either recurrent respiratory infections or symptomatic malabsorption not clearly explained otherwise (e.g., immunoglobulin deficiency and other diseases) should routinely have a sweat test as part of their diagnostic evaluation.

Assay of duodenal content for determination of pancreatic enzyme activity usually need not be done unless the diagnosis is unsettled after a quantitative sweat test. From a practical standpoint, determination of the proteolytic enzymes by one of the chemical procedures is sufficient. In particular, the new, rapid spectrophotometric methods are especially useful (9,10). Cystic fibrosis accounts for virtually all pancreatic deficiency in childhood, although other rare causes of pancreatic achylia do exist (e.g., hypoplasia of exocrine pancreas, familial pancreatitis, and others). In all of the latter patients, sweat test results are normal.

Other laboratory tests. Most other laboratory tests are noncontributory. In particular, serum electrolytes are within the normal range in patients with cystic fibrosis when they are reasonably well clinically. When there is severe pulmonary disease, the serum electrolyte pattern is apt to be that of compensated—or at times uncompensated—respiratory acidosis. There is hypoelectrolytemia in patients with heat prostration and shock resulting from the massive outpouring of electrolytes in sweat during hot weather, although this sequence is not apt to occur in young infants. We have, however, observed a number of infants who gradually developed negative salt balance, even in winter, and eventually developed severe dehydration and a very low serum-sodium value. Indeed, if this clinical situation is encountered (11), the possibility of cystic fibrosis (in addition to that of adrenal insufficiency) should be contemplated. Hypoprothrombinemia and hypoalbuminemia are especially likely to occur in young infants. The usual limited tests of liver function frequently give no evidence of hepatic impairment. However, a recent study of 49 patients with cystic fibrosis (12), age 3 to 41 years, revealed that about a third had serological evidence of hepatobiliary disease before clinical signs were evident. The transaminases (EC 2.6.1.1, 2.6.1.2), α-glutamyltransferase (EC 2.3.2.2), and the liver isoenzyme of alkaline phosphatase (EC 3.1.3.2) appear to be the most reliable indicators of this complication.

Roentgenograms of the chest are usually not helpful in the perinatal period. However, in an occasional patient within the first few days of life, generalized emphysema is present to a varying degree and suggests the possibility of cystic fibrosis. This disease is also the most frequent single cause of lobar atelectasis (especially right upper and right middle lobe) during the first few months of life, but after the neonatal period. Again, cystic fibrosis should be thought of under such circumstances.

Newborn Screening Tests

In recent years, there has been considerable interest in developing a simple and reliable method that could be applied to population surveys or to mass testing of newborns for cystic fibrosis. None of the methods proposed so far has withstood the test of time. For a screening test to be truly effective it must be simple, reliable, and inexpensive. Specifically, in cystic fibrosis its importance is to assess more precisely the true incidence of the disease and to allow for proper genetic counseling as well as recognition and early initiation of treatment.

Specific-ion electrodes.   These have been tried for determining sodium and chloride on the skin's surface. However, many disadvantages have been noted (*13*), including the failure of some subjects to sweat sufficiently, leading to a requirement for artificial sweat stimulation. The method is expensive and personnel require special training. Therefore, skin electrodes to measure sweat electrolytes have not found acceptance as a method for mass screening of newborns and have not replaced the usual sweat test done after three weeks of age.

Screening tests based on albumin in meconium.   The best possibility for mass screening of newborns is based on the fact that albumin in meconium is increased in cystic fibrosis patients, if they have pancreatic deficiency. Presumably, this occurs because albumin ingested with amniotic fluid is not degraded adequately because pancreatic enzymes are absent. Several methods are available (*14*), but the best one seems to be the test-tape determination developed in Germany, which is commercially available.[1] With ascending chromatography on a paper test strip and tetrabromophenolphthalein-ethylester as an indicator, it measures protein concentrations in meconium of more than 20 mg/g dry weight, resulting in an intense ink-blue coloration; the end-point is thus easy to read. It is important to use the first portion of meconium, or the second, as it is known that albumin concentration decreases with consecutive meconium specimens. The test takes only 10 min and the training of personnel is considered to be relatively simple. In Europe, each test has been estimated to cost between fifteen cents and one dollar.

Several different countries in Western Europe, as well as a few groups in the United States, have collaborated in trials of this test (*15*). So far, 34 000 newborn infants, chosen without conscious bias, have been examined, among whom 19 neonates had positive results for this test. Apparently, few falsely positive tests were obtained if properly trained personnel were applying the test strip; but three infants later found to have cystic fibrosis had negative tests. It should be realized that there are serious theoretical limitations to this test, leading to both false negatives and false positives. Patients with cystic fibrosis who do not have pancreatic deficiency will not be detected with this method because their digestion of ingested albumin is normal. This category accounts for at least 10 to 15% of all patients with cystic fibrosis in childhood; but as previously mentioned, the frequency may be higher at birth. Conversely, because this and other similar screening tests measure total protein rather than albumin specifically, other infants who have conditions leading to increased protein content of meconium may also be positive, the commonest case being that of occult gastrointestinal bleeding. It has been suggested (*14*) that meconium samples that give positive tests should be followed up in the same hospital with protein electrophoresis to determine whether albumin is increased or if other protein fractions are responsible for the positive result. It is, of course, essential to evaluate all patients who give positive tests with a pilocarpine iontophoresis sweat test after the age of three to four weeks. In the meantime, these patients should be considered as possible fibrocystics, on the reasonable assumption that proper dietary or antibiotic measures will do the patient no harm if he has clinical symptoms of either malabsorption or pulmonary disease, while on the other hand a great deal might be lost if such a patient is not properly treated, but really does have cystic fibrosis.

In summary, the Boehringer Mannheim test appears to be the best method presently available for screening of newborns because it meets two of the previously mentioned

---

[1] Boehringer Mannheim Corp., Mannheim, West Germany (in U.S.A.: 219 E. 44th St., New York, N.Y. 10017).

criteria for a screening test: It is simple and inexpensive. However, it may fail to meet the third criterion, because it is only moderately reliable.

Diagnosis of Cystic Fibrosis in Adults

Even though the focus of this monograph is the newborn, the present discussion would be incomplete if the special difficulties of diagnosis in adolescents and young adults were not mentioned. Clinical chemists will occasionally encounter this situation, and may have to give some evaluation as to the merits of the sweat test in comparison to the other diagnostic criteria. The diagnosis of cystic fibrosis may be especially difficult in patients seen for the first time as adolescents or young adults because they often do not present what physicians visualize as the classic textbook picture of the disease, i.e., a small, wasted, chronically-ill-appearing patient. Indeed, some of them are tall, well nourished, and relatively healthy looking. Under these circumstances, the criteria required for a definitive diagnosis should be more rigid than in children, especially in view of the moderately increased values for mean sweat electrolytes that occur after age 15 to 20 years. There are virtually no conditions other than cystic fibrosis that give values above 80 to 90 mmol chloride or sodium/litre, even in the older age group. Therefore, if the sweat test is abnormal (especially if values exceed these) and there is a combination of chronic pulmonary symptoms and malabsorption, the correct diagnosis may be ascertained even in this age group. Although duodenal drainage for measurement of tryptic and other pancreatic enzyme activities is no longer done routinely in children, it is recommended in these older individuals.

As an aid to diagnosis in adult patients, the "dynamic test" has been advocated (2), in which the difference in response of sweat electrolytes to administration of salt-retaining steroids is assessed between normal subjects and fibrocystic patients. However, the more recent findings of a significant and variable decrease in sweat sodium in patients with cystic fibrosis after exogenous administration of aldosterone makes it difficult, if not impossible, to use this test as a diagnostic aid (1,2).

Other Tests for Diagnosis

For the sake of completeness, it should be mentioned that characteristic pathological changes in specimens of rectal mucosa obtained by rectal biopsy and of labial salivary glands obtained by punch biopsy have been advocated as diagnostic aids, especially in patients beyond the first few months of life. We have not found it necessary so far to use either of these two methods. Assay of nail clippings for sodium content also seemed like a useful possibility in distinguishing between cystics and other patients, especially as they can be sent by mail. However, the results have been very variable in and among various laboratories and the increased sodium content of the nails is presumably due merely to a "sponge" effect of the sweat. The method, therefore, has not found wide acceptance.

PROGNOSIS

During the perinatal period, the major problem is intestinal obstruction (meconium ileus or small intestinal atresia), owing to the nature of the complication and the possibility of additional surgical or postsurgical complications. Infants who survive neonatal intestinal obstruction have essentially the same prognosis as do other patients with cystic fibrosis. There are generally no respiratory symptoms in the first few days or even in the first few weeks of life; however, the possibility of an early onset of chronic pulmonary disease, even in the first few days of life, exists.

Later the pulmonary involvement usually dominates the clinical picture and determines the fate of the patient. The effects of pancreatic deficiency are less important to the ultimate outlook and usually not difficult to manage with dietary measures, especially after the first few months of life.

Ninety per cent or more of patients, after a prolonged illness, eventually die of pulmonary insufficiency; however, uncontrollable bleeding attributable to portal hypertension and massive loss of salt in hot weather occasionally are fatal hazards in this disease.

No precise figures are available on survival; a reasonable estimate is a mean life-span of 15 to 20 years. Some patients with cystic fibrosis die in infancy or early childhood, but an increasingly large number survive 20 or 30 years or longer. Although early diagnosis, early treatment, and aggressive therapy during serious pulmonary complications are effective in prolonging the life of patients, the natural variation in the severity of cystic fibrosis—and especially in the degree of pulmonary involvement—is an equally important factor in determining the outcome. As in other genetic diseases, differences in penetration or variations in the genetic error may account for these findings.

TREATMENT

It should be appreciated that until the basic defect is uncovered, a fully effective and lasting treatment cannot be devised. At present, therapy is mainly palliative, aimed at combating, slowing, or preventing some of the secondary or tertiary complications of this disease.

Principles of treatment (1,16) that should be kept in mind are as follows:

Therapy should be individualized.

Active therapy of pulmonary involvement deserves the major emphasis.

Dietary measures are needed only when pancreatic deficiency is present and especially in the young age group.

Additional salt intake is required by all patients exposed to hot weather (unless contraindicated by cor pulmonale) regardless of the pancreatic status.

All routine immunizations (e.g., diphtheria, tetanus, measles, polio) should be given at the usual times.

Therapy of pulmonary involvement. As previously mentioned, in the neonatal period or first few weeks of life, respiratory disease is usually not a problem. But if there is an early onset of pulmonary infection, antibiotic therapy is mandatory. Some small infants with cystic fibrosis may have a considerable degree of bronchiolitis which has been improved at times by the administration of steroids.

In general, treatment of pulmonary involvement is based on: (*a*) evacuation of mucopurulent secretions by physical methods and at times by use of aerosol solutions and (*b*) appropriate and timely use of antimicrobial agents to combat infection. Both of these modes of therapy are essential to therapeutic success.

It is generally agreed that physical therapy to relieve bronchial obstruction due to accumulated secretions is needed continuously by patients with even minimal pulmonary involvement. Clapping, cupping, postural drainage, deep breathing, assisted coughing, thoracic squeezing, and vibration are used. Inhalational therapy by "interrupted" aerosol therapy (if the patient's age permits) or the mist tent is used at times to hydrate secretions and thus assist other physical therapy methods.

Therapeutic courses of intensive antibiotic therapy (usually for not less than one to three weeks) are indicated in an attempt to halt progressive deterioration during acute exacerbation of pulmonary disease. To be effective, it is important that these drugs be carefully chosen and given in sufficient dosage over an adequate period (16). The routes of administration selected depend on severity and acuteness of the disease and on the type of antibiotic agent to be used. Whenever possible, the choice of the antimicrobial drug should be based on the results of sputum or nasopharyngeal cultures and tests of susceptibility to antibiotics of the isolated bacterial pathogens. Based on the most frequent flora of the respiratory tract in patients with cystic fibrosis, as previously mentioned, an anti-staphylococcus agent is usually selected together with one or both of the anti-pseudomonas drugs—gentamicin and carbenicillin—for treatment of acute exacerbations.

Aerosol antibiotic therapy is to be regarded as a form of topical treatment, but only as an adjunct to systemic administration during periods of intensive antibiotic therapy. In many clinicians' experience, most severely ill patients cannot be effectively controlled without continued antibiotic therapy for months or even years, and a broad-spectrum antibiotic agent is frequently needed.

Dietary therapy. The consequences of pancreatic deficiency can be readily obviated with dietary therapy in conjunction with administration of one of the pancreatic extracts. The patient's appetite should be a guide to the intake and the diet should be high in protein and calories and moderate in fat content. Fairly strict dietary measures usually are needed in infancy and early childhood when commercially available powdered high-protein milk preparations can be used to advantage. Subsequently, skim milk is advised until later childhood when homogenized milk can be given if the patient tolerates it. Soybean milk preparations should not be used in infancy as they may lead to hypoproteinemia and edema. Supplementation with medium-chain-length triglycerides has been used with some success. Anabolic steroids are of some use in increasing appetite and promoting weight gain; but to avoid side effects, only short, repeated courses are recommended. There is no substantial evidence that they improve respiratory disease. If lactase (β-galactosidase, EC 3.2.1.23) deficiency is present and symptomatic, it may be necessary to limit the dietary lactose intake.

Dietary measures appear to become less necessary with advancing age, although individual variations are found. In general, the nutritional state is more closely correlated to the severity of the pulmonary infection than to the pancreatic function.

Treatment of abnormal salt loss. Additional sodium chloride (1–4 g/day, according to weight) should be given to all patients exposed to hot weather (regardless of pancreatic status), if cor pulmonale does not contraindicate it. Massive salt depletion through prolonged sweating in hot weather may present a real medical emergency. As much as 10 ml of isotonic saline solution i.v. per kilogram body weight, administered in 15 min, may be needed in infant patients whose extracellular fluid volume is severely depleted and who are in imminent danger of cardiovascular collapse. This is to be followed by appropriate fluid and electrolyte replacement therapy.

Other treatment may be needed but usually only after a few months or years of life. Various surgical and medical methods are used to treat the many complications of this protean disease, including those resulting from chronic pulmonary disease (hemoptysis, pneumothorax, cor pulmonale, etc.), portal hypertension, glycosuria, nasal polyps, and many others (1).

SUMMARY

Cystic fibrosis, the most common semilethal generalized hereditary disease in the United States, is characterized clinically by a triad of symptoms: chronic pulmonary disease, pancreatic deficiency, and elevated sweat electrolytes. It is transmitted as a mendelian recessive trait and may be a symptom complex that is the result of more than one genetic error.

The basic pathological lesion consists of obstruction and dilatation of the secretory gland by abnormal secretions. The most striking manifestations are in the pancreas, but localized foci of biliary obstruction and fibrosis are frequently found at autopsy in the newborn. Lungs appear normal in most infants who have died of complications other than chronic lung disease in the first few days of life.

The unknown basic defect in cystic fibrosis leads to (*a*) high sweat-electrolyte concentrations and (*b*) abnormal behavior of "mucous secretions" with consequent obstruction of organ passages resulting in most clinical and pathological manifestations of the disease. The sweat-electrolyte defect is present at birth and throughout life and unrelated to either severity of the underlying disease or involvement of various organs. Tissue culture abnormalities, the "circulating CF factors," and altered blood polyamine concentrations have been found in homozygotes and heterozygotes for this gene. However, none of these findings can be applied as yet to either genetic counseling or antenatal diagnosis.

Cystic fibrosis is not strictly a disease of neonates, but often manifests itself at birth or during the first few weeks of life. A typical timetable for development of the clinical manifestations in this disease is presented. Meconium ileus, small intestinal atresia, pancreatic achylia, and the sequence of events in chronic pulmonary disease are described in some detail. The flora of the respiratory tract consists primarily of *Staphylocossus aureus hemolyticus* or *Pseudomonas aeruginosa*. Patients with cystic fibrosis are immunologically competent.

If death occurs in the neonatal period, diagnosis is necessarily based on autopsy findings. If the typical pancreatic changes are not present, it is frequently possible to make the diagnosis based on ancillary clinical and pathologic lesions.

After birth, the criteria for diagnosis of cystic fibrosis are: elevated sweat electrolytes, chronic pulmonary disease, and pancreatic deficiency. After the patient is three weeks of age, a quantitative sweat test by pilocarpine iontophoresis is the cornerstone of the laboratory diagnosis of this disease. It is difficult to obtain a reliable test in the first three to four weeks of life because the sweat glands do not appear to function adequately. Qualitative sweat tests and measures of conductivity of sweat are not reliable. Biopsies of the rectum and of labial salivary glands and analysis of nail clippings for sodium content have been advocated as diagnostic aids, but are not recommended. All infants, children, adolescents, and young adults with either recurrent respiratory infections or symptomatic malabsorption not clearly explained otherwise should routinely have a quantitative sweat test as part of their diagnostic evaluation. Even though this is a symposium on newborns, a brief discussion is given of the special difficulties of diagnosis in adolescents and young adults.

Assays of duodenal content for determination of pancreatic enzyme activity need not usually be done unless there is a question as to the diagnosis. In such cases new, rapid spectrophotometric methods for determination of proteolytic enzyme activity are useful. With few exceptions most other laboratory tests are noncontributory. Roentgenograms of the chest are usually not helpful in the perinatal period.

Few of the procedures proposed so far for newborn screening for cystic fibrosis have withstood the test of time. The best method at present seems to be based on a test tape that detects the high albumin content of meconium in most infants with cystic fibrosis. This test appears to be fairly simple and moderately inexpensive; however, it is only moderately reliable as it will not detect patients who have cystic fibrosis without pancreatic deficiency. Conversely, other infants may give a falsely positive result if they have conditions leading to increased protein content of meconium (e.g., gastrointestinal bleeding).

Prognostically, during the perinatal period the major problem in cystic fibrosis is intestinal obstruction. Later, the pulmonary involvement dominates the clinical picture and determines the fate of the patient. The effects of pancreatic deficiency are less important to the ultimate outlook. The mean life-span is estimated to be 15 to 20 years, although many patients with cystic fibrosis die in infancy or early childhood while an increasing number live to 30 years of age or even longer. As in other genetic diseases, difference in penetration or variation of the genetic error may account for these differences.

Principles of treatment are given. Dietary therapy, as well as treatment of abnormal salt loss, and especially therapy of pulmonary involvement are briefly outlined.

ADDENDUM: SWEAT TEST BY PILOCARPINE IONTOPHORESIS

An electric current source should supply direct current at 0–22 V. The current passing between electrodes is measured with a milliamperemeter that accurately records variations between 0 and 5 milliamperes. A simple wiring diagram for a battery-operated machine has been given by Gibson and Cooke (*17*); various models are also commercially available.

The area to be iontophoresed is washed with distilled water and dried. The flexor surface of the forearm is used except in small infants, in whom the thigh may be substituted. Two milliliters of pilocarpine nitrate (2 ml/litre) is pipetted onto a 2 × 2 inch gauze square placed on a positive copper electrode (1.8 × 1.8 inches), which is then applied to the washed area. A negative copper electrode of similar size (permanently covered with gauze) is placed elsewhere on the same extremity, its gauze covering wet with isotonic sodium chloride solution. Both electrodes are firmly attached with rubber straps of the kind used for electrocardiography. The lead wires are then connected and the current is gradually raised to 4 mA in 15 to 20 s. Iontophoresis is continued for 5 min. A current of 4 mA passing through a 25-cm^2 area of skin is barely detectable, but if the positive electrode is not completely covered with gauze or if the contact with the skin is poor, the current passes through a much smaller area and gives rise to a burning sensation. In this case, momentary pressure should be applied to the offending electrode, or the strap should be tightened.

After completion of iontophoresis, the electrodes are removed, the gauze with pilocarpine solution is discarded, and the area of skin under the positive electrode is washed with distilled water and dried. A thin pad of dry gauze, 2 inches square (a brand with low sodium content), or a low-ash filter paper of similar size, is removed from a flask (in which it was previously weighed) and placed over the area of skin in which the pilocarpine was iontophoresed. The gauze or filter paper is then covered with a plastic square (1.5 $\times$ 2.5 inches) and sealed at the edges with waterproof adhesive tape to prevent evaporation. The collection gauze or filter paper is left in place for 30 to 45 min and then reweighed in the same flask. The difference between the second and the first weights represents the amount of sweat collected (usually 100–600 mg). To avoid contamination of the gauze or filter paper by fingers, one should use a forceps for all steps.

The sweat is then eluted from the gauze or filter paper with distilled water or other appropriate solution and analyzed for chloride by one of the titration methods (Cotlove Chloride Titrator preferred), and for sodium by flame photometry or atomic-absorption spectrophotometry.

Main Cautions in Performing and Interpreting a Sweat Test

1. The quantity of sweat for analysis should not be less than 100 mg.

2. If the gauze or filter paper collecting sweat is not sealed adequately evaporation may cause the electrolyte values to be higher than they are in reality.

3. The dilutions used to elute sweat and analyze for sodium are markedly different from those used to determine serum sodium. This is perhaps the most frequent cause of error.

4. The subject to be tested must be in stable clinical condition when the test is done. Otherwise, interpretation of results may be erroneous.

REFERENCES

1. di Sant'Agnese, P. A., The pancreas. In *Nelson Textbook of Pediatrics*, 10th ed., V. C. Vaughan, III and R. J. McKay, Eds., W. B. Saunders Co., Philadelphia, 1975.

2. di Sant'Agnese, P. A. and Talamo, R. C., Pathogenesis and physiopathology of cystic fibrosis of the pancreas, *N. Engl. J. Med.* 277, 1287–1295, 1343–1352, 1399–1408 (1967).

3. Oppenhiemer, E. H. and Esterly, J. R., Pathology of cystic fibrosis. In *Perspectives in Pediatric Pathology*, H. S. Rosenberg, Ed., Yearbook Publishers, Chicago.

4. Editorial: Developments in cystic fibrosis research. *Lancet* ii, 307–308 (1973).

5. Polly, M. J. and Bearn, A. G., Cystic fibrosis: Current concepts, *J. Med. Genet.* 11, 249–252 (1974).

6. Lundgren, D. W., Farrell, P. M., and di Sant'Agnese, P. A., Polyamine alterations in blood of homozygotes and heterozygotes for cystic fibrosis, *Clin. Chim. Acta* 62, 357 (1975).

7. Oppenheimer, E. H. and Esterly, J. R., Cystic fibrosis of the pancreas. *Arch. Pathol.* 96, 149–154 (1973).

8. Taussig, L. M. et al., Fertility in males with cystic fibrosis, *N. Engl. J. Med.* 287, 586–589 (1972).

9. Schwert, G. W. and Takenaka, Y., A spectrophotometric determination of trypsin and chymotrypsin, *Biochim. Biophys. Acta* 16, 570 (1955).

10. Hummel, B. C. W., A modified spectrophotometric determination of chymotrypsin, trypsin and thrombin, *Can. J. Biochem.* 37, 1393 (1959).

11. di Sant'Agnese, P. A., Salt depletion in cold weather in infants with cystic fibrosis of the pancreas, *J. Am. Med. Assoc.* 172, 2014-2021 (1960).

12. Kattwinkel, J., Taussig, L. M., Statland, B. E., and Verter, J. I., The effects of age on alkaline phosphatase and other serologic liver function tests in normal subjects and patients with cystic fibrosis, *J. Pediatr.* **82,** 234–242 (1973).

13. Kopito, L. and Shwachman, H., Studies in cystic fibrosis: Determination of sweat electrolytes in situ with direct reading electrodes, *Pediatrics* **43,** 794 (1969).

14. Prosser, R. et al., Screening for cystic fibrosis by examination of meconium, *Arch. Dis. Child.* **49,** 597–601 (1974).

15. Stephan, U., Busch, E. W., Kollberg, H., and Hellsing, K., Cystic fibrosis detection by means of a test-strip, *Pediatrics* **55,** 35–38 (1975).

16. di Sant'Agnese, P. A., Cystic fibrosis. In *Current Pediatric Therapy*, 6th ed., S. S. Gellis, and B. M. Kagan, Eds., W. B. Saunders Co., Philadelphia, Pa., 1973, pp. 229–236.

17. Gibson, L. E. and Cooke, R. E., A test for concentration of electrolytes in sweat in cystic fibrosis of the pancreas utilizing pilocarpine by iontophoresis, *Pediatrics* **23,** 545–549 (1959).

18. di Sant'Agnese, P. A. and Powell, G. F., The eccrine sweat defect in cystic fibrosis of the pancreas (mucoviscidosis), *Ann. N. Y. Acad. Sci.* **93,** 555–599 (1962).

Immunological Responses
of the Newborn

JOSEPH A. BELLANTI, M.D.

During its nine-month gestation, the mammalian fetus is not ordinarily called upon to demonstrate immunological capabilities. Protected in its intrauterine environment from infectious agents and antigens, the fetus is in a sense immunologically pristine. Nonetheless, the cells that go to make up the immunological system appear early in fetal life, even though they are fully activated only after birth when the neonate has begun to interact with his environment. Several observations now support the view that the human fetus and neonate, though capable of responding, have an impaired state of resistance to a wide variety of microorganisms. The devastating effects of congenital infection with rubella in the fetus (as contrasted with the disease in the older child) and the overwhelming sepsis caused by relatively noninvasive Gram-negative bacteria are but two examples of how the stage of immunological development at the time of infection may dramatically affect disease expression. In this presentation, the relationship of normal physiological and biochemical processes to disease states will be emphasized, together with the necessity for an understanding of the relationship between the results of tests performed in the clinical laboratory and underlying pathological processes.

COMPONENTS OF THE IMMUNOLOGIC SYSTEM

Resistance to infectious diseases involves all of the host's immunological capability, which is implemented by a variety of cell types and cell products that interact in the recognition and disposal of microbial agents (1,2). For ease of discussion, these components may be subdivided into primary (nonspecific), secondary (specific), and tertiary (tissue-injuring) responses (Figure 1).

Primary (Nonspecific) Immune Responses

Primary responses consist of the inflammatory response and phagocytosis (Figure 1). In the adult, these responses are carried out primarily by polymorphonuclear leukocytes,

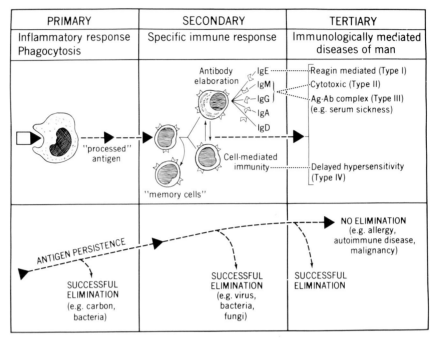

Figure 1. Schematic representation of the total immunological capability of the host, based upon efficiency with which foreign matter is eliminated. From Bellanti, J. A., *Immunology*, W. B. Saunders Co., 1971.

macrophages (monocytes), and eosinophils, either alone or in concert with the complement system and specific antibody (opsonins).

In the immunologically competent host, most foreign substances, including nonvirulent organisms (e.g., certain bacteria and viruses), are effectively cleared by phagocytic processes alone. In the case of organisms that have acquired virulent or pathogenic characteristics, however, phagocytosis alone may be ineffective, and antibody and complement (opsonins) must supplement phagocytosis for the complete destruction of the organism. In the case of the developing fetus and neonate, several maturational deficiencies of both phagocytosis and inflammatory response exist, and these may explain not only the unusually great susceptibility to infection at this time of life but also the different pathological expressions of disease.

The complement system. The complement system consists of 11 discrete serum proteins that can be activated by a variety of stimuli as a consequence of the antigen-antibody reaction or by a number of other alternative systems such as the clotting system. During this activation, several biologically active products are generated (Figure 2). These factors include anaphylatoxin activity (C3a, C5a), which enhances vascular permeability; chemotactic factors (C3a, C5a and $C\overline{567}$), which attract a variety of cell types to the activation site; a phagocytosis-promoting activity (C3b); and lytic activity when the entire sequence is activated. Recently, it has been shown that the complement system can be activated by several nonimmune mechanisms, such as the coagulation system and by polysaccharides in the absence of antibody, in what has been called the bypass mechanism, which is actually the properdin system originally described by Pillemer.

BIOACTIVE PRODUCTS OF THE COMPLEMENT SYSTEM GENERATED IN SEQUENCE AND IN BYPASS

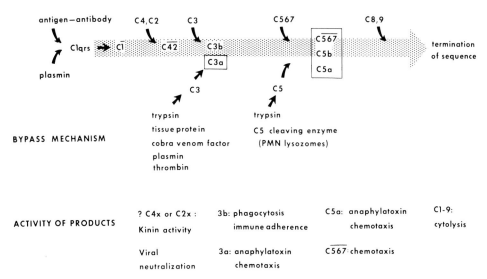

Figure 2. Composite of biological functions of the complement system, and methods by which biologically active products can be generated. From Bellanti, J. A., *Immunology*, W. B. Saunders Co., 1971.

If an organism is completely eliminated at this stage, the host's immune response ends. However, in most cases, products of the primary interaction, called antigens or immunogens, are formed, and these then stimulate the secondary (or specific) immune response.

Secondary (Specific) Immune Responses

The secondary immune responses consist of two effector mechanisms—(*a*) the elaboration of specific antibody, products of the humoral or B-cell system, and (*b*) cell-mediated immunity, expressions of delayed hypersensitivity, or the T-cell system (Figure 1).

Humoral immunity. This term refers to those manifestations of the specific immune response that are affected by products of the thymic-independent or bursal (B) system. The specific effector molecules of humoral immunity that contain specific antibody activity are called the immunoglobulins. In the adult, five major classes of immunoglobulins are known to exist, each with discrete chemical and biological properties (Table 1). The immunoglobulins are designated by the letters G, A, M, D, and E, placed after either the symbol γ (for gamma globulin) or the abbreviation Ig (for immunoglobulin).

The IgG globulins, the most abundant of the immunoglobulins, are found in substantial concentrations in both intravascular and extravascular spaces. They have relatively long biological half-lives (about 20 to 30 days), they cross the placenta, and they can fix complement. This class of immunoglobulins is responsible for most of the immunity to most of those infecting agents that are spread by way of the bloodstream, including bacteria, viruses, parasites, and fungi. These antibodies also function as opsonins, enhancing phagocytosis, or they may exert their effects directly by neutralizing complement-mediated reactions.

Table 1. Comparison of Immunoglobulin Classes

	IgG	IgA	IgM	IgD	IgE
Physiochemical					
Molecular weight	150 000	170 000	890 000	150 000	196 000
Sedimentation rate (S_{20w})	7	7 (10, 14)	19	7	8
Biological					
First detectable antibody	0	0	+	0	0
Major part of secondary response	+	0	0	0	0
Bind complement	+	0	+	0	0
Active placental transport	+	0	0	0	0
Reaginic activity	0	0	0	0	+
Local synthesis	0	+	0	0	+
Mean half life (days)	23	6	5	2.8	1.5
Upper limit (in mg/l) of normal adult concns in serum	12400	2800	1200	30	0.3

The IgA globulins, the second most abundant serum immunoglobulins in the adult, attain high concentrations in the external secretions, where they are referred to as the secretory IgA immunoglobulins (3). They are produced in high concentrations by those lymphoid cells that are contiguous with the gastrointestinal, respiratory, and urinary tracts. Here the IgA globulins are combined with an additional protein produced in epithelial cells (termed the secretory component or transport piece), which endows the molecule with physicochemical resistance against deleterious effects found in these areas, such as proteolytic enzymes. This class of immunoglobulins has been shown to be particularly beneficial in localized types of infections such as respiratory viral infections (4); however, it is believed that because they do not fix complement by the classical means, the IgA immunoglobulin antibodies function by binding directly to the foreign substance. Their unique properties also allow them to function particularly well in the gastrointestinal tract. The well-known association of decreased incidence of enteric bacterial infections and respiratory infections in the breast-fed neonate may be explained in part by the presence of this unique immunoglobulin in colostrum and breast milk.

The IgM immunoglobulins are the largest of the immunoglobulin molecules; their size restricts them almost entirely to the intravascular space (Table 1). These molecules are efficient agglutinators of particulate antigens such as bacteria and can also fix complement with great efficiency. They are formed early in the immune response and are believed to be of greatest importance during the earliest phases of infection. These macroglobulin antibodies also characterize the fetal and neonatal immune responses and their detection in cord serum has been suggested as a screening method for the diagnosis of intrauterine congenital infections (5).

The precise biological function of the IgD globulins has not yet been described, although some antibody activity has been reported in cases of penicillin hypersensitivity in the human. Recently, IgD was shown to be present on the membranes of a large proportion of human peripheral blood lymphocytes of adults and newborns. It was proposed that IgD may function as a lymphocyte antigen receptor (6).

The reaginic (skin sensitizing) antibody, IgE globulin, is the only immunoglobulin normally present in only trace amounts in serum and secretions. There is a striking increase in the serum IgE globulins in patients with parasitic diseases and allergic disorders of the atopic variety. These antibodies have the unique ability to attach to receptors on various cells of the body and to initiate aspects of the immediate hypersensitivity reaction through the release of vasoactive amines from mast cells. The IgE globulins, like those of secretory IgA, are produced chiefly in cells lining the respiratory and gastrointestinal tracts and are encompassed within the external secretory system of antibody. Under normal circumstances, the only immunoglobulins that gain access to the fetus across the placenta are the IgG globulins. This transfer occurs mostly during the third trimester of intrauterine life and explains the relatively low concentrations of IgG globulins in premature infants (7). Although gamma globulin synthesizing cells appear in the human fetus by the 12th week of gestation (8), these proteins are not ordinarily detected in the serum of the embryo until the 38th day of gestation (9,10). IgG globulin concentrations in serum were shown to remain under 1.0 g/litre (100 mg/100 ml) until about the 17th week of gestation, when they begin to increase gradually. At term, gamma globulin concentrations in the infant usually exceed the concentrations in the mother's serum by 5 to 10%.

Manifestations of the antigen-antibody interaction. The presence of antibody is usually detected by an antigen-antibody interaction. For ease of discussion these interactions can be divided into three categories: primary, secondary and tertiary (Table 2).

Table 2. Manifestations of the Antigen-Antibody Interactions

Type	Technique of measurement or biologic expression of antigen-antibody interactions
Primary	Ammonium sulfate precipitation method (Farr technique) Direct immunofluorescence
Secondary	Precipitation Agglutination Complement-dependent reactions Neutralization
Tertiary	Beneficial: toxin neutralization Deleterious: serum sickness

The primary or initial interaction of antigen with antibody is the basic event. It consists of the binding of antigen with the two or more available sites on any given antibody molecule. The measurement of primary antigen-antibody interactions can be assessed by one of several techniques, such as the ammonium sulfate precipitation method (11) or by direct immunofluorescence. These techniques measure directly the reaction of antigen with antibody and are sometimes useful in the diagnosis of infectious diseases. The primary interaction of antigen with antibody is rarely visible, however, and the primary event is usually ascertained only through secondary and tertiary interactions (Table 2).

The secondary manifestations of the antigen-antibody interaction include precipitation, agglutination, complement-dependent reactions, and neutralization. These reactions are of practical importance to the physician since they form the basis of a number of laboratory tests used in the detection and identification of antigens and antibodies involved in infectious disease processes, for example, complement fixation tests, bentonite flocculation tests, among others (Table 2).

The antigen-antibody interaction is sometimes expressed as tertiary manifestations which are the in vivo expressions (Table 2). At times these reactions may be beneficial (e.g., toxin neutralization); at other times, they may lead to disease through immunologic injury (as in serum sickness).

Cell-mediated (delayed hypersensitivity) immunity. Cell-mediated immunity or delayed hypersensitivity refers to those manifestations of the specific immune response that are stimulated by antigen-sensitized lymphocytes which come under the influence of the thymus during differentiation as described below, and are referred to as the thymic-dependent (T) system, independent of circulating antibodies. Generation of the immune response requires interaction between stimulating antigen and the specific receptors on the surfaces of immunocompetent cells. Immunoglobulins appear to play a role in one type of immunocompetent cells, the so-called B cells, which carry intact immunoglobulin receptors on their surface. The T cells of the immune system do not carry complete immunoglobulin markers, and the nature of these receptors is unclear. For most of the immunological reactions, interaction between B and T cells is required; however, there are certain antigens that stimulate T cells preferentially, others B cells, and still others that require prior processing by macrophages (*12*). Evidence is now accumulating that cellular hypersensitivity takes a large share in protecting against a wide variety of infectious agents, including intracellular bacteria, viruses, fungi, and protozoa. In these situations, the antigen-antibody interaction appears to be relatively less effective than cell-mediated immunity. The cellular effector mechanism seems to be stimulated in those infections in which antigen is either inaccessible or persistent—that is, intracellular. The presence of delayed hypersensitivity is the in vivo expression of cellular immunity and forms the basis of one of the oldest and most useful diagnostic procedures, the delayed-type skin reaction.

Several techniques for identifying T lymphocytes, B lymphocytes, and macrophages have been under intensive study during the past few years. The distinguishing features of these three cell types are shown in Table 3.

Components of the cell-mediated reaction. Like the antigen-antibody reaction, the lymphocyte-antigen interaction may also be divided into three categories: primary, secondary, and tertiary reactions (Table 4).

The primary reaction of antigen with the sensitized lymphocyte is the basic event and consists of the binding of antigen to a receptor on the cell surface. Some cellular hypersensitivity reactions involve both immunologically specific and nonspecific cellular components. The sensitive cells are lymphocytes of the thymus-dependent system and the nonspecific cells are macrophages originating from a rapidly dividing pool of bone marrow promonocytes (*13*). After the antigen reacts with the sensitized cell, a sequence of events occurs that comprises the secondary manifestations.

The secondary (in vitro) manifestations of the cell-mediated reaction are detected indirectly, from morphologic, biochemical, or biological effects. The morphologic changes

Table 3. Distinguishing Characteristics of T Lymphocytes, B Lymphocytes. and Macrophages

Membrane markers	T lymphocytes	B lymphocytes	Macrophages
IgG	−	+	−
Receptor for C3 (erythrocyte-antibody-complement rosettes)	−	+	+
Receptor for immunoglobulin or antibody-antigen complexes (Fc)	−	+	+
Thymus-specific antigens (θ, mouse thymocyte leukemia antigen, etc.)	+	−	−
Reactors for sheep red blood cells (erythrocyte rosettes)	+	−	−
In vitro stimulation of DNA synthesis by mitogens			
Phytohemagglutinin	+	−[a]	−
Concanavallin A	+	−	−
Lipopolysaccharide (bacterial endotoxin)	−	+	−
Anti-immunoglobulin	−	+	−
Specific binding to antigen-coated beads	−	+	−
Mixed lymphocyte culture reactivity	+	−	−
Graft-versus-host reaction-inducing capacity	+	−	−
Adherence to surfaces (glass, plastic)	−[b]	−[c]	+
Phagocytic	−	−	+

[a] Some B lymphocytes may be recruited to divide secondarily because of factors elaborated by activated T lymphocytes. B cells may also be stimulated when the mitogen is attached to solid support.

[b] Except for blast cells.

[c] Except for mature plasma cells or when immune complexes are attached to B cells.

Table 4. Manifestations of the Cell-Mediated (Delayed Hypersensitivity) Reaction

Type	Techniques of measurement or biological expression of antigen-antibody interactions
Primary	Binding of antigen with receptor on lymphocyte
Secondary	Morphologic (blast transformation)
	Biochemical (incorporation of precursors into DNA or RNA)
	Biologic (elaboration of low-molecular-weight substances)
Tertiary	Beneficial: antimicrobial immunity
	Deleterious: autoimmune diseases

of lymphocytes in tissue culture consist of blast-cell transformation with subsequent mitosis. Several agents, such as specific antigen or nonspecific mitogens, have been shown to induce these changes, and several biochemical techniques of labeling DNA or RNA may be used to measure them in lymphocyte reactivity, for example, uptake of tritiated thymidine (*14*). After sensitized lymphocytes interact with antigen, the lymphocytes elaborate an array of diverse proteins of low (as compared to most proteins) molecular weight, which are believed to be the effectors of cell-mediated immunity (*1,15*) (Table 5). Recognition of these effector molecules has attracted considerable interest recently, from both the diagnostic and the therapeutic standpoints. Measurement of the specific effector substances is useful in diagnosing a variety of diseases associated with specific immunological deficits—for example, congenital thymic aplasia (Di George's syndrome), chronic mucocutaneous candidiasis, and ataxia telangiectasia. It is also assuming increasing importance in the immunological approaches to malignancy. Many of these diseases have been corrected by immunological reconstitution, and it seems reasonable to assume that an increasing number of infectious diseases may respond to replacement therapy with any one of several of these effector substances.

The tertiary effects of cell-mediated reactions consist of in vivo manifestations (Table 4). In the past, these tertiary manifestations, such as delayed hypersensitivity, formed the majority of observations of the cell-mediated event. As knowledge of the effector molecules has increased, however, the basis of these in vivo expressions is becoming more

Table 5. Effector Molecules of Cell-Mediated Immunity

	Molecular weight	Physical properties	Activities	
			In vitro	In vivo
Transfer factor	<10 000	Heat labile; dialyzable polypeptide	Unknown	Transfer of reactivity to uncommited lymphocytes
Macrophage inhibitory factor (MIF)	35 000-70 000	Nonheat stable; nondialyzable	Prevents random migration of macrophages	May lead to accumulation of macrophages
Lymphotoxin	80 000	Heat labile; nondialyzable	Target cell injury	No known effect
Skin-reactive factor	70 000			Localized cutaneous reaction
Chemotactic factors	60 000		Attact macrophages; attract PMNs	
Mitogenic factors	25 000		Enhance cell transformation	
Interferon	25 000	Heat stable	Inhibits viral replication	Inhibits viral replication
Antibody	160 000	Heat stable; nondialyzable	Reactive with antigen	Varied

clear. Tertiary manifestations can be either beneficial or deleterious (Table 4). They form the basis of antimicrobial immunity against acute and chronic infectious agents, as well as surveillance against malignancy. In some diseases, tuberculosis for example, the clinical manifestations of hyperactivity of cell-mediated immunity (delayed hypersensitivity) are readily apparent. In other clinical states, there is an inability to express cell-mediated responsiveness, a state termed "anergy." This lack of responsiveness occurs in the very young, owing to developmental immaturity; in the aged; in many infectious diseases and in other diseases of unknown etiology, for instance, sarcoidosis; as a secondary response to certain malignancies, such as lymphoma; and in patients receiving immunosuppressive therapy. In all of these disorders, there is a marked susceptibility to infections, particularly opportunistic infections caused by viral, fungal, and parasitic agents. Of particular importance are those infections transmitted congenitally in which a depression of cell-mediated immune responses occurs. In congenital rubella syndrome, for example, a depression in both the lymphoproliferative responses to phytohemagglutinin (16), as well as a depression in specific cell-mediated immunity to rubella virus (17), has been described. In addition, a depression of specific cell-mediated immunity to rubella virus during normal pregnancy has been reported (18). Immune-deficiency diseases that may present in the newborn period are described below.

Tertiary Immune Responses (Immunologically Mediated Diseases)

If antigen still persists, the tertiary responses are called into play. These are no longer beneficial to the host, and thus are immunologically mediated diseases (Figure 1). It has been postulated that antigen persistence may result from the nature of the antigen itself or from a genetic or developmental defect in antigen processing (19). If antigen persists, four types of immunological interactions can be elicited: types I, II, III, and IV (Table 6). These manifestations may be either temporary or permanent, depending upon the efficiency with which antigen is eliminated (19). If antigen can be removed successfully, the adverse effects of the antigen persistence are transient, but if the antigen persists, the host may respond with maximal immune reactivity, which of itself may cause a sustained injury such as that seen in autoimmune diseases. Immunologically mediated diseases rarely occur in the fetus and newborn but can result from maternal sensitization during pregnancy, as in Rh sensitization, or as a secondary manifestation of an intrauterine infection, for example, congenital syphilis.

DEVELOPMENTAL ASPECTS OF IMMUNITY

The maturation of both nonspecific and specific immune responsiveness in the human begins in utero during the eighth to twelfth week of gestation (8,20,21). The differentiation of cells destined to perform these functions appears to arise from a population of progenitor stem cells that are located within the yolk sac, fetal liver, and bone marrow of the developing fetus. Depending upon the microchemical environments surrounding these cells, they will differentiate along at least two avenues, the hematopoietic and the lymphopoietic.

Hematopoietic Differentiation

One type of microchemical environment leads to the proliferation and differentiation of stem cells into the myeloid, erythroid, and megakaryocyte precursors. Granulocytopoiesis

Table 6. Types of Immunologic Interactions Contributing to Tertiary Immune Responses

Type	Target organs	Clinical examples	Mechanism	Comment
I. (Anaphylactic)	Gastrointestinal tract Skin Lungs	Milk allergy Urticaria Asthma	IgE reaginic antibody	A rare result of intrauterine sensitization
II. (Cytotoxic)	Circulating blood elements Gamma globulin	Hemolytic disease of newborn Transient hypogamma-globulinemia	Transplacental transfer of maternal IgG	The result of isoimmunization of pregnancy
III. (Immune complex)	Blood vessels Skin Joints Kidneys Lungs	Serum sickness Glomerulonephritis	Antigen-antibody complexes	May account for disease manifestations of congenital infections, e.g., nephritis
IV. (Delayed hypersensitivity)	Skin Lungs Nervous system Thyroid Other organs	Contact dermatitis Tuberculosis Allergic encephalitis Thyroiditis	Sensitized lymphocytes	May account for disease manifestations of congenital infections, e.g., tuberculosis, syphilis

first takes place in the liver of the fetus, at about the second month of gestation. This site is gradually replaced by the bone marrow, which assumes increasing activity at about the fifth month.

Lymphopoietic Differentiation

Cells destined to differentiate into lymphopoietic cells come under two separate inductive influences: the thymus (T) and the bursa (B) or bursal equivalent tissues.

T-cell system. The thymus gland is derived from the epithelium of the third and fourth pharyngeal pouches at about the sixth week of fetal life; the parathyroid glands also begin their development at this time from the same pouches. As further differentiation proceeds, a caudad migration of epithelium occurs, and, beginning at about the eighth week, blood-borne stem cells enter the gland and are drawn into lymphoid differentiation. As the lymphocytes continue to infiltrate the thymus, it differentiates into a dense cortex containing many small lymphocytes and a less dense, loose, central medulla with relatively more epithelial components. Recent evidence suggests that a hormone (thymosin) (22) is produced by these epithelial cells and may be operative in the expansion of the peripheral lymphocyte populations. Although the characterization of this hormone is only preliminary (23), its use has intriguing possibilities for clinical medicine in replacement therapy (24).

A more rapid mitotic activity occurs in the thymus gland than in any other lymphatic organ. Curiously, however, more than 70% of the lymphoid cells die within the substance of the gland. The precise explanation for this is unknown, but it has been suggested that it may be related to a censorship function of the thymus in which potentially harmful clones of lymphocytes are eliminated. After they emerge from the thymus gland, the thymus-dependent (T) lymphocytes acquire new surface antigen markers, such as the theta antigen in the mouse. Although these receptors are now being intensely investigated, their nature and function remain unclear; they are believed by some to be related to antigen-recognition units on the surface membranes of T cells.

After the T cells leave the gland, they circulate through the lymphatic and vascular systems as long-lived lymphocytes (the recirculating pool), which then populate certain restricted regions of lymph nodes, forming thymic-dependent areas in the subcortical regions of lymph nodes and periarterial regions of the spleen. Thymectomy in the neonatal animal renders the animal deficient in the numbers of these recirculating T cells and depletes the thymic-dependent areas in lymphoid tissue. The long-lived nature of these lymphocytes and their degree of competence in the human may explain why, after thymectomy, immediate deficits are not usually apparent in the newborn, although they may become apparent in later life.

The clinical importance of the simultaneous embryogenesis of the parathyroid gland and thymus to the neonatologist is evident in one of the immunologic deficiency disorders, Di George's syndrome (1,20). In this disorder, the infant lacks not only thymic function but also parathyroid activity. Thus the patient presents with repeated infections caused by fungus or virus, and with hypocalcemic tetany. The successful immunological reconstitution of the patient can be accomplished by using thymic transplants, either naked (25,26) or encased in Millipore chambers (27). A major involvement of the second and third pharyngeal pouch has also been described in association with absence of the thyroid gland and thymus (28). Thus, if a newborn infant shows either tetany or hypothyroidism, defects in thymic function should also be diligently sought.

B-cell system. If the progenitor cells are influenced by a second type of microchemical environment, differentiation will occur that produces a population of lymphocytes and plasma cells concerned with humoral immunity or antibody synthesis. This population (8) is influenced by and is expanded within a second anatomical site that has been located with certainty only in birds, in which it is called the bursa of Fabricius. This population of cells, termed B cells, comprises a much smaller part of the recirculating pool. The lymphocytes populate other regions of lymphoidal tissues, the thymic-independent regions, which include the germinal centers and medullary cords of lymph nodes. The B cells can be identified by the presence of surface immunoglobulin markers as described above. Removal of the bursa or its mammalian equivalent leads to a profound deficiency of gamma globulin with little or no effect on cell-mediated immunity. Antibody provides a major bulwark of defense against the highly encapsulated high-grade pyogenic pathogens such as pneumococci, *Hemophilus influenzae*, and meningococci. In the human, B cells, as identified by individual immunoglobulin surface markers, make their first appearance at differing ages according to the same sequence of appearance of the serum immunoglobulins (29).

The function of this two-compartment system is important for an understanding of the primary immune deficiency disorders, as well as for a framework of a more logical approach to the management of maturational deficiencies in the fetus and newborn. Selective deficiencies of the B system, so-called agammaglobulinemias, appear in patients as recurrent bacterial infections. Selective deficiencies of the T system are associated with fungal infections such as mucocutaneous candidiasis and infections caused by viruses, including both the DNA and RNA viruses. Combined B- and T-cell defects are the most serious of the immunological deficiency syndromes; the patients have profound deficiencies in both cell-mediated and antibody functions combined with a diversity of infections. The developing fetus and newborn infant are compromised in many aspects of B- and T-cell function. These will be described in subsequent sections.

FACTORS IN DEVELOPMENTAL ASPECTS OF IMMUNITY WHICH MAY AFFECT RESPONSES TO INFECTION

The three compartments of man's immunological system are maximally functional only in the adult. At various times in the life-span of the individual, some of these systems function with reduced efficiency.

Nonspecific Immunity

A number of abnormalities of nonspecific immunity may affect the newborn infant. They involve the movement of phagocytic cells toward a foreign substance (chemotaxis) and the subsequent inflammatory response, the preparation of such substances for ingestion by cells (opsonization), and the intracellular destruction of substances (digestion). Most of these impairments of nonspecific immunity occur as expressions of developmental immaturity and may affect function during this period of life (46–47).

Bactericidal activity and metabolic activity. After phagocytes ingest foreign particles, oxygen consumption increases because glucose utilization by the hexose monophosphate pathway is increased (48–49). Hydrogen peroxide formed as the result of increased activity by this pathway is believed to be highly important in the killing of many bacteria through activation of the myeloperoxidase/halide system (50). The nitroblue tetrazolium test is a screening method for the measurement of activity in the hexose monophosphate pathway and depends on the formation of a blue formazan pigment during the phagocytic event (51). Defective activity is exemplified by chronic granulomatous disease and is associated with recurrent infections caused by Gram-negative organisms and staphylococci (52). In this disorder, defective activity in this pathway is combined with diminished nitroblue tetrazolium reduction. The newborn, who also shows defective shunt activity, is plagued by the same spectrum of infection as an adult with chronic granulomatous disease (47). Thus, in a sense, the newborn may show maturational defects similar to those present in cases of this disease. Published data concerning metabolic activity of leukocytes in the newborn, however, are inconsistent. Some investigators have found decreased metabolic activity via the hexose monophosphate pathway, others have found normal activity (43). Nitroblue tetrazolium dye reduction is normal or increased in the newborn, but decreases as maturation occurs during the first six months of life. Afterward it increases continuously with age (53).

The results for quantitative nitroblue tetrazolium dye reduction and assay of glucose-6-phosphate dehydrogenase (EC 1.1.1.49) and 6-phosphogluconate dehydrogenase (EC 1.1.1.43) activity in 122 infants and 24 adults are given in Table 7. A stepwise increase in nitroblue tetrazolium dye reduction and leukocyte phosphate-dehydrogenase activity is seen with maturation, leukocyte gluconate dehydrogenase did not show this stepwise increase. These data provide further evidence for an increase in functional activity of the immunological system and systems intrinsic to the neutrophilic leukocyte (intracellular systems) or extrinsic to it (extracellular systems).

The inflammatory response of the neonate. Injury of tissue or invasion by microorganisms triggers a sequence of systemic and local events. The febrile response is believed to reflect enhanced metabolic activity and to be related to the release of endogenous pyrogens from the host leukocytes and the resulting hypothalamic response (30). This response is not, however, particularly well developed in the neonate, and fever is not a reliable sign of infection in this period. Similarly, leukocytosis and the increased rate of erythrocyte sedimentation that is commonly associated with bacterial infections in the older infant and child are not particularly useful diagnostic signs during the neonatal period. However, other signs of inflammatory response such as an increase in α- and β-globulins combined with an elevation of C-reactive protein do occur in the neonatal period and are helpful in diagnosing infectious diseases. Moreover, although it is well recognized that an abnormally high total neutrophil count is an inconsistent and unreliable index of neonatal sepsis, recent evidence suggests that an increase in total numbers of nonsegmented (band) forms may be a more significant and valuable diagnostic aid (31).

Chemotaxis. Several localized events also occur in the inflammatory response. For example, after a foreign substance is introduced into the skin, a number of inflammatory cells move in an organized fashion toward the foreign configuration, a process referred to as chemotaxis. In the sequence of cellular events in the adult, a prominent polymorphonuclear leukocyte infiltration occurs during the first 4 to 12 h, followed by a predominantly mononuclear response (macrophages and lymphocytes). The skin of the neonatal infant, however, is relatively deficient in manifesting the expressions of nonspecific immunity (32). In the newborn, the shift from a granulocytic to a mononuclear cell response is slower and less intense than in the adult, reflecting a maturational deficiency. Furthermore, in some studies a curiously high percentage of eosinophils has

Table 7. Changes in Leukocyte NBT Dye Reduction G-6-PD and 6-PGD Activities with Maturation

Age	Newborn	1–6 months	6–12 months	12–18 months	1.5–4 years	4–10 years	10–14 years	Adult years
No. tested	23	13	21	18	20	19	8	18
NBT (mean ΔA) ±S.E.	0.127 ±0.011	0.090 ±0.008	0.098 ±0.008	0.123 ±0.011	0.148 ±0.013	0.139 ±0.007	0.175 ±0.024	0.206 ±0.025
No. tested	9	8	10	14	17	14	6	24
G-6-PD (μmol/mg protein) mean ±S.E.	78.2 ±10.4	21.2 ±5.5	7.8 ±0.7	44.6 ±11.2	52.3 ±10.6	98.1 ±12.5	147.7 ±17.3	141 ±3.6
6-PGD (μmol/mg protein) mean ±S.E.	82.2 ±7.6	39.0 ±3.0	44.1 ±3.6	50.6 ±2.4	44.4 ±2.9	45.5 ±2.6	43.7 ±2.8	34.6 ±1.5

been observed in the 2- and 4-h exudate of newborns older than 24 h but not in those less than 24 h old (33,34). It is of interest that the lesions of erythema toxicum, well known to neonatologists, consist primarily of eosinophilic leukocytes (35).

Complement.   A maturational development of the complement components is seen in the human. These are reviewed in several recent reports (37–39).

Phagocytosis.   Once mobilized, the cells mount an attack on their target by a process of phagocytosis (literally, "cell-eating"). In the adult, many foreign substances such as nonvirulent organisms may simply be ingested by phagocytic cells, whereas virulent organisms must first be prepared for such ingestion by specific antibody or complement. Because only the IgG globulins are transmitted across the placenta and because complement activity is low in the neonate, the newborn is thus compromised in opsonic functions (35,40).

There have been conflicting reports concerning the adequacy of phagocytosis in the neonate. These differences probably reflect methodologic differences in technique. In some studies it has been shown that phagocytosis by leukocytes from the neonate is abnormal when cells are suspended in serum from newborns (41). Normal activity is restored when the same cells are suspended in serum from adults, suggesting that the primary defect may reside in extracellular factors (42–45). However, other studies have shown that more subtle cellular defects may occur when the cells are tested in various concentrations of serum. It is probable that a maturational defect of both cellular and extracellular factors accounts for the diminished phagocytic activity, and this underscores the need for the clinical laboratory to age-adjust such values in interpreting immunological responses in the newborn.

Humoral Immunity

Maternal-fetal relationships.   One of the challenging problems in developmental biology is the question of how a fetus, who inherits one half of its antigens from paternally controlled genes foreign to the mother, can be tolerated successfully during pregnancy. This has been attributed largely to the barrier function of the placenta. By acting as a mechanical barrier, the placenta usually effectively separates the formed elements of the blood between the mother and the fetus. There are elements (antibodies), however, that do gain access to the fetus and provide protection.

There are different pathways by which maternal antibody is transmitted to the fetus in different species (54) (Table 8). In species with large numbers of membranes intervening between the maternal and fetal circulations, the colostral route seems to be a more important route of transfer of antibodies, and newborns absorb these antibodies from the gastrointestinal tract. Conversely, in mammals with fewer such layers, as is the case in humans, the transplacental route of antibody delivery seems to have assumed greater importance. The IgG molecule possesses two end groupings. Studies performed with enzymatic splitting have demonstrated that one ending, called the Fab fragment, is responsible for antibody activity and specific binding with antigen. The other portion, called the Fc fragment, displays more nonspecific functions, such as binding to cellular receptors or the activation of complement (55–56).

Thus, in the human, the predominant transfer of antibody occurs via the passage of IgG immunoglobulins from the maternal circulation to that of the fetus. This involves an active transport of the immunoglobulin by virtue of a receptor located on the Fc

Table 8. Relationship of Type of Placentation with Character of Maternal-Fetal Transfer of Antibody in Various Species

Animal	Number of placental membranes	Relative importance[a] of route	
		Placental	Colostral
Horse	6	0	+++
Sheep, cow	5	0	+++
Cat, dog	5	+	++
Rat, mouse	4	+	++
Rabbit, guinea pig	3	+++	±
Man, monkey	3	+++	0

[a] The relative importance is indicated arbitrarily from 0 (unimportant) to +++ (very important).

fragment. This is the manner by which the fetus receives a library of preformed antibody from his mother, reflecting most of her experiences with infectious agents. The secretory IgA immunoglobulins found in breast milk also provide local protection on the mucous membranes of the gastrointestinal tract. Although these antibodies are not absorbed significantly in the human, their unique structure renders them more effective in these sites and may explain the lower incidence of enteric and respiratory infections seen in breast-fed infants.

The development of serum immunoglobulins during intrauterine life and postnatally is shown schematically in Figure 3. The concentrations of immunoglobulin, almost

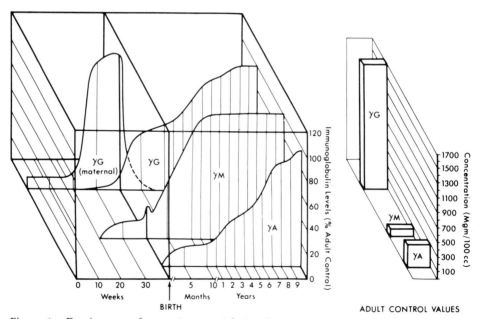

Figure 3. Development of serum immunoglobulins during maturation. From Bellanti, J. A., *Immunology*, W. B. Saunders Co., 1971.

exclusively IgG, at birth are equivalent to those of the mother. There are few or no IgA and IgM globulins present in cord sera, because these immunoglobulins do not cross the placenta. In addition, the fetus is usually protected in utero from antigenic stimuli and therefore is not called upon to synthesize these immunoglobulins actively under normal circumstances. However, if the fetus is challenged in utero as a consequence of immunization or infection (e.g., congenital rubella, cytomegalic inclusion disease, toxoplasmosis), he will respond with antibody production, largely of the IgM variety (5,57–59). This exclusion of other classes of antibody benefits the fetus in many cases. For example, the exclusion of the IgM isohemagglutinins, leukoagglutinins, or the IgE antibodies of allergy forestalls disease that may be produced by these antibodies. But it also precludes the passage of other maternal antibodies that would be beneficial to the newborn, such as the IgM antibodies, which are important in defense against Gram-negative bacteria (opsonins, agglutinins, and bactericidal antibodies). This may explain in part the increased susceptibility of the newborn to infection with Gram-negative organisms such as *Escherichia coli* (40).

The types of antibodies that the fetus obtains in this manner vary greatly (Table 9). This, in part, reflects the quantity of antibodies in the maternal circulation as well as their molecular size. For example, low-molecular-weight IgG antibodies, such as rubeola antibody, that are present in high concentrations in maternal serum are readily transferred. IgG antibodies that are present in lower concentrations, such as *Bordetella pertussis*, are poorly transferred, whereas macroglobulin antibodies, such as Wasserman antibody, are excluded.

Table 9. Relationship of Antibody Type with Transplacental Transfer

Good passive transfer	Poor passive transfer	No passive transfer
Diphtheria antitoxin	*Hemophilus influenzae*	Enteric somatic (o).
Tetanus antitoxin	*Bordetella pertussis*	antibodies (*E. salmonella*,
Antierythrogenic toxin	*Shigella flexneri*	shigella, *E. coli*)
Antistaphylococcal antibody	Streptococcus MG	Skin-sensitizing antibody
Salmonella flagella (H)		Heterophile antibody
antibody		Wasserman antibody
Antistreptolysin		
All the antiviral antibodies		
present in maternal circula-		
tion (rubeola, rubella,		
mumps, poliovirus)		
VDRL antibodies		

Because the IgG immunoglobulins are passively transferred, they have a half-life of only 20 to 30 days; their concentration in serum therefore declines rapidly within the first few months of life, and is the lowest between the second and fourth months. During this period, referred to as physiological hypogammaglobulinemia, the infant may be susceptible to recurrent infections. During the course of the first few years, gamma globulin concentrations increase because the maturing infant is exposed to antigens in his environment. There appears to be a sequential development in gamma globulin at different rates: the IgM globulins attain adult concentrations by one year of age, the

IgG globulins by five to six years of age, and the IgA globulins by ten years of age. This pattern of appearance of immunoglobulins recapitulates that which is seen in phylogeny and also appears to parallel the pattern observed after an antigenic exposure during the primary immune response (*1*).

Cell-Mediated Immunity

Evaluation of cell-mediated immunity is somewhat more difficult because only limited studies are available. The homograft rejection phenomenon has been studied in a variety of animal species and is present early in gestation. In humans, the homograft reaction is thought to be present because maternally acquired competent lymphocytes passing to the fetus might be expected to mount a graft-versus-host reaction if these were not rejected by a competent fetal response. There has been one example of such an event, which followed intrauterine transfusion in an Rh incompatibility (*60*). The ability of fetal thymocytes to react to stimulation with phytohemagglutinin has been shown to be present as early as the 14th week of gestation (*61*).

Cellular immunity at the time of or after birth has been studied in many species. In the human it is present at birth. The human neonate responds with delayed hypersensitivity responses that provide a useful indication of certain clinical diseases, for instance, tuberculosis. In one study (*62*), cord blood lymphocytes were found to respond to the nonspecific effects of phytohemagglutinin, pokeweed mitogens, and staphylococcal filtrate. Thus the normal neonate has a well-developed capacity to manifest responses, both in vivo and in vitro. The expression of in vivo responses may be somewhat diminished, owing to the immaturity of nonspecific (inflammatory) responses.

OPERATIONAL CLASSIFICATION OF INFECTIOUS DISEASES

For ease of discussion, we may speak of four modes of infection by organisms: (*a*) acute, fulminating infections of relatively short duration, (*b*) chronic infections capable of intracellular parasitism, (*c*) latent infections (primarily viral), part of whose genome may be integrated into that of the host, and (*d*) toxigenic infections (primarily bacterial) in which the production of toxin accounts for many of the disease manifestations (Table 10) (*1*).

Acute Infections

The first type of infection is exemplified by bacteria (e.g., staphylococci or *E. coli*) and by viruses (e.g., enteroviruses) that may gain access to the body either through the hematogenous route in the fetus or through any of the natural portals of entry such as the gastrointestinal tract, the respiratory tract, or the skin of the neonate. These infections are characterized by a rapid, acute, fulminating course in which the outcome of the host-parasite relationship is quickly determined. Multiplication of the organisms is limited, and they may cause a localized lesion accompanied by abscess formation; other organisms are effectively killed by polymorphonuclear leukocytes, and others may be killed only in the presence of antibody and complement. If host defense mechanisms are sufficient to contain these organisms locally, resolution and healing will occur. On the other hand, if the mechanisms are insufficient, the infection can spread regionally or gain access to the systemic circulation, resulting in either fulminating sepsis or viremia. These organisms

Table 10. Classification of Immune Mechanisms in Infectious Diseases

Type	Example	Primary		Secondary	
		Phagocytosis	Inflammatory response	Antibody	Cell-mediated
Acute	Bacterial: staphylococcus *Escherichia coli*	++	++	+	±
	Viral: enterovirus	+	±	++	±
Chronic	Bacterial: Tbc, syphilis	++	++	±	++
	Viral: rubella, CMV	±	±	++	++
	Fungal: candida	+	+	±	++
	Parasitic: *Toxoplasma gondii* *Pneumocystis carinii*	++	+	±	++
Latent	Viral: herpes simplex	±	±	+	++
Toxigenic	Bacterial: diphtheria, tetanus cholera	±	+	++	0

[a] The relative importance of the mechanisms are indicated arbitrarily from 0 (relatively unimportant) to ++ (very important).

that cause acute infection may be completely eliminated or they may persist in a chronic infection.

Chronic Infections

The second type of host-parasite interaction is that characterized by a protracted or chronic course of infection in which the ingested organisms can survive within the phagocyte and establish an intracellular parasitism (1). These include agents such as the tubercle bacillus, viruses such as rubella, fungi such as *Candida*, and protozoal agents such as *Toxoplasma gondii*. Paradoxically, such parasites may even be carried by phagocytes into deeper tissues where they may be capable of infecting surrounding tissues or existing as intracellular parasites within macrophages. A heightened reactivity of phagocytes toward the infecting as well as the nonrelated organisms has been shown by these parasitized macrophages ("activated macrophages"). Delayed hypersensitivity is a prominent feature of these types of interactions.

Latent Infections

The third type of host-parasite interaction is most commonly exemplified by viruses that become integrated into host cells (1). The viral particles are not always released from the cell. However, under certain circumstances such as immunosuppression, trauma, fever, endocrine, or environmental factors, the virus may be released. Periods of cyclic exacerbations in chronically infected host cells are exemplified by such viruses as herpes simplex and herpes zoster. In other circumstances, depending upon the nature of the virus host-cell interaction, the cells are transformed, and although complete virus particles may not be released from the infected cell, a number of other changes occur and new antigens appear on the cell surfaces. Oncogenic viruses are related to such cell transformation. Cell-mediated immunity appears to have a prominent role in the control of these complex interactions (2).

Toxigenic Infections

The fourth type of host-parasite interaction is that involving toxin production, primarily bacterial. These toxins are of two types, exotoxins and endotoxins. Exotoxins are proteins elaborated by bacteria as extracellular products that function as cell poisons (e.g., diphtheria and tetanus toxins). Endotoxins are constituents of cell walls of Gram-negative bacteria and are released only after the bacterial cell is destroyed or autolyzed. Endotoxins are composed of a lipid polysaccharide complex. The salient differences between exotoxins and endotoxins are illustrated in Table 11.

Table 11. Differences between Exotoxins and Endotoxins

	Exotoxins	Endotoxins
Production	Released extracellularly	Part of cell wall of bacteria
Bacteria	Gram-positive	Gram-negative
Stability	Labile	Stable to heating
Composition	Protein	Lipopolysaccharide
Relative toxicity	More potent	Less potent
Biologic activity	Inhibit protein synthesis, cytotoxic, neurotoxic, salt and water effects	Fever, intravascular coagulation, leukopenia, Schwartzman phenomenon
Clinical importance	Toxoid for vaccines	Associated with shock, Waterhouse-Friderichsen syndrome, intravascular coagulation

INTERRELATIONSHIPS BETWEEN THE VARIOUS COMPARTMENTS OF THE IMMUNOLOGICAL RESPONSE IN INFECTIOUS DISEASES

The compartments of the immunological system work in concert, so that when the primitive defense mechanisms have been surmounted and the specific immunological responses are stimulated, the products of the latter are used to enhance the former. When the specific immune responses are stimulated, the resultant production of opsonins and simultaneous cell-mediated events results in products that can enhance phagocytosis by macrophages or polymorphonuclear leukocytes. Although both responses are stimulated in all infections, it must be emphasized that one or the other predominates, depending upon the type of infection, and that there is a quantitative relationship between the mechanisms expressed and the infective characteristics of the pathogen. The responses in each of the four types of infection exemplify these relationships.

Acute Infections

In an acute infection by a nonencapsulated, nonvirulent bacterium, the organism will be readily phagocytosed. In contrast, in the case of an encapsulated organism, after the subsequent production of antibody and the initiation of the complement cascade, phagocytosis by polymorphonuclear leukocytes will be enhanced. Simultaneously, cell-mediated immunity is stimulated, which enhances phagocytosis by macrophages. Because these organisms are not regularly phagocytosed by macrophages, this scheme appears to be of relatively lesser importance. However, in clinical situations in which the polymorphonuclear leukocytes are deficient, as in the newborn or in chronic granulomatous disease, a prominent but low-efficiency macrophage interaction occurs, indicating that this mechanism can be utilized.

Chronic Infections

The chronic type of infection is best exemplified by infection with the tubercle bacillus. In the initial encounter between the organism and the polymorphonuclear leukocytes, a paradoxical situation arises. The polymorphonuclear leukocyte can ingest the organism but cannot degrade the lipid capsule. Thus the invading microorganism is transported to deeper tissues where the short-lived polymorphonuclear leukocytes provide only a limited period for intracellular parasitism. The major cellular response in this type of infection is subsequent phagocytosis by macrophages, in which the organisms survive for even longer periods of time. In addition, upon ingestion, there is a simultaneous stimulation of cell-mediated events with the elaboration of lymphocyte products such as macrophage inhibitory factor and chemotactic factors, which can further enhance the activity of macrophages. If these pathogens remain viable, further response of the host is manifested through an immune granuloma formation, which serves to further wall off or localize the infected area. Recent evidence indicates that the termination of intracellular parasitism coincides with the development of increased macrophage efficiency, which appears to be under the control of the effector molecules released from sensitized lymphocytes. Such an increase in efficiency also increases the ability of the macrophage to kill nonrelated organisms.

Latent Infections

The latent type of interaction is best exemplified by infection with certain viruses such as herpes simplex. In such infections, the stimulation of cell-mediated immunity appears to be of paramount importance in terminating infection. Interaction of the virus-infected cell with sensitized lymphocytes releases the diverse array of effector molecules described above. For example, the released cytotoxin can destroy infected cells, chemotactic factors are generated that recruit phagocytes to remove debris, and the released interferon may prevent viral multiplication and, thereby, the spread of virus to adjacent cells. Recently it has been shown that the macrophage and the polymorphonuclear leukocytes are also very important in preventing the spread of herpes virus from cells or between cells. Thus, there appears to be in all infections an interaction and interdependence between the various components of the immunological response that confers a survival advantage to the host.

Toxigenic Infections

The fourth type of host-parasite interaction involves the production of toxin. The first defense of the host is through neutralization of the toxin by the production of specific antibody (antitoxin). This detoxification process leads to the production of toxin-antitoxin complexes, which are removed by phagocytic degradation. The endotoxins exhibit a more generalized effect on the host, including pyrogen release by polymorphonuclear leukocytes resulting in fever, leukopenia, and the initiation of the coagulation sequence with intravascular coagulation and shock (Schwartzman phenomenon). Although antibodies are formed to endotoxin, they do not appear to be of protective value as in the case of exotoxin.

APPLICATION OF IMMUNOLOGICAL PRINCIPLES IN THE PREVENTION, DIAGNOSIS, AND THERAPY OF INFECTIOUS DISEASES IN THE NEONATAL PERIOD

Immunologic principles can also be used successfully in the prevention, diagnosis, and therapy of infectious diseases in the neonatal period. Diseases such as pertussis, tetanus, varicella, and measles have been either prevented or attenuated in the newborn through the judicious use of immune serum globulin or specific immune globulin. Moreover, immunotherapy may be applied in the prevention of other diseases, as for instance the use of specific hepatitis B immune serum globulin (63) in the prevention of neonatal hepatitis. Infectious diseases can also be prevented by active immunization. Since it is now established that the neonate is immunocompetent, he can be successfully immunized against a variety of infectious agents, for example, tuberculosis. In clinical trials of BCG vaccine in the newborn, there has been a significant reduction in subsequent complications of tuberculosis such as miliary tuberculosis or tuberculous meningitis (64).

A number of immunological testing procedures that may be performed in the neonatal period may be useful in the diagnosis of intrauterine or perinatal infections. Particularly important are the quantitation of the immunoglobulins and the determination of specific IgM antibody responses. The measurement of IgA and IgM immunoglobulins in cord sera is of particular interest, because these gamma globulins are not transported from the mother to the fetus by the placenta. Under ordinary circumstances, IgM globulins are present in cord sera in concentrations approximately one tenth those of normal adult values (<200 mg/litre) and IgA is essentially nondetectable. Both proteins reportedly are increased in cord sera from documented cases of intrauterine infections (65,66). Rubella virus, cytomegalovirus, herpes simplex, toxoplasma, *Treponema pallidum*, *Trypanosoma cruzi*, and even infections with bacterial agents can elicit IgM responses as a consequence of infection (5). Several studies have now shown that quantitation of IgM globulins is a good screening test during the newborn period for the diagnosis of intrauterine or associated infections. In these studies, not only false positives but also false negatives have been documented. For example, the presence of high values of IgM or IgA may be the consequence of maternal bleeding into the fetal circulation (67). Increased IgM globulin concentrations caused by maternal bleeding can be differentiated from IgM produced by active antibody synthesis by performing serial immunoglobulin determinations. In maternal bleeding, there is a rapid fall in IgM concentrations within the first week and usually a parallel decrease in IgA due to the short half-life of these immunoglobulins. In infections, on the other hand, the concentrations may stay high unless effective therapy is instituted. The true incidence of maternal bleeding or placental leakage seems to be high. It has been reported that placental leaks occurred in 11% of pregnancies studied (65) and were noted at the time of delivery in 60% of infants with abnormally high concentrations of IgM or IgA (67). Increased concentrations of IgM were found in 4.1% and 4.2% of newborns, respectively, by two groups of authors (66,67), and the incidence of clinical or subclinical infections in the group with abnormally high concentrations of IgM at birth was 34% (66).

Specific Anti-Immunoglobulin M Fluorescence in the Diagnosis of Congenital Infections

Detection of high titers of antibodies by use of such techniques as neutralization and complement fixation will provide information regarding the specificity of the reactions, but these positive reactions can be given by the IgG, IgA, or IgM classes of antibody. Because only the IgG globulins cross the placenta in appreciable amounts, a positive test will not distinguish between intrauterine infection and passive transfer of antibody from the mother.

The use of fluorescence to detect specificity of IgM antibodies against *Toxoplasma gondii* has become popular recently and has been extended to the diagnosis of other infectious diseases (68). This technique has been used successfully for the diagnosis of congenital infection with toxoplasma, rubella, cytomegalovirus, herpes simplex, and syphilis ("TORCHS" group) (5).

The procedure is simple, and rapidly and specifically answers the problem at hand. The serum of the newborn is incubated with specific antigen. After washing, an anti-IgM fluorescein-tagged antiserum is applied to the slide. If IgM antibodies are present, they will remain as antigen-antibody complexes and can be detected by their pattern of fluorescence. Serial dilutions of newborns' sera with a positive reaction will allow the quantitation of the reaction. The titer seems to correlate well with the concentration of IgM globulins. The principal problem encountered in this technique is obtaining a good fluorescein-conjugated specific-antibody reagent for the detection of IgM-associated antibodies. In spite of this, however, it seems to be the most promising diagnostic tool currently available for the diagnosis of intrauterine and neonatal infections.

DIAGNOSIS OF IMMUNE-DEFICIENCY DISORDERS

A number of diagnostic clues available in the newborn period should alert the physician to the possibility of immune-deficiency disorders. Table 12 lists some of the major classes of immune deficiency that can be diagnosed in the newborn period, together with their times of onset and the types of infection that are commonly seen in these disorders. Table 13 lists some of the pertinent clinical and historical information that could be useful in the diagnosis of these disorders.

A knowledge of immunological principles may also be applied to the treatment of infectious diseases in the newborn. The judicious use of fresh whole blood, for example, can be a helpful adjunct in the treatment of neonatal sepsis caused by Gram-negative organisms because it provides such factors as IgM antibody and complement. Use of fresh blood may also help correct a deficiency of those cellular elements necessary for a

Table 12. Immune Deficiency Disorders Which Can Be Diagnosed in the Newborn Period

Disorder	Example	Genetics	Time of onset	Type of infection
Phagocytic function				
quantitative	Neutropenia	Variable	At birth	Virulent bacteria, e.g., staphylococcus
qualitative	Chronic granulomatous disease	X-linked, autosomal recessive	At birth	Less virulent bacteria, e.g., *E. coli*
Antibody	Agammaglobulinemia Dysgammaglobulinemia	Variable	>6 months	Virulent bacteria
Cell-mediated (delayed hypersensitivity) function	Congenital aplasia of thymus (Di George's syndrome)	Variable	At birth	Fungal, viral
Combined antibody and cell-mediated function	"Swiss" agammaglobulinemia	X-linked, autosomal recessive	At birth	Bacterial, viral, fungal
Variable	Ataxia telangiectasia Wiskott-Aldrich syndrome	Autosomal recessive X-linked recessive	>6 months >6 months	Fungal, viral

Table 13. Diagnostic Clues in Suspecting Immune Deficiency Disorders in the Newborn Period

Finding	Comment
Hypocalcemic tetany	Di George's syndrome—can be diagnosed by skin tests for delayed hypersensitivity and in vitro lymphocyte stimulation phytohemagglutinin
History of immune deficiency in other family members	
Agammaglobulinemia	Quantitative immunoglobulins not useful because of passive transfer of IgG; determination after 2 to 4 months helpful in establishing diagnosis
Chronic granulomatous disease	NBT test not helpful because it may be nonspecifically elevated. Tests of bactericidal function helpful, if infections occur
Thymic disorders	Tests of cell-mediated immunity (e.g., phytohemagglutinin) helpful

successful defense against other microorganisms (for instance, viruses). Because cell-mediated immunity is so important in antiviral defense, the immunocompetent lymphoid cells provided by fresh blood can be helpful in treatment. However, caution must be observed in administering immunocompetent lymphoid cells to the neonate, who, for other reasons, may not be immunocompetent; theoretically, such treatment could result in a fatal graft-versus-host reaction (60). These reactions have been described in infants who received intrauterine transfusions for treatment of Rh incompatibility, but they may also be a potential risk after simple transfusions. Finally, immunological principles may also be applicable to therapy in other ways, such as the use of transfer factor of inducers of interferon.

SUMMARY

The human newborn infant is compromised immunologically in both nonspecific and specific immunity. During the newborn period the infant is deficient in all the major nonspecific immune responses: the inflammatory response, the movement of cells toward an area of injury (chemotaxis), and the capacity of macrophages to engulf and subsequently destroy a foreign substance. The specific immune responses of the bone marrow derived or bursal (B) system and the thymic-dependent (T) system likewise show maturational deficiencies.

Accompanying the process of phagocytosis is an increased metabolic activity of the polymorphonuclear leukocyte, which involves primarily the hexose monophosphate pathway. The H_2O_2-myeloperoxidase–halide system, which is subsequently activated, is importantly involved in bactericidal activity and can be assessed either by use of functional tests of bacterial killing or through the reduction of nitroblue tetrazolium dye to a blue formazan pigment. In a study of 122 infants and children, both reduction of this dye and activities of glucose-6-phosphate dehydrogenase and phosphogluconate dehydrogenase in the leukocyte were assessed. All of these increased as the infant matured, in a manner similar to that described for the specific immunological system (e.g., gamma globulin production).

It is against this developmental backdrop of immunological immaturity and maturation that laboratory tests of the neonate must be requested and evaluated.

REFERENCES

1. Bellanti, J. A. (Ed.), *Immunology*, W. B. Saunders Co. Philadelphia, Pa., Neonate Book Chapter 21, 1971.

2. World Health Organization: Cell-mediated immunity and resistance to infection, *Technical Report Series No. 519*, Geneva, 1973.

3. Tomasi, T. B., Jr. and Bienenstock, J., Secretory immunoglobulins. *Adv. Immunol.* **9,** 1 (1968).

4. Bellanti, J. A.: Biologic significance of the γ A secretory immunoglobulin, *Pediatrics* **48,** 715 (1971).

5. Sever, J. L., Immunoglobulin determinations for the detection of perinatal infections, *J. Pediatr.* **75,** 1111 (1969).

6. Rowe, D. S., Hug, K., Forni, L. and Pernis, B., Immunoglobulin D as a lymphocyte receptor, *J. Exp. Med.* **138,** 965 (1973).

7. Hobbs, J. R. and Davis, J. A., Serum γ G-globulin levels and gestational age in premature infants, *Lancet* **i,** 757 (1967).

8. Lawton, A. R., Self, K. S., Royal, S. A. and Cooper, M. D., Ontogeny of B-lymphocytes in the human fetus, *Clin. Immunol. Immunopath.* **1,** 84 (1972).

9. Giltin, D. and Biasucci, A., Development of gamma G, gamma A, gamma M, beta 1_a, beta 1_c, C'1 esterase inhibitor, ceruloplasmin, transferrin, hemopexin, haptoglobin, fibrinogen, plasminogen, alpha-1-antitrypsin, orosomucoid, beta-lipoprotein, alpha-2-macroglobulin and prealbumin in the human conceptus, *J. Clin. Invest.* **48,** 1433 (1969).

10. Hyvarinen, M., Zeltzer, P., Oh, W. and Stiehm, R., Influence of gestational age on serum levels of alpha-1 fetoprotein, IgG globulin, and albumin in newborn infants, *J. Pediatr.* **82,** 430 (1973).

11. Farr, R. S., A quantitative immunochemical measure of the primary interaction between ^{131}I BSA and antibody, *J. Infect. Dis.* **103,** 239 (1958).

12. Playfair, J. H. L., Cell cooperation in the immune response, *Clin. Exp. Immunol.* **8,** 839 (1971).

13. Van Furth, R. and Cohn, Z. A., The origin and kinetics of mononuclear phagocytes, *J. Exp. Med.* **128,** 415 (1968).

14. Hirschhorn, K. et al., Immune response and mitosis of human peripheral blood lymphocytes in vitro, *Science* **142,** 1185 (1963).

15. David, J. R., Lymphocyte mediators and cellular hypersensitivity, *N. Engl. J. Med.* **288,** 143 (1973).

16. Montgomery, J. R. et al., Viral inhibition of lymphocyte response to phytohemagglutinin, *Science* **157,** 1068 (1967).

17. Fuccillo, D. A. et al., Impaired cellular immunity to rubella virus in congenital rubella, *Infect. Immunol.* **9,** 81 (1974).

18. Thong, Y. H. et al., Impaired in vitro cell-mediated immunity to rubella virus during pregnancy, *N. Engl. J. Med.* **289,** 604 (1973).

19. Bellanti, J. A. and Green, R. E., Immunological reactivity expression of efficiency in elimination of foreignness, *Lancet* **ii,** 526 (1971).

20. Stiehm, R. and Fulginiti, V. A., *Pediatric Immunologic Diseases*. W. B. Saunders Co., Philadelphia, 1973, 1.

21. August, C. S., Berkel, A. I., Merler, E., and Driscoll, S. Onset of the lymphocyte function in the developing human fetus, *Pediatr. Res.* **5,** 539 (1971).

22. Goldstein, A. L., Asanuma, Y., and White, A., The thymus as an endocrine gland: properties of thymosin, a new thymus hormone, *Recent Prog. Horm. Res.* **26**, 550 (1970).

23. Goldstein, A. L. et al., Purification and biological activity of thymosin, a hormone of thymus gland, *Proc. Nat. Acad. Sci. U.S.A.* **69**, 1800 (1972).

24. Small, M. and Trainin, N., Contribution of a thymic humoral factor to the development of immunologically competent population from cells of mouse bone marrow, *J. Exp. Med.* **134**, 786 (1971).

25. August, C. S. et al., Implantation of a foetal thymus, restoring immunological competence in a patient with thymic aplasic (Di George's syndrome), *Lancet* **ii**, 1210 (1968).

26. Cleveland, W. W., Fogel, B. J., Brown, W. T. and Kay, H. E. M., Foetal thymic transplant in a case of Di George's syndrome, *Lancet* **ii**, 1211 (1968).

27. Steele, R. W. et al., Familial thymic aplasia. Attempted reconstitution with fetal thymus in a Millipore diffusion chamber, *N. Engl. J. Med.* **287**, 787 (1972).

28. Hong, R., Gatti, R., Rathbun, J. C. and Good, R. A., Thymic hypoplasia and thyroid dysfunction, *N. Engl. J. Med.* **282**, 470 (1970).

29. Cooper, M. D. and Lawton, A. R., Circulating B-cell in patients with immunodeficiency, *Am. J. Pathol.* **69**, 513 (1972).

30. Atkins, E. and Bordel, P., Fever, *N. Engl. J. Med.* **286**, 27 (1972).

31. Akenzua, G., Hui, Y. T., Zipursky, A., and Milner, R., Neutrophil and band counts in the diagnosis of neonatal infections, *Pediatrics* **54**, 38 (1974).

32. Eitzman, D. V. and Smith, R. T., The nonspecific inflammatory cycle in the neonatal infant, *Am. J. Dis. Child.* **97**, 326 (1959).

33. Bullock, J. D. et al., Inflammatory response in the neonate re-examined, *Pediatrics* **44**, 58 (1969).

34. Sheldon, W. H. and Caldwell, J. B. H., The mononuclear cell phase of inflammation in the newborn, *Bull. Johns Hopkins Hosp.* **112**, 258 (1963).

35. Miller, M. E. and Stiehm, E. R., Phagocytic, opsonic and immunoglobulin studies in newborns, *Calif. Med.* **119**, 43 (1973).

36. Adinolfi, M., Ontogeny of components of complement and lysozyme. In *Ontogeny of Acquired Immunity*, R. Porter and J. Knight, Eds. Ciba Foundation Symposium. American Elsevier Pub. Co., New York, N.Y., 1972.

37. Pillemer, L. et al., The properdin system and immunity, *Science* **120**, 279 (1954).

38. Colten, H. R., Ontogeny of the human complement system: In vitro biosynthesis of individual complement components by fetal tissues, *J. Clin. Invest.* **51**, 725 (1972).

39. Kohler, P. F., Maturation of the human complement system, *J. Clin. Invest.* **52**, 671 (1973).

40. Gotoff, S. P., Neonatal immunity, *J. Pediatr.* **85**, 149 (1974).

41. Gluck, L. and Silverman, W. A., Phagocytosis in premature infants, *Pediatrics* **20**, 951 (1957).

42. Matoth, Y. Phagocytic and ameboid activities of the leukocytes in the newborn infant, *Pediatrics* **9**, 748 (1952).

43. Park, B. H., Holmes, B., and Good, R. A., Metabolic activities in leukocytes of newborn infants, *J. Pediatr.* **76**, 237 (1970).

44. Miller, M. E., Phagocytosis in the newborn infant: Humoral and cellular factors, *J. Pediatr.* **74**, 255 (1969).

45. Pearson, H. A., Phagocytosis by leukocytes of newborn infants, *J. Pediatr.* **74**, 329 (1969) (Editorial).

46. Coen, R., Grush, O., and Kauder, E.: Studies of bactericidal activity and metabolism of the leukocyte in full-term neonates, *J. Pediatr.* **75**, 400 (1969).

47. Bellanti, J. A., Cantz, B. E., Maybee, D. A., and Schlegel, R. J., Defective phagocytosis by newborn leukocytes: A defect similar to that in chronic granulomatos disease? *Pediatr. Res.* **3**, 376 (1969). (Abstract).

48. Cline, M. J., Metabolism of the circulating leukocyte, *Physiol. Rev.* **45**, 674 (1965).

49. Brant, L., Studies on the phagocytic activity of neutrophilic leukocytes, *Scand. J. Haematol.* Suppl. 2 (1967).

50.   Klebanoff, S. J., Myeloperoxidase-halide-hydrogen peroxide antibacterial system, *J. Bacteriol* **95**, 2131 (1966).

51.   Baehner, R. L. and Nathan, D. G., Quantitative nitroblue tetrazolium test in chronic granulomatous disease, *N. Engl. J. Med.* **278**, 971 (1968).

52.   Bridges, R. A., Berendes, H., and Good, R. A., A fatal granulomatous disease of childhood: The clinical, pathological and laboratory features of a new syndrome, *Am. J. Dis. Child.* **97**, 387 (1959).

53.   Bellanti, J. A. et al., Biochemical changes in human polymorphonuclear leukocytes during maturation. In *The Phagocytic Cell in Host Resistance*, J. A. Bellanti and D. H. Dayton, Eds. Raven Press, New York, N.Y. 1975.

54.   Vahlquist, B., Transfer of antibodies from mother to offspring, *Adv. Pediat.* **10**, 305 (1958).

55.   Porter, R. R., The hydrolysis of rabbit γ-globulin and antibodies with crystalline papain, *Biochem. J.* **73**, 119 (1959).

56.   Franck, F. and Neslin, R. S., Recovery of antibody-combining activity of interaction of different peptide chains isolated from purified horse antitoxin, *Folia Microbiol. (Parah.* 2) **8**, 128 (1963).

57.   Alford, C. A., Jr., Studies on antibody in congenital rubella infections. I. Physicochemical and immunologic investigations of rubella neutralizing antibody. *Am. J. Dis. Child.* **110**, 455 (1965).

58.   Bellanti, J. A. et al., Congenital rubella, *Am. J. Dis. Child.* **110**, 464 (1965).

59.   Alford, C. A., Jr., Immunoglobulin determinations in the diagnosis of fetal infection, *Pediatr. Clin. N. Am.* **18**, 99 (1971).

60.   Naiman, J. L. et al., Possible graft-versus-host reaction after intrauterine transfusion for Rh erythroblastosis fetalis, *N. Engl. J. Med.* **281**, 697 (1969).

61.   Hayward, A. R. and Soothill, J. F.: Reaction to antigen by human foetal thymus lymphocytes. In *Ontogeny of Acquired Immunity*, R. Porter and J. Knight, Eds., Ciba Foundation Symposium. American Elsevier Pub. Co., New York, N.Y., 1972.

62.   Leikin, S., Mochir-Fatemi, F. and Park, K., Blast transformation of lymphocytes from newborn human infants, *J. Pediatr.* **72**, 510 (1968).

63.   Krugman, S., Giles, J. P., and Hammond, J., Viral hepatitis, type B (MS-2 strain): Prevention with specific hepatitis B immune serum globulin, *J.A.M.A.* **218**, 1665 (1971).

64.   Rosenthal, S. R. (Ed.): *BCG Vaccination against Tuberculosis*. Boston, Little, Brown & Co., Boston, Mass., 1957.

65.   Stiehm, E. R., Ammann, A. J. and Cherry, J. D., Elevated cord macroglobulins in the diagnosis of intrauterine infections, *N. Engl. J. Med.* **275**, 971 (1966).

66.   Alford, C. A., Jr., Immunoglobulin determinations in the diagnosis of fetal infection, *Pediatr. Clin. N. Am.* **18**, 99 (1974).

67.   Miller, M. J., Sunshine, P. J., and Remington, J. S., Quantitation of cord serum IgM and IgA as a screening procedure to detect congenital infection: Results in 5,006 infants, *J. Pediatr.* **75**, 1287 (1969).

68.   Remington, J. S., Miller, M. J., and Brownlee, L., IgM antibodies in acute toxoplasmosis I. Diagnostic significance in congenital cases and a method for their rapid demonstration, *Pediatrics* **41**, 1082 (1968).

The Biochemical and Clinical Aspects of Genital Ambiguity in the Neonate

MELVIN E. JENKINS, M.D.

The biochemical processes that determine sexual differentiation of the internal and external genital structures are not fully understood, despite the early classic experiments of Jost (1–3) and extensive subsequent research on genital differentiation. Here I will review current concepts of genital differentiation from the standpoint of control mechanisms in health and derangements in disease. Some clinical experiments in nature demonstrating profound masculinizing influences on the genetic female fetus and feminizing influences on the male fetus will be presented. The role of the clinical chemist in problems related to genital ambiguity will also be considered.

Genetic sex determines gonadal sex, which, in turn, determines body sex as it relates to internal-duct structures (Figure 1). One might look upon the progressive control systems as stages of sexual determination of differentiation between early fetal age and birth.

In terms of genetics, it has long been apparent that fertilization of a normal X-chromosome-bearing ovum by an X-chromosome-bearing sperm produces an XX female, and by a Y sperm produces an XY male. However, neither the control mechanisms nor the precise chemical compounds that determine whether a primitive gonad will differentiate into an ovary or into a testis have yet been identified.

The primitive gonad can be identified as early as the fourth week of intrauterine life, in the coelomic epithelium in the genital ridges of the dorsal mesentery. The early gonadal primordium proliferates sex cords into the underlying mesenchyme (Figure 2). The first set of cords is assumed to have testicular potentialities, and these cords become future testicular components in the male, while in the female they form the ovarian cortex. It should be emphasized that proliferation of the sex cords from the germinal epithelium has never been demonstrated experimentally by any type of study, including measurement of mitotic turnover rates. Moreover, there are animals (the rat, for example), in which successive proliferation of sex cords has never been observed.

As early as 1914, Witschi (4) postulated that the undifferentiated gonad in animals consists of two components of opposing significance: the internal medulla and the

247

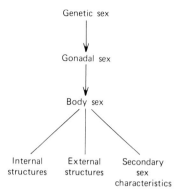

Genetic sex

Gonadal sex

Body sex

Internal structures   External structures   Secondary sex characteristics

Figure 1. Stages and sequences of morphologic differentiation of sexual structures.

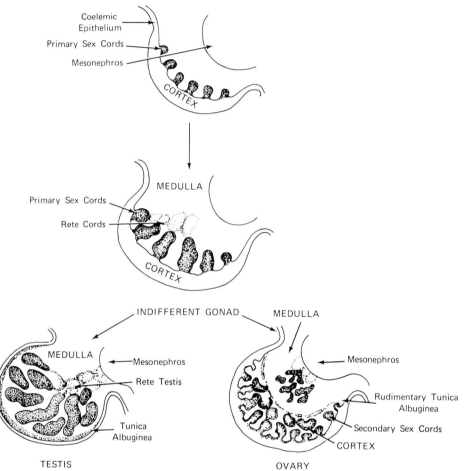

Coelemic Epithelium
Primary Sex Cords
Mesonephros
CORTEX

MEDULLA
Primary Sex Cords
Rete Cords
CORTEX

INDIFFERENT GONAD   MEDULLA

MEDULLA
Mesonephros
Rete Testis
Tunica Albuginea

TESTIS

Mesonephros
Rudimentary Tunica Albuginea
Secondary Sex Cords
CORTEX

OVARY

Figure 2. Gonadal differentiation. *Top:* Gonad at indifferent stages of sexual differentiation: the
primary sex cords represent the male or medullary component, whereas the germinal epithelium represents, potentially, the cortical component. *Middle:* Differentiation of a testis consists in the further
development of the primary sex cords, and the reduction of the germinal epithelium to a thin, serous
membrane, accompanied by development of the tunica albuginea. *Bottom:* Differentiation of an ovary
consists in reduction of the primary sex cords to medullary cords of the ovary, whereas the cortex is
formed by continued development of cortical cords from the germinal epithelium. From R. K. Burns,
In *Sex and Internal Secretions*, 1, 3rd ed., W. C. Young, Ed. Williams and Wilkins Co., Baltimore, Md.,
1961, p 76, by permission.

superficial cortex. He further postulated that these two gonadal components were antagonistic and secreted opposing inductive substances, which he called medullarine and cortexine. Whether or not the resulting gonad was a testis or an ovary depended, he thought, on the prevalence of one inducer over the other. This theory has been extended to suggest that most of the testis derives from medullary components of the primitive gonad and most of the ovary, including its germ cells, is derived from the primitive cortex (Figure 2).

Regardless of the mechanisms of differentiation of the gonad into ovary or testis, two points remain quite clear. First, the testis differentiates into a functional organ at an earlier stage of fetal development than does the ovary. The testis becomes fully functional in terms of the capacity of Leydig cells to secrete testosterone and dihydrotestosterone as early as the sixth to eighth fetal week. The ovary is not fully developed until about 18 weeks of gestation, and continues to differentiate, as well as to shed primordial ova, throughout fetal life. Secondly, it is now known that the testis is the sex differentiator of the internal-duct structures and the external genitalia. This concept supports Jost's experiments (1), which demonstrated that when male or female rabbits were surgically castrated in utero before the onset of genital differentiation, they uniformly acquired a female genital tract. Normal uteri and female internal-duct structures developed, as well as normal female external genitalia, indicating that the fetal ovary is dispensable for genital organogenesis in the female. This concept also indicates that the fetal testis prevents the genital tract from becoming feminine and thereby imposes masculinity on the fetus. Furthermore, this function appears to influence the primordial internal genital structures locally (i.e., unilaterally) if a testis is present on one side but absent on the other; on the side where there is a testis, feminine internal-duct structures are suppressed, but they develop on the contralateral, nonstimulated side.

Fetal testes secrete testosterone and dihydrotestosterone during fetal life and also produce a second type of substance, an as-yet-unidentified polypeptide. This polypeptide is responsible for suppression of the müllerian duct system, preventing uterine and fallopian tube development, and also assists in the development of the male internal-duct structures—the vas deferens, seminal vesicles, and prostate (Figure 3). Testosterone or dihydrotestosterone, on the other hand, is responsible for the masculinization of the external genitalia in progressive stages (Figure 4).

Jost's original experiments (1–3) have been supported by a number of subsequent experimental observations, as well as by clinical disorders in which either the ovary or the testis is dysgenic or absent at an early critical stage of fetal genital differentiation. For example, if a fetal rabbit is exposed to the antiandrogen, cyproterone acetate, the male rabbits are abnormal with female external genitalia, but the uterus and tubes will be absent (5). This concept further supports the existence of two hormones in the sense that cyproterone acetate only suppresses androgenic effects, therefore the postulated organizer, testicular polypeptide, remains potent enough to suppress female internal-duct structures. Figure 3 summarizes the differentiation of the internal-duct structures in most mammalian species. As illustrated on the left, normal uterus and tubes develop in the presence of ovaries. On the right, the presence of a testis has suppressed the development of the uterus and tubes but has participated in the formation of male internal sex structures. In the center, a neutral situation is demonstrated, in which either ovaries or testes are absent in either the male or female, resulting in the formation of a normal uterus and tubes. These concepts are tabulated in Table 1, which summarizes the effects of the müllerian regression factor (inhibitor) and testosterone secreted by the fetal testis on the masculinization of the male fetus.

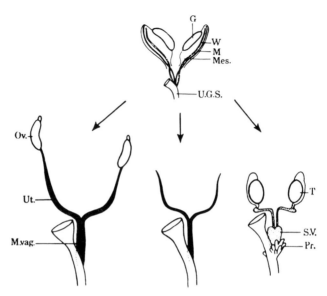

Figure 3. Internal genital differentiation. From Jost, A., *Johns Hopkins Med. J.* **130**, 42 (1972), by permission.

Table 1. Influences of Hormonal Substances on Genital
Differentiation of Male Fetus

Process	Factor needed	
	Müllerian regression factor	Testosterone
Müllerian inhibition	+	
Wolffian stimulation	+	+
External virilization		+

FOUR CLINICAL EXAMPLES OF GENITAL AMBIGUITY

Luteoma of pregnancy.   The first patient (Figure 5) is a three-day-old female with almost completely masculinized external genitalia and an enlarged clitoris, a phallic urethra with completely fused labioscrotal folds comprising the apparent scrotum. A clue to the diagnosis in this patient was the fact that the mother had shown some virilizing signs during her pregnancy, including increased facial hair, deepening of her voice, and enlargement of the clitoris. This infant was delivered by cesarean section, at which time a large left ovarian tumor was found and removed. Histologically, the tumor was categorized as a pregnancy luteoma; on in vitro incubation studies with radioactively tagged pregnenolone or progesterone, it demonstrated a significant capacity to produce androgens, including testosterone. A buccal smear, done on this infant at two days of age, was more than 20% chromatin positive and her chromosomal karyotype was 46 XX. A normal uterus was palpated on rectal examination. She underwent corrective surgery of her external genitalia at age seven months. Figure 6 illustrates her completely feminized external genitalia one month after corrective surgery.

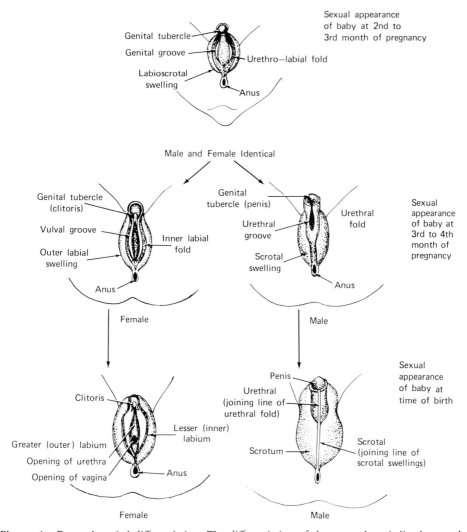

Figure 4. External genital differentiation. The differentiation of the external genitalia along male lines depends on androgen stimulation, which results in increased growth of the genital tubercle and fusion of the labial folds into the penis and scrotum, respectively. From Wilkins, L., In *The Diagnosis and Treatment of Endocrine Disorders in Children and Adolescents*, 3rd ed. Charles C Thomas, Springfield, Ill., 1966, p 302, by permission.

Virilizing adrenal hyperplasia. This eight-day-old female was admitted to the pediatric service in a salt-losing crisis with moderately severely masculinized external genitalia (Figure 7). Note that the clitoris is substantially enlarged and that there is fusion of the labioscrotal folds, with a common opening for the urethra and vagina. This second patient, like the first, had completely normal internal female genitalia—normal ovaries, uterus, and tubes. This patient demonstrates the effect of androgens produced by the fetus on the external genitalia of the developing female during the eighth to twelfth fetal week.

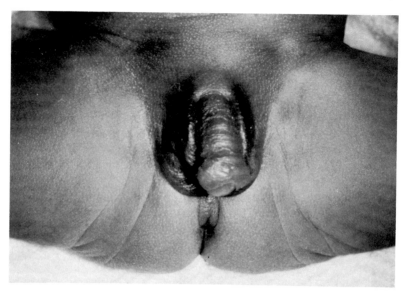

Figure 5. Patient 1, age 3 days. Note the extreme masculinization of the external genitals. Mother was also virilized by a pregnancy luteoma necessitating cesarean section for delivery. From Jenkins, M. E. et al., Ambiguity genitalia in a female infant associated with luteoma of pregnancy, *Am. J. Obstet. Gynecol.* **101**, 924 (1968), by permission.

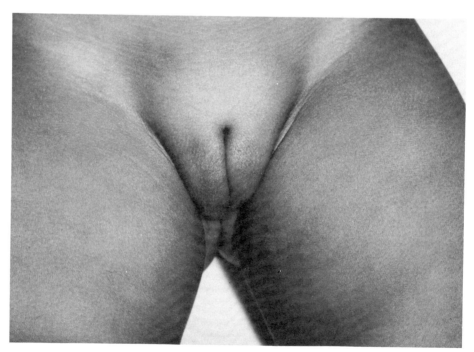

Figure 6. Patient 1, age 8 months, after corrective surgery of genital ambiguity. From Jenkins, M. E., *Am. J. Obstet. Gynecol.* **101**, 926 (1968), by permission.

252

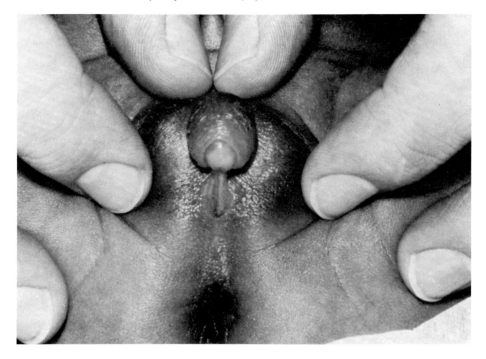

Figure 7. Patient 2. Moderately severe virilization in female with congenital adrenal hyperplasia (21 hydroxylation block). Note clitoral enlargement and labial fusion.

XO/XY mosaicism. This third patient (Figure 8), age one month, had a testis and hydrocele on the right side with an ovarian streak on the left side. At surgery, one half of a uterus and fallopian tube were demonstrated on the side of the ovarian streak. No female internal-duct structures were demonstrated on the side of the testis. This experiment in nature supports the idea of a lateralizing effect on genital differentiation of compounds produced by the testis.

Testicular feminization. This phenotypic female (Figure 9) had an XY chromosomal pattern and normal testes but an insensitivity of all peripheral tissues, including the hypothalamus, to testosterone. Therefore, the external genitalia are normally female at birth and such patients feminize at puberty, because the hypothalamus is also insensitive to androgen (8). When gonadotropin, follitropin (follicle-stimulating hormone), and lutropin (luteinizing hormone) increase at puberty, the testis, which has estrogen-producing capacity, begins to produce more estrogen, which ultimately establishes a feedback relationship with pituitary gonadotropin. When serum estrogen concentrations characteristic of the normal adult are reached, normal feminization occurs. Unfortunately, the testes in these patients must be removed after secondary sexual characteristics are complete because of their increased tendency to malignant degeneration after the third decade. This patient, as would be suspected, had no uterus or female internal-duct structures, because the testicular organizer substance could suppress the müllerian ducts, but androgens produced by these testes had no effect because of the genetically acquired peripheral resistance to testosterone.

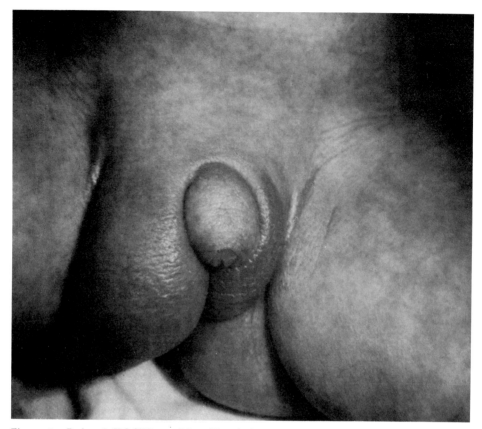

Figure 8. Patient 2, XO/XY mosaicism. Note bulge representing hydrocele on the right.

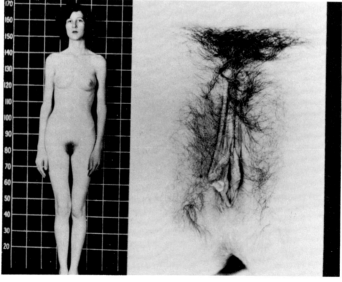

Figure 9. Patient 4. Genetic male with testicular feminization. Note normal female phenotype despite XY chromosomal pattern. From Wilkins, L. In *The Diagnosis and Treatment of Endocrine Disorders in Children and Adolescents*, 3rd ed. Charles C Thomas, Springfield, Ill., 1966, p 322, by permission.

These are but a few of many examples of clinical experiments in nature that support the experimental observations of Jost (1) and others that the testes are essential to masculinization of the fetus and that genetic sex plays no role except as a determinant of differentiation of the primitive gonad into either an ovary or a testis.

ROLE OF THE CLINICAL CHEMIST

The clinical chemist must appreciate the urgency of an early diagnosis and decision on sex of rearing that the physician must make when the newborn has ambiguous genitalia. Parental and extended family anxiety over the ambiguity can only be successfully approached by a team of health providers—pediatrician, psychiatrist, psychologist, health educators, clinical chemists, and others. Because many of the females virilized at birth have adrenal hyperplasia and because most of the patients with adrenal hyperplasia are losing salt, there are significant risks of shock and potential death during the first few days or weeks after birth. Clinical tests to determine this condition are, in fact, emergency procedures. Table 2 outlines the diagnostic steps and tests that are essential for an early diagnosis. The clinical chemist in a hospital setting must familiarize himself with the indicated procedures in newborns with genital ambiguity and must become a member of the total team to fully participate in the early management of this emergency health problem. The chemist provides the objective diagnostic clues that are essential for total patient care.

Table 2. Diagnostic Steps in Evaluation of Newborns with Ambiguous Genitalia

Buccal smear (sex chromatin)
Chromosomal studies
Urinary 17-ketosteroids
Urinary 17-hydroxycorticosteroids
Plasma androgens
Serum sodium, potassium, chloride, CO_2 (may need frequent repeats)
Blood pH
Urethal cytology
Exploratory laparotomy to view internal structures and for gonadal biopsy, when indicated.

SUMMARY

Genital ambiguity can occur in an otherwise normal female who has been exposed to excessive androgen during the critical stages of external genital differentiation and in the male who experiences insufficient exposure to either organizer substance or androgens between the eighth and twelfth fetal week. Chemical control mechanisms of sexual differentiation have been reviewed and illustrative cases are presented that support the experimental basis for normal sexual differentiation. The role of the clinical chemist is emphasized, and this important member of the health-care team must participate in the total management of the infant with genital ambiguity if appropriate and effective management is to be achieved.

REFERENCES

1. Jost, A., Sur les effets de la castration précoce de l'embryon mâle de lapin, *Compt. Rend. Soc. Biol.* (Paris) 141, 126 (1947).

2. Jost, A., Sur le rôle des gonades foetales dans la differenciation sexuelle somatique de l'embryon de lapin, *Compt. Rend. Assoc. Anat.* 51, 255 (1947).

3. Jost, A., Researches sur la differenciation sexuelle de l'embryon de lapin, III. Role des gonades foetales dans la differenciation sexuelle somatique, *Arch. Anat. Microsc. Morphol. Exp.* 361, 271 (1947).

4. Witschi, E., Biochemistry of sex differentiation in vertebrate embryos. In *The Biochemistry of Animal Development*, R. Webeb, Ed., Academic Press, Inc., New York, N.Y. 1967, pp 193–225.

5. Jost, A., Steroids and sex differentiation of the mammalian foetus, Proc. 11nd Internat. Congr. Hormonal Steroids, Milano, 1966. *Excerpta Med. Int. Cong. Ser. No. 132*, 74, 1966 (Amsterdam).

6. Jenkins, M. E., Surano, R. B., and Russel-Cutts, C., Ambiguous genitalia in female newborns associated with luteoma of pregnancy. *Am. J. Obstet. Gynecol.* 101, 923 (1968).

7. Wilkins, L., *The Diagnosis and Treatment of Endocrine Disorders in Childhood and Adolescence*, 3rd ed, Charles C Thomas, Springfield, Ill. 1965, pp 321–322.

8. Polani, P. E., Hormonal and clinical aspects of hermaphroditism and the testicular feminizing syndrome in man, *Philos. Trans. R. Soc. Lond.* Biol Sci., 259, 187 (1970).

Respiratory Distress Syndrome

MARILYN RENFIELD, M.D.

Probably no other illness of the newborn has been the object of as much intense research and devoted clinical care as has hyaline membrane disease, respiratory distress syndrome. In the United States alone, about 25,000 infants die from hyaline membrane disease each year (1). But the magnitude of this disease is only partly revealed by mortality statistics. Each infant, struggling to breathe and live with this illness, should receive intensive care provided by a devoted staff of nurses, physicians, inhalation therapists, and laboratory personnel. There follow days of intense medical care and years of pediatric follow-up for the survivors. Although no one has yet delineated the precise causes and means of preventing hyaline membrane disease, we are near a breakthrough in our understanding of this syndrome.

Hyaline membrane disease is not so much a disease as it is a consequence of developmental immaturity. It occurs primarily in the premature infant who is not yet ready for extrauterine life, with its requirement for air breathing. Indeed, the term "prematurity" might best be defined in terms of pulmonary maturation, for little else matters if the newborn infant cannot adequately aerate his lungs.

During intrauterine life, the pulmonary system has a developmental sequence of its own that is in part independent of gestational age. It is when this maturation sequence is not complete at the time of birth that hyaline membrane disease is likely to occur.

THE MATURATION SEQUENCE OF THE LUNGS

Pulmonary maturation can be assessed from both the cellular and the biochemical aspects.

Cellular Maturation (2,3,4)

Before 16 weeks of gestation, the lungs consist of cuboidal glandular cells, derived from the primitive gut endoderm. There are no air spaces and no capillaries. By 16 to 20 weeks of gestation, alveolar ducts and early capillary ingrowth are seen. The alveolar epithelium has not yet differentiated into its distinct cell types. By term, a remarkable differentiation has occurred. Type I alveolar lining cells form a thin barrier lying next to the capillary endothelial cells. It is across this small barrier that gas exchange occurs in the lungs—O_2 moves from the alveolus into the capillary, where it is bound to hemoglobin within erythrocytes, and CO_2 from hemoglobin and plasma into the alveolar air space, where it is exhaled. Type II alveolar lining cells appear within each alveolus. They are relatively thick cells and contain osmiophilic inclusions, also called lamellar inclusion bodies. These inclusions appear to be the pulmonary surfactant. Type II cells serve as the storage site for surfactant; it is from these cells that surfactant is discharged into the alveolar air space. Whether or not type II cells also manufacture surfactant is still not known (2,5). Therefore, the capacity for surfactant production and release depends upon the differentiation of the type II cell.

Why is surfactant production important in hyaline membrane disease (2)? At autopsy, lungs of infants who succumb to hyaline membrane disease are found to lack the capacity to reduce surface tension on compression. The lungs are totally atelectatic. Normally, the presence of a surface-active complex (surfactant) lining the alveoli prevents atelectasis and allows the lungs to keep a residual volume at the end of expiration (1,5,6). Gas exchange can then occur during both the inspiratory and the expiratory phases of the respiratory cycle. In hyaline membrane disease, there is an absence or delayed appearance of pulmonary surfactant to serve as this antiatelectasis factor.

Biochemical Maturation of the Lungs (7)

Two major kinds of pulmonary surfactant are produced in the fetal lung. The first is via the methyltransferase or "fetal" pathway, and the end product is a lecithin that contains an α-palmitic acid and β-myristic acid (Figure 1). This lecithin is first made during the 22nd to 24th weeks of gestation and is produced to term in human and primate fetuses. Other animals lack this methylation pathway and die of respiratory insufficiency if born prematurely. In human fetuses born prematurely, it is this methylation pathway that offers a hope of survival. However, it is a fragile pathway, with a rapid turnover rate. Synthesis of this "fetal" lecithin is easily inhibited by acidosis, hypothermia, hypoxia, and hypercapnia (1). An infant may be born with this pathway functioning, but these deleterious events may occur during labor, delivery, or the early hours of life, and result in cessation of surfactant production, initiating the chain of events that results in hyaline membrane disease.

The second pathway is called the phosphocholine transferase reaction or "mature" pathway. The end product is a lecithin with palmitic acid on both the α- and the β-carbons of choline (Figure 2). This dipalmityl lecithin begins to be produced at about 35 weeks of gestation in the human fetus, and it allows for mature alveolar stability. Its synthesis is usually not inhibited by acidosis, hypoxia, hypercapnia, or hypothermia. It allows the more mature fetus and term infant to survive the normally acidotic process of labor and delivery, without cessation in pulmonary surfactant production.

Figure 1. The methyl transferase reaction (fetal pathway) (From 7).

Phosphatidylethanolamine + 2 $CH_3\rightarrow$ phosphatidyldimethylethanolamine + $CH_3\rightarrow$ lecithin containing palmitic acid and myristic acid

↑

3-S-adenosyl-L-methionine

1. Made from 22–24 weeks of gestation; allows humans and primates to be born prematurely.
2. Rapid turnover rate.
3. Synthesis inhibited by acidosis, hypothermia, hypoxia, hypercapnia.

Figure 2. Phosphocholine transferase reaction (mature pathway). (From 7).

Cytidine-PO$_4$-PO$_4$-choline + D-α-diglyceride lecithin containing α-palmitic acid and β-palmitic acid

1. Lecithin synthesis for mature alveolar stability.
2. Matures at about 35 weeks of gestation in humans.
3. Synthesis not easily inhibited by acidosis, hypothermia, hypoxia, of hypercarbia.

LABORATORY TESTS FOR ASSESSING PULMONARY MATURATION

The pulmonary fluid that fills the lungs in utero before air breathing has occurred leaves the lungs and enters the amniotic fluid. Analysis of amniotic fluid, obtained by amniocentesis, for the presence of dipalmityl lecithin serves as a diagnostic tool to assess pulmonary maturation. The two most widely used tests are the lecithin/sphingomyelin (L/S) ratio (7,8), and the shake (or bubble) test (9).

An L/S ratio >2 is evidence of pulmonary maturity and the absence of hyaline membrane disease in almost all cases. Unfortunately, a ratio <2 has a high false-negative predictability. In a study by Spellacy, 57.1% of cases with an L/S ratio <2 did not get hyaline membrane disease (10) (Table 1).

Table 1. Accuracy of the L/S Ratio in Predicting the Occurrence of Hyaline Membrane Disease[a]

	L/S ratio <2	L/S ratio >2
No. of cases	14	128
Respiratory distress syndrome	6(42.9%)	1(0.8%)
False-negative rate	57.1%	—
False-positive rate	—	0.8%

[a] From ref. 10.

The same commonness of false-negative results is seen for the bubble test; 76% of cases that give a negative test do not get hyaline membrane disease. On the other hand, a positive bubble test also indicates pulmonary maturity in essentially all cases, with no hyaline membrane disease occurring (11) (Table 2). When an obstetrician tries to assess

Table 2. Accuracy of Bubble Stability Test in Predicting the Occurrence of Hyaline Membrane Disease[a]

Total no. of cases		No. cases with normal respiration	No. with RDS[a]	Accuracy of prediction (%)
Bubble stability				
Negative	25	19	6	24.0
Intermediate	18	16	2	11.1
Positive	37	37	0	100.0

[a] From ref. 11.

pulmonary maturity by these two tests, he can be reasonably sure that the baby will not have hyaline membrane disease if the results indicate maturity. Unfortunately, an "immature" L/S ratio or negative bubble test is unreliable in predicting the occurrence of hyaline membrane disease.

CHARACTERISTICS OF HYALINE MEMBRANE DISEASE

Infants at Risk and Diagnostic Signs and Symptoms

Infants especially at risk for the development of hyaline membrane disease are those infants in whom the process of pulmonary surfactant maturation is not yet completed at the time of birth or in whom insults have occurred that inhibit further synthesis of surfactant.

Those most at risk are immature infants (prematures and infants of diabetic mothers), asphyxiated preterm infants (asphyxiation caused by, e.g., bleeding, hypotension, delayed second stage of labor), and infants delivered by cesarean section necessitated by some obstetrical complication. Rarely, asphyxiated term infants may be affected. As in most neonatal illnesses, males are affected twice as often as females (*12*).

Infants so afflicted show signs of illness within the first hours of postnatal life, often while still in the delivery room. Physical signs of respiratory distress include tachypnea, tachycardia, see-saw respiration, intercostal and xiphoid retractions, flaring of the alae nasi, expiratory grunting, and cyanosis.

The roentgenogram of the chest reveals a classic triad of findings upon which the diagnosis is based: a ground-glass appearance, air bronchograms, and a fine reticulogranular pattern. These findings are the result of widespread alveolar atelectasis, associated with collapse of terminal alveoli, fluid exudation, and some capillary hemorrhage. Hence bronchi and bronchioles are seen as air-filled passages, which contrast with the relatively solid lung surrounding these structures (*12*).

Physiological Derangements in Hyaline Membrane Disease (*13–17*)

Some insult occurs to initiate a chain of events resulting in the disorder called hyaline membrane disease. The precise nature of this insult or series of insults is not now fully understood, but may include asphyxia of the fetus. Asphyxia results in hypercarbia, hypoxia, and acidosis, which in turn cause intense pulmonary vasoconstriction. The consequences of pulmonary vasoconstriction are profound, producing a vicious cycle that perpetuates the illness (*13*) (Figure 3). Pulmonary vasoconstriction results in hypoperfusion of alveolar cells, which in turn causes the following sequence of events:

- anaerobic metabolism of alveolar cells with acidosis and further damage to alveolar cells;
- deficient cellular metabolism with decreased surfactant synthesis, leading to alveolar atelectasis and poor lung compliance;
- membrane fragility, breakdown of alveoli, and alveolar cell death;
- fibrin effusion into alveolar ducts and air spaces when alveolar cell integrity is lost;
- right-to-left intrapulmonary shunting with unoxygenated venous blood entering the systemic circulation;
- further decrease in gas exchange with increasing hypoxia and acidosis; and
- greater pulmonary vasoconstriction and further alveolar cell death.

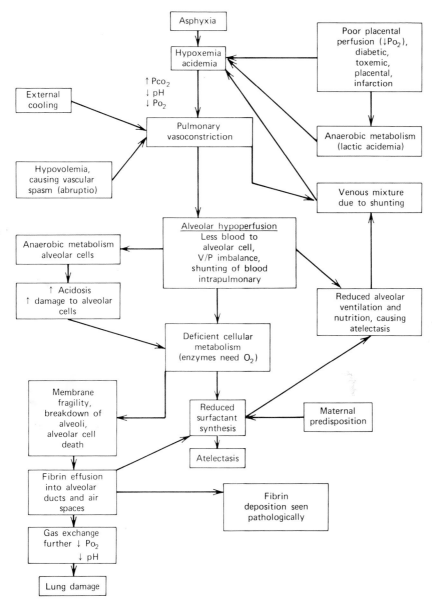

Figure 3. Mechanisms of respiratory distress. (After D. W. Tooley, Cardiovascular Research Institute, University of California at San Francisco, California 94122.)

The cycle continues unless hypoxia, acidosis, and hypercarbia can be reversed and pulmonary perfusion restored.

Other possible causes of pulmonary vasoconstriction—in addition to acidosis, hypercarbia, and hypoxia—are external cooling and hypovolemia.

Pathologically, one sees widespread alveolar atelectasis, hyaline membranes formed by fluid exudation and fibrin deposition in alveolar ducts and air spaces, dilated lymphatics, and intense arteriolar constriction (*14*).

Infants are often in systemic circulatory collapse because of the high pulmonary vascular resistance, high pulmonary artery pressure, low aortic blood pressure, and large right-to-left intrapulmonary shunting of unoxygenated blood (*18*).

Correction of acidosis, hypoxia, hypothermia, and hypovolemia serves to reverse the pulmonary vasoconstriction, thereby lowering toward normal the pulmonary vascular resistance and elevating toward normal the aortic blood pressure. Pulmonary blood flow and arterial oxygenation are improved significantly.

THERAPY OF HYALINE MEMBRANE DISEASE (*13*)

A thermoneutral environment is provided by use of incubators. By keeping the body temperature of the infant normal, O_2 consumption is kept at its lowest, and the infant is under no demand to utilize O_2 to maintain body heat (*19*).

Fluids are provided to meet fluid and basal caloric needs. Very small infants may also be given supplemental protein, minerals and vitamins, and high concentrations of glucose in an attempt to provide more calories. Blood ammonia, osmolality, electrolytes, glucose, and protein, and urinary specific gravity and pH must be monitored during this therapy (*20*).

Acid-base Balance

Oxygen. So that aortic blood gases can be accurately monitored, aortic catheterization is performed. The catheter remains in place as long as the need to monitor blood gases exists. Oxygen is delivered to the infant to try to keep the arterial p_{O_2} between 6.7 and 10.7 kPa (50 and 80 mmHg). The higher the arterial p_{O_2}, the greater the risk of retrolental fibroplasia, although there is no specific value at which toxicity can be expected. In view of the fact that a fetus exists in utero with p_{O_2} of 2.7 to 4.7 kPa (20–35 mmHg) in the umbilical vein, any p_{O_2} greater than this may be potentially toxic to the retina of an immature infant. On the other hand, an arterial p_{O_2} much below 5.3 to 6.7 kPa (40–50 mmHg) is on the very steep part of the hemoglobin dissociation curve, and small changes in arterial p_{O_2} can rapidly desaturate hemoglobin. By virtue of having fetal hemoglobin, the infant has better hemoglobin-carrying capacity than does the adult for any given arterial p_{O_2} (hemoglobin saturation curve shifted toward the left); he also has a higher hemoglobin concentration in his blood.

As with any use of O_2 in greater than ambient concentrations, pulmonary toxicity may occur. This complication is related both to breathing higher than ambient concentrations of O_2 and to the arterial p_{O_2}.

Alkali (buffer). The acidosis found in hyaline membrane disease is usually a mixed metabolic and respiratory acidosis. In the early stages of the disease, the lungs can still ventilate rather effectively, and the hyperventilating infant lowers his arterial p_{CO_2}. Poor peripheral circulation, hypoxia, and birth asphyxia combine to cause a metabolic acidosis secondary to lactic acid accumulation. Measurement of arterial blood gases (pH, p_{O_2} and p_{CO_2}) allows one to determine the base deficit. To correct the base deficit, sodium bicarbonate (or in rare cases, tromethamine [THAM]) is then administered according to the formula: base deficit $\times$ body weight (kg) $\times$ 0.3 = mEq buffer to be given. Inspired O_2 concentrations are adjusted according to the arterial p_{O_2} to achieve the desired arterial oxygen tension.

Later in hyaline membrane disease, as the infant becomes exhausted from his labored breathing and as the lungs become progressively more damaged, the arterial p_{CO_2} begins to increase. The acidosis at this point is often mixed, being both respiratory and metabolic in origin. In practice, one would first attempt to correct the respiratory acidosis and afterward, by use of sodium bicarbonate, any metabolic acidosis component that remained.

First and foremost, correction of respiratory acidosis requires adequate ventilation. In an infant who is not very fatigued, self-induced hyperventilation by crying is often effective in lowering the arterial p_{CO_2}. When this fails, intermittent bag-and-mask ventilation may be used. If, despite these efforts, hypercarbia, hypoxia, or both, continue to worsen or if apnea becomes frequent, artificial ventilation with a respirator is advised.

Obviously, frequent and precise measurements of arterial blood gases are mandatory as a guide to how much buffer or how much ventilation to provide. The stakes are high, for the vicious cycle that perpetuates the illness begins with asphyxia (hypercarbia, hypoxia, acidosis) and the resulting pulmonary vasoconstriction. Correction of disordered acid-base balance is among the top priorities in treating the disease. Unfortunately for the patient, the laboratory, and the clinician, the disease gets worse before getting better, and the infant's condition can change rapidly hour by hour. Arterial blood gases must be measured frequently and after each therapeutic maneuver.

What if the physician is not successful in catheterizing the umbilical artery and threading the catheter into the aorta? Obviously, measurements of central arterial blood gases from the aorta are the most meaningful. The peripheral circulation is vasoconstricted for about a week after birth, making measurements of capillary blood gases, obtained from a warmed heel stick, less than ideal—but they are better than no measurement at all, and the capillary pH and p_{CO_2} so obtained are reasonably accurate (*21*). This is also the case with venous blood pH and p_{CO_2}. From capillary or venous blood gases, a base deficit may be determined, and the amount of buffer to be given can be calculated. The clinician must simply judge the arterial p_{O_2} by whether or not cyanosis is present in the infant—often a difficult judgment to make!

Antibiotics. As treatment for possible congenital pneumonia—which may or may not be present—antibiotics are given by some physicians. In some cases diagnosed clinically as hyaline membrane disease, congenital pneumonia is found at postmortem examination. Prophylactic antibotics may also be given to "cover the umbilical catheter," although this practice is open to considerable question (*21*). Nonetheless, bacterial cultures should be made from blood, umbilical catheter, tracheal secretions, isolette, respiratory therapy equipment, endotracheal tubes, and the like.

Shock

Some infants with hyaline membrane disease appear to be in shock, with pallor, cool extremities, falling aortic blood pressure, and falling hematocrit. The hypovolemia that may be present in some infants (*22*) is treated by administering whole blood or packed erythrocytes.

At birth, acute hypovolemia secondary to birth asphyxia, fetoplacental bleeding, or early cord clamping must be treated vigorously. Hypovolemia causes pulmonary vasoconstriction and thus contributes to the pathological cycle of the disease. Physiological signs of hypovolemia found in hyaline membrane disease are increased left ventricular output, decreased aortic blood pressure, and increased peripheral vascular resistance.

Actual measurements of erythrocytes and total blood volume in hyaline membrane disease showed that mortality is highest in those infants with the lowest erythrocyte volume (23).

Whole blood is given to replace that withdrawn for laboratory testing. It is important to remember that the total blood volume of an infant is only 80 ml/kg of body weight, and daily or twice-daily volume replacement is often necessary.

A pale, cold infant, tending toward shock, whose systemic aortic blood pressure is low or falling, and in whom the hematocrit is less than 45% or is falling, must receive treatment to expand the blood volume. Salt-poor albumin may be given until appropriately matched donor blood is available. The preferred blood to use is fresh, heparinized blood from a compatible ambulant donor. Fresh blood without acid citrate-dextrose solution eliminates the problems caused by blood that is acidotic and depleted of calcium.

Immediate determination of blood type and Rh, and direct and indirect Coomb's tests on the infant's blood are necessary. Hematocrit must be serially measured, to judge whether or not hypovolemia is present, as revealed by a declining hematocrit during the first few hours of life. (In normal infants, the hematocrit usually increases slightly during the first 12 hours of postnatal life.)

Use of End-Expiratory Pressure and Respirators

Before the use of respirators, the average rate of survival for hyaline membrane disease was about 48%. If an infant weighed less than 1.00 kg at birth, his chances of surviving the disease were virtually nil.

Beginning in the 1960s, artificial ventilation was used for infants with hyaline membrane disease, with variable results (24–28). Overall survival when respirators were used was about 61%—an increase of 13% in the salvage rate. Strict criteria were used before placing an infant on a respirator. In general, if an infant has an arterial p_{O_2} of less than 4.0 to 5.3 kPa (30–40 mmHg) while breathing 100% O_2, one can predict a 90 to 100% chance of mortality (29).

A similar grim outcome could be expected if the arterial p_{CO_2} increased to greater than 9.3 to 10.7 kPa (70–80 mmHg) despite attempts to ventilate the infant without a respirator, or if the blood pH was <7.0 to 7.1 despite buffer therapy (30).

There are many kinds of respirators now available. The outcome depends not so much on the type of machine used as on the personnel and support teams caring for the infant. Needless to say, respirator therapy for hyaline membrane disease is an heroic and maximum mode of therapy. Although one often can save infants whose lives would end without such therapy, survival rates are still low for infants whose birth weight is less than 1.00 to 1.20 kg. The quality of life in survivors, according to follow-up studies, seems to be good (31,32).

Complications seen with use of respirators include hemorrhage into the central nervous system, pneumothorax, complications with the endotracheal tube (obstruction, tracheal stenosis and edema, infection), chronic lung disease, and pulmonary oxygen toxicity.

Serial chest roentgenograms will show whether or not the disease is improving or whether pulmonary complications are appearing.

One of the more significant breakthroughs in therapy has been the application of end-expiratory pressure—either positive or negative pressure applied at the end of the expiratory phase of respiration. Positive end-expiratory pressure is applied via endotracheal tubes or through a snug-fitting nosepiece, transmitting positive pressure through the oropharynx into the trachea and bronchi (33). Alternatively, negative end-expiratory pressure is administered via a sealed negative pressure tank surrounding the infant's thorax, with the head and oropharynx outside the tank at atmospheric pressure. Negative pressure applied around the thorax causes air to be aspirated in through the nose and mouth, and the amount of negative thoracic pressure applied is directly related to the amount of positive airway pressure. This technique eliminates the need for endotracheal intubation or other invasive procedures (*34*).

It is thought that application of either positive or negative pressure at the end of the infant's expiratory phase of respiration prevents collapse of the alveoli and terminal bronchioles at the end of expiration. Because infants with hyaline membrane disease have a deficiency or absence of pulmonary surfactant, the surface tension in the alveoli is very high at the end of expiration, causing widespread alveolar atelectasis. End-expiratory pressure mechanically holds open these alveoli, permitting effective ventilation to continue during the expiratory phases of respiration. Pressures of from 30 to 150 mm H_2O are usually applied (*35*).

By holding open terminal bronchioles and alveoli at end expiration, the therapy increases functional residual capacity and significantly decreases functional right to left intrapulmonary shunting of blood (*35*).

Once this procedure is begun, the arterial p_{O_2} usually increases significantly (the average increase is about 4.6 kPa (35 mmHg), with little if any effect on arterial p_{CO_2}, aortic blood pressure, or central venous pressure.

The marked increase in p_{O_2} with the infant still breathing high concentrations of oxygen allows one to significantly lower the ambient concentration of oxygen required to maintain a satisfactory arterial p_{O_2}. Hence, the infant is less often exposed to a high concentration of oxygen, and the concomitant pulmonary oxygen toxicity is often thus prevented or minimized.

Because this technique is relatively simple and without undue risks, it is used long before the criteria for respirator therapy are met. Most physicians will begin to use end-expiratory pressure when the arterial p_{O_2} is about 8.0 to 9.3 kPa (60–70 mmHg) while inhaling 60 to 70% (by volume) O_2.

More than any other therapeutic advance, this sort of therapy has significantly improved the overall survival rate for infants with hyaline membrane disease and obviated the need for using cycling respirator therapy in many cases.

Future Therapies in Hyaline Membrane Disease

Research continues on means to prevent this disease and improve its therapy. While one could comment on many ideas being researched, I will limit myself to two.

Exchange transfusions with use of adult blood (Table 3).   In adults, hemoglobin contains 2,3-diphosphoglycerate, which acts to release oxygen for cellular metabolism. Fetal hemoglobin contains less 2,3-diphosphoglycerate. Hence, fetal hemoglobin binds oxygen more tenaciously, and at any partial pressure less oxygen is released to the peripheral tissues. The question under study is whether replacing fetal hemoglobin with hemoglobin from adults, by an exchange transfusion of adult blood, would help the infant to oxygenate his peripheral tissue better, thereby minimizing asphyxia and lactic acidosis (*36*).

Prevention of hyaline membrane disease by inducing pulmonary surfactant production in utero. In those infants in whom hyaline membrane disease is caused by a lack of surfactant

Table 3.　Exchange Transfusions with Blood from Adults

Adult hemoglobin	Fetal hemoglobin
↑ 2, 3-Diphosphoglycerate	↓ 2, 3-Diphosphoglycerate
↑ O_2 release to tissues	↓ O_2 release to tissues
↓ O_2 bound to hemoglobin	↑ O_2 bound to hemoglobin

(i.e., extreme immaturity of the fetus), it might be helpful to stimulate pulmonary surfactant production before birth. Once born, this immature newborn would then have enough pulmonary surfactant to maintain alveolar stability and prevent atelectasis and its physiological consequences.

In experimental animals, administration of glucocorticoids before birth seems to initiate and/or enhance pulmonary surfactant production, especially that of dipalmityl lecithin, and hyaline membrane disease is avoided more often than in control animals. Limited studies in the human fetus likewise suggest encouraging results. Preliminary results (Tables 4 and 5) show a beneficial effect only with fetuses of less than 32 weeks gestation when their mothers were given betamethasone from 24 to 7 days before delivery (37,38). The precise mechanism of action of the glucocorticoid is not yet known, nor is it known whether infants over 32 weeks of gestation will be helped by this form of in utero therapy. Of course, hyaline membrane disease that may be due to other causes is probably not preventable by glucocorticoid therapy of the fetus.

Table 4.　Incidence of RDS Related to Gestational Age in Live-born Infants of Unplanned Deliveries 24 Hours to 7 Days after Entry to Trial

	Betamethasone treated			Controls			P
	No.	RDS	%RDS	No.	RDS	%RDS	
Gestational age at delivery							
26 to < 32 wk.	33	7	21.2	38	24	63.2	.01
32 to < 37 wk.	80	3	3.8	60	2	3.3	—
> 37 wk.	2	0	0.0	1	0	0.0	—
	115	10	8.7	99	26	26.3	< .01

From ref. *38.*

Monitoring of General Physiological Status

This complex physiology requires continuous surveillance of the newborn throughout the course of the illness, including the following additional clinical chemical monitoring:

Calcium.　Hypocalcemia is frequent in infants who have hyaline membrane disease, have poor oral intake of calcium, and receive alkali to buffer their acidosis. Daily determination of calcium is important. Infants with hypocalcemia may exhibit symptoms such as apnea, hypotonicity, jitteriness, seizures, and poor suck (39).

Table 5. Occurrence of RDS as Related to Interval between Treatment and Delivery in Live-born Infants Delivered after Unplanned Premature Labor

	Betamethasone treated			Controls			P
	No.	RDS	%RDS	No.	RDS	%RDS	
Entry-delivery interval							
< 24 h	55	14	25.5	56	15	26.8	NS[a]
Between 1 and 7 days	115	10	8.7	99	26	26.3	0.005
> 7 days	109	7	6.4	98	5	5.1	NS
All live-born infants	279	31	11.1	253	46	18.2	0.04

[a] Not significant.

From ref. *38*.

Bilirubin. There are many reasons why jaundice occurs so commonly in infants with hyaline membrane disease; this problem is beyond the scope of this paper. Almost all of these infants are premature, with immature liver conjugating-enzyme activity and poor caloric intake. Increased bilirubin production is caused by erythrocyte hemolysis, which is increased by acidosis, use of donor blood, and use of arterial catheters. In addition, with high hemoglobin concentration at birth, fetal erythrocytes normally undergo accelerated hemolysis in the weeks after birth. Increased production of bilirubin and poor liver conjugation of bilirubin—with the consequent poor excretion of bilirubin—serve to cause significant jaundice.

Exchange transfusions, to prevent brain damage caused by bilirubin toxicity to the central nervous system (kernicterus), are performed when bilirubin concentrations in the serum are still relatively low, because even modest increases in bilirubin are toxic to the premature infant who has had acidosis, hypothermia, hypercarbia, or hypoxia (*40,41*). Knowledge of the total serum-protein value helps the clinician determine when exchange transfusions may be needed because bilirubin is bound to the albumin in the plasma, and only unbound bilirubin may enter the central nervous system and cause kernicterus. Hence, repeated determinations of bilirubin and total protein and liberal use of exchange transfusions are necessary.

Other. Measurements of blood electrolytes, sugar, ammonia, total protein and osmolality, and measurements of the urinary specific gravity, pH, and glucose are necessary. Infants with this disease receive fluids, electrolytes, calories, and protein parenterally. Some of these parenteral solutions are highly concentrated and may cause a glucose-induced diuresis, dehydration, hyperammonemia, and electrolyte imbalance. For these reasons, the above-mentioned measurements are helpful (*20*).

SUMMARY

Hyaline membrane disease is the most common fatal pulmonary disorder of the premature infant. The presumed cause is developmental immaturity of the lungs. Pulmonary surfactant is low or absent as revealed by immature L/S ratios and negative shake tests.

Physical signs of respiratory disease and a characteristic roentgenogram allow the clinician to make a presumptive diagnosis of hyaline membrane disease. Some physiological derangements in the disease are: lactic acidosis, hypoxia, hypercarbia, deficiency of pulmonary surfactant, diminished lung compliance, intense pulmonary vasoconstriction with pulmonary hypoperfusion, functional right-to-left shunts, alveolar transudation of fluid with alveolar edema, atelectasis, and fibrin deposition.

Therapy for hyaline membrane disease is directed to correction of these derangements. It includes: (*a*) maintenance of the thermoneutral environment; (*b*) fluids and nutrients; (*c*) correction of acid-base balance with oxygen, alkali, and respiratory support; (*d*) antibiotics; (*e*) correction of hypovolemia with transfusions; and (*f*) use of end-expiratory pressure or artificial ventilation with respirators.

Monitoring the infant's physiological status is an ongoing obligation and includes frequent laboratory measurements of arterial blood gases, calcium, bilirubin, hemoglobin, hematocrit, electrolytes, glucose, ammonia, total protein, and osmolality, and bacterial cultures in those infants receiving parenteral alimentation or respiratory support.[1]

REFERENCES

1.   Gluck, L., Pulmonary surfactant and neonatal respiratory distress, *Hospital Practice* 6, No. 11, 45–56 (November, 1971).

2.   Morgan, T., Pulmonary surfactant, *N. Engl. J. Med.* 284, 1185–1193 (1971).

3.   Towers, B., The fetal and neonatal lung. In *Biology of Gestation*, N. S. Assali, Ed., Academic Press, New York, N.Y., 1968, pp 189–223.

4.   Avery, M. E., Developmental considerations in neonatal respiratory adaption. In chapter on "Prematurity as a Contributing Factor," *Idiopathic Respiratory Distress Syndrome*. U.S. Public Health Service, National Institutes of Health, Bethesda, Md., 1967–1968, pp 37–55.

5.   Scarpelli, E. M., Pulmonary surfactants and their role in lung disease, *Adv. in Pediatr.* 16, 177–210 (1969).

6.   Adams, F. H., Fujiwara, T., Emmanouilides, G. C., and Räihä, N., Lung phospholipids of human fetuses and infants with and without hyaline membrane disease, *J. Pediatr.* 77, 833–841 (1970).

7.   Gluck, L. and Kulovich, M., Measuring the functional maturation of the fetus with the lecithin-sphingomyelin ratio. *Yearbook of Obstetrics and Gynecology*, J. P. Greenhill, Ed. Yearbook Med. Publishers, Chicago, Ill., 1972, pp 256–267.

8.   Gluck, L. et al., Diagnosis of the respiratory distress syndrome by amniocentesis, *Am. J. Obstet. Gynecol.* 109, 440–445 (1971).

9.   Clements, J. A. et al., Assessment of the risk of the respiratory distress syndrome by a rapid test for surfactant in amniotic fluid, *N. Engl. J. Med.* 286, 1077–1081 (1972).

10. Spellacy, W. N. and Buhi, W. C., The usefulness of amniotic fluid lecithin/sphingomyelin ratio in predicting neonatal respiratory problems, *South Med. J.* 66, 1090–1093 (1973).

11. Bhagwanani, S. G., Fahmy, D., and Turnbull, A. C., Bubble stability test compared with lecithin assay in prediction of respiratory distress syndrome, *Br. Med. J.* i, 697–700 (1973).

12. Avery, M. E. and Fletcher, B. D., Hyaline membrane disease. In *The Lung and Its Disorders in the Newborn Infant,*—3rd ed., Saunders, Philadelphia, Pa., pp 191–233 (1974).

13. Klaus, M. and Fanaroff, A., Respiratory problems. In *Care of the High Risk Neonate*. Saunders, Philadelphia, Pa., 1973, pp 119–151.

14. Stahlman, M. et al., Pathophysiology of respiratory distress in newborn lambs: Circulatory, biochemical, and pathological considerations, *Am. J. Dis. Child.* 108, 375–393 (1964).

[1] *Ed. note:* The reader may wish to refer also to the chapters on the L/S ratio by Nelson and Forman in *Amniotic Fluid—Physiology, Biochemistry, and Clinical Chemistry* (vol. 1 in this series; Wiley, New York, N.Y., 1974, pp 221–258).

15. Chu, J. et al., The pulmonary hypoperfusion syndrome, *Pediatrics* **35**, 733–742 (1965).

16. Stahlman, M., Perinatal circulation, *Pediatr. Clin. N. Am.* **13**, (3) 753–767 (1966).

17. Chu, J. et al., Neonatal pulmonary ischemia. Part I: Clinical and physiologic studies, *Pediatrics* **40**, 709–782 (1967).

18. Stahlman, M. et al., Assessment of the cardiovascular status of infants with hyaline membrane disease. In *The Heart and Circulation in the Newborn and Infant*, D. Cassels, Ed., Grune & Stratton, New York, N.Y., 1966, pp 121–129.

19. Bruck, K., Temperature regulation in the newborn infant, *Biol. Neonate.* **3**, 65–119 (1961).

20. Sinclair, J. C., Driscoll, J. M., Heird, W. C., and Winters, R. W., Supportive management of the sick neonate: Parenteral calories, water, and electrolytes. *Pediatr. Clin. N. Am.* **17**(4), 863–893 (1970).

21. James, S. L., Complications arising from catheterization of the umbilical vessels. In *Problems of Neonatal Intensive Care Units*, Report of the 59th Ross Conference on Pediatric Research. Ross Laboratories, Columbus, Ohio, 1969, pp 36–43. (Discussion by Usher, R.)

22. Faxelius, G. et al., Comparison of red cell volume in infants with hyaline membrane disease and infants with other forms of respiratory distress. Abstracts of the American Pediatric Society, Inc. and the Society for Pediatric Research, Atlantic City, 1970, p 237.

23. Usher, R. et al., Red cell volume in respiratory distress syndrome. Abstracts of the American Pediatric Society, Inc. and the Society for Pediatric Research, Atlantic City, 1971, p 104.

24. Stahlman, M. et al., Negative pressure assisted ventilation in infants with hyaline membrane disease, *J. Pediatr.* **76**, 174–182 (1970).

25. Hesse, H., Harrison, V., Klein, M., and Malan, A., Intermittent positive pressure ventilation in hyaline membrane disease, *J. Pediatr.* **76**, 183–193 (1970).

26. Gruber, H. and Klaus, M., Intermittent mask and bag therapy: An alternative approach to respirator therapy for infants with severe respiratory distress, *J. Pediatr.* **76**, 194–201 (1970).

27. Helmrath, T., Hodson, A., and Oliver, T., Positive pressure ventilation in the newborn infant: The use of a face mask. *J. Pediatr.* **76**, 202–207 (1970).

28. Dietrich, E. W., Roloff, W., and Stern, L., Continuous negative pressure in the management of severe respiratory distress syndrome, *J. Pediatr.* **81**, 384–391 (1972).

29. Swyer, P. R., An assessment of artificial respiration in the newborn. In *Problems of Neonatal Intensive Care Units*. Report of the 59th Ross Conference on Pediatric Research. Ross Laboratories, Columbus, Ohio, 1969, pp 25–35.

30. Klaus, M., Artificial ventilation: Review of published results. In *Idiopathic Respiratory Distress Syndrome*. U.S. Public Health Service, National Institutes of Health, Bethesda, Md., pp 93–103 (1967–1968).

31. Stahlman, M., What evidence exists that intensive care has changed the incidence of intact survival? In *Problems of Neonatal Intensive Care Units*, Report of the 59th Ross Conference on Pediatric Research, Ross Laboratories, Columbus, Ohio, 1969, pp 17–24.

32. Johnson, J. D. et al., Prognosis of children surviving with the aid of mechanical ventilation in the neonatal period. Abstracts of the American Pediatric Society, Inc. and the Society for Pediatric Research, Washington, D.C., 1972 p 144.

33. Gregory, G. et al., Treatment of the idiopathic respiratory distress syndrome with continuous positive airway pressure, *N. Engl. J. Med.* **284**, 1333–1340 (1971).

34. Vidyasagar, D. and Chernick, V., Continuous positive transpulmonary pressure in hyaline membrane disease: A simple device, *Pediatrics* **48**, 296–299 (1971).

35. Llewellyn, A. and Swyer, P., Assisted ventilation. In *Care of the High Risk Neonate*. M. Klaus and A. Fanaroff, Eds., W. B. Saunders Co., Philadelphia, Pa., 1973, pp 152–167.

36. Oski, F. A., The unique fetal red cell and its function: E. Mead Johnson Award address, *Pediatrics* **51**, 494–500 (1973).

37. Liggins, G. C. and Howie, R. N., A controlled trial of antepartum glucocorticoid treatment for prevention of the respiratory distress syndrome in premature infants, *Pediatrics* **50**, 515–525 (1972).

38. Howie, R. N. and Liggins, G. C., Prevention of respiratory distress syndrome in premature infants by antepartum glucocorticoid treatment. In *Respiratory Distress Syndrome.* C. A. Villee, D. B. Villee, and J. Zuckerman, Eds., Academic Press, Inc., New York, N.Y., 1973, pp. 369–380.

39. Tsang, R. C. and Oh, W., Neonatal hypocalcemia in low birth weight infants, *Pediatrics* 45, 773–781 (1970).

40. Boggs, T. R., Hardy, J. B., and Frazier, T. M., Correlation of neonatal serum total bilirubin concentrations and developmental status at age eight months, *J. Pediatr.* 71, 553 (1967).

41. Gartner, L. M., Snyder, R. N., Chabon, R. S., and Bernstein, J., Kernicterus: High incidence in premature infants with low serum bilirubin concentrations, *Pediatrics* 45, 906–917 (1970).

Pathogenesis of Neonatal Hyperbilirubinemia

GERARD B. ODELL, M.D.

JULIO O. CUKIER, M.D.

APOLO C. MAGLALANG, M.D.

PATHOPHYSIOLOGY OF NEONATAL HYPERBILIRUBINEMIA

Hyperbilirubinemia is probably the rule in infants during their first week of life if one accepts that serum concentrations of bilirubin greater than 26 μmol/litre (1.5 mg/100 ml) are abnormal. About 15% of the newborn population develop serum bilirubin concentrations that exceed 120 μmol/litre (7.0 mg/100 ml) and such concentrations are associated with visible jaundice (1). Because visible jaundice is so common and is apparently harmless to most neonates, the term "physiological jaundice" has been applied (2). However, the development of jaundice is often attributable either to disorders in bilirubin metabolism itself or, secondarily, to diseases that impair the clearance of bilirubin (3). Consequently, the occurrence of jaundice during neonatal life should be regarded as a very useful clinical sign, and when it is properly interpreted, it can lead to early diagnosis of underlying disease.

Here, we describe the production, distribution, and clearance of bilirubin, with emphasis on those diseases affecting particular steps in the metabolism of bilirubin that are associated with jaundice during neonatal life (Table 1).

FORMATION OF BILIRUBIN

Bilirubin is formed as a result of the catabolism of porphyrin-containing proteins, primarily hemoglobin (4). It has been estimated that 85% of bilirubin formation is derived from the catabolism of hemoglobin in senescent erythrocytes and the remainder from nonhemoglobin proteins ("shunt bilirubin") (5,6). The cyclic tetrapyrrole is normally opened at the α-position of the ring, and the cleavage of the porphyrin is considered a

Table 1.   Causes of Hyperbilirubinemia during Neonatal Life

Overproduction	Undersecretion	Mixed
A. Fetal-maternal blood group incompatibility—Rh, ABO, others	G. Metabolic–endocrine 1. Familial nonhemolytic jaundice, types 1 and 2 2. Galactosemia 3. Hypothyroidism 4. Tyrosinosis 5. Hypermethioninemia 6. Drugs and hormones 1. Novobiocin b. Pregnanediol c. Certain breast milks d. Lucey-Driscoll syndrome 7. Infants of diabetic mothers 8. Prematurity 9. Hypopituitarism & anencephaly 10. Cardiac failure	I. Sepsis J. Intrauterine infections 1. Toxoplasmosis 2. Rubella 3. Cytomegalic inclusion-body disease 4. Herpes simplex 5. Syphilis 6. Hepatitis (HAA) K. Epidemic hepatitis
B. Hereditary spherocytosis		
C. Nonspherocytic hemolytic anemias 1. G6PD deficiency & drug 2. Pyruvate kinase defic. 3. Other erythrocyte enzyme defic. 4. α-Thalassemia 5. γ-Thalassemia 6. Vitamin K_3-induced hemolysis		
D. Extravascular blood— petechiae; hematomata; pulmonary, cerebral or occult hemorrhage	H. Obstructive 1. Biliary atresia a. Trisomy 18 2. Choledochal cyst 2. Cystic fibrosis 4. Tumor or *band* (extrinsic obstruction) 5. Cholestatic syndromes a. Progressive: elevated serum bile acids b. Nonprogressive: normal serum bile acids c. Intermittent	
E. Polycythemia 1. Maternal–fetal or feto-fetal transfusion 2. Delayed clamping of the umbilical cord		
F. Increased enterohepatic circulation 1. Pyloric stenosis 2. Intestinal atresia or stenosis including annular pancreas 3. Hirschsprung's disease 4. Meconium ileus or meconium plug syndrome 5. Fasting and/or other cause for hypoperistalsis 6. Drug-induced paralytic ileus (hexamethoniums) 7. Swallowed blood		

mixed-function oxidation that requires the microsomal enzyme heme oxygenase (decyclizing) (EC 1.14.99.3) and cytochrome P 450 (7). The products of the reaction are the linear tetrapyrrole biliverdin (as its IX α-isomer) and carbon monoxide (Figure 1).

The biliverdin is further reduced to bilirubin by hydrogenation of the central α-methine bridge; this reaction is catalyzed by the cytosol enzyme, biliverdin reductase (EC 1.3.1.24) (7).

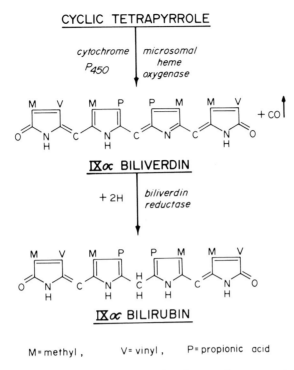

CYCLIC TETRAPYRROLE

Figure 1. Formation of bilirubin from cyclic tetrapyrroles.

Measurements of the carbon monoxide formed in the catabolism of the porphyrin ring provide quantitative measurements of the rate of bilirubin formation. Such studies demonstrate that 100 to 140 μmol (6–8 mg) of bilirubin is produced per day per kilogram body weight by infants, in contrast to rates of 34 to 51 μmol (2–3 mg) per kilogram per day for adults (8). This twofold greater formation of bilirubin is largely the result of the shorter life span of fetal erythrocytes (9) and obviously is a factor contributing to hyperbilirubinemia during neonatal life. This greater load of bilirubin in neonatal life may also explain why so many diseases are often associated with hyperbilirubinemia during the neonatal period. The greater requirements for hepatic excretion of bilirubin would be more likely to result in retention of bilirubin whenever liver function is impaired.

IN UTERO CLEARANCE OF FETAL BILIRUBIN

The subsequent clearance of bilirubin formed by the catabolism of heme is schematically diagrammed in Figure 2. In the extracellular fluids, bilirubin is tightly bound to albumin, which is a carrier for bilirubin in the circulation (10).

During intrauterine life the clearance of bilirubin from the fetal circulation can proceed by at least two different mechanisms. The fraction of bilirubin that is dissociated from fetal albumin in the placental circulation can diffuse across the placental membranes and enter the maternal circulation (11–13). The albumin in the maternal circulation can bind the bilirubin and transport it away from the placenta; the maternal liver thus clears fetal bilirubin. The higher concentration of albumin in the maternal circulation favors such a dialytic clearance of bilirubin from the fetus.

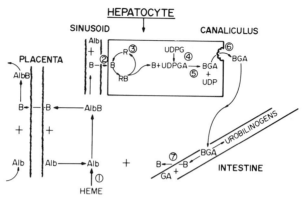

Figure 2. The intrauterine clearance of fetal bilirubin by the maternal placenta and fetal liver. *Alb*, albumin; *B*, bilirubin, *AlbB*, albumin–bilirubin complex; *R*, receptor-carrier proteins of hepatic cytosol; *UDPG*, uridine diphosphate glucose; *UDPGA*, uridine diphosphate glucuronic acid; *BGA*, bilirubin glucuronide.

The encircled numerals *1–3* refer to the steps in formation, hepatic uptake, and binding of bilirubin in the liver cytosol. Steps *4–6* refer to the formation of the substrate UDPGA, the conjugation of bilirubin by glucuronosyl transferase, and the secretion of conjugated bilirubin by the canaliculus. Step 7 indicates the intralumenal hydrolysis of conjugated bilirubin and its absorption re-entry into the fetal circulation.

The other mechanism by which bilirubin clearance occurs is the action of the fetal liver itself. Some of the bilirubin that enters the sinusoidal circulation of the fetal liver comes into close proximity to the plasma-membrane surface of the hepatocyte in the spaces of Dissé. That fraction of the bilirubin dissociated from albumin can enter the hepatocyte and be bound by the receptor carrier proteins of the cytosol as indicated at points 2 and 3 in Figure 2.

HEPATIC UPTAKE OF BILIRUBIN

Compromise of the sinusoidal circulation will decrease the amount of bilirubin delivered to the hepatocytes; this is a particularly important factor after delivery of the fetus, when clearance of bilirubin via the placenta is no longer possible. Neonatal illnesses associated with hypoperfusion of the liver are likely to delay the hepatic clearance of bilirubin and lead to increased bilirubin concentrations in serum. Persistence of the fetal circulation, such as is seen in the "respiratory distress syndrome" of prematurely born infants, is particularly relevant, because the ductus venosus remains patent (*14,15*). When this happens, much of the portal blood flow is shunted from the portal vein directly to the hepatic vein and bypasses the sinusoidal circulation of the liver.

Transfer of bilirubin from extracellular fluid into the cytosol of the hepatocyte is believed to be influenced by the concentration gradients across the cell. The concentration of the receptor-carrier proteins in the membranes and cytosol of the hepatocytes could, therefore, influence the clearance of bilirubin from the sinusoidal circulation (*16,17*). The receptor-carrier proteins (Y and Z) of the cytosol transport many organic anions that undergo subsequent metabolism by the liver and, therefore, prior saturation of the receptor proteins with them could diminish the sites available for clearance of bilirubin (*18–20*). Studies of primates indicate that the concentration of one of the major receptor-carrier proteins ("Y-protein" or "ligandin") in the cytosol of the liver is low in the fetus and during the first week of extrauterine life as compared with later life (*21*). Induction of higher concentrations of ligandin has also been observed when animals are treated with phenobarbital (*22*).

INTRAHEPATIC METABOLISM OF BILIRUBIN

Once bilirubin has gained access to the hepatocyte, its eventual excretion depends on its being converted to more polar derivatives that can be secreted by the canalicular apparatus, as schematically shown at the right-hand side of Figure 2. The conjugation of bilirubin involves the formation of glycosides of bilirubin by esterification of the propionic acid sidechains, primarily with the hexuronic acid, glucuronic acid (*23,24*). The precursor of this substrate is uridine-5'-diphosphate glucose (UDPG), which is catalytically dehydrogenated to uridine diphosphate glucuronic acid (UDPGA), step 4 in Figure 2 (*25*). Availability of UDPGA depends not only on the functional maturation of the UDPG-dehydrogenase (EC 1.1.1.22), which perhaps is relatively deficient in newborns (*26*), but also on a sufficient supply of glucose from the circulation or glycogen stores within the liver. A common clinical finding is that illness associated with hypoglycemia during neonatal life is often attended by a more pronounced hyperbilirubinemia. Galactosemia and prolonged fasting are conditions that are associated with exaggerated hyperbilirubinemia in the neonatal period that may represent examples of substrate deficiency of UDPGA for bilirubin conjugation (*3*). This may also be the situation in the infant of the diabetic mother who develops hypoglycemia in the neonatal period. There are also experimental data indicating that whenever glucagon concentrations are abnormally high, microsomal heme oxygenase activity also increases (*27*). Bilirubin production may be accelerated by more rapid conversion of available heme to bilirubin in hypoglycemic syndromes, and the deficiency in the hepatic conjugation of bilirubin caused by substrate deficiency of UDPGA is intensified. Although not shown in Figure 2, UDPGA also serves as a substrate for pyrophosphatases and sugar hydrolases, which catalyze the production of glucuronic acid-1-phosphate from the UDPGA for use in cell membrane synthesis (*28*).

Conversion of bilirubin to its more polar glucuronide is catalyzed by the microsomal enzyme, bilirubin UDP glucuronosyltransferase (EC 2.4.1.17) (step 5, Figure 2) (*29*). Studies of rodents and of recently expired premature infants suggest a pronounced deficiency in the activity of this enzyme in fetuses and newborns (*26,30–32*). The identification of an absolute deficiency of this enzyme in the lifetime jaundice of Gunn rats and of humans with familial nonhemolytic icterus (Crigler-Najjar syndrome) emphasized the critical relationship of the conjugation of bilirubin to its hepatic clearance (*33,34*). In most neonates who develop jaundice, the increased serum bilirubin is almost exclusively attributable to "indirect" reacting [<17 μmol/litre (<1.0 mg/100 ml) "direct" reacting] and, therefore, unconjugated bilirubin. Consequently, neonatal jaundice could represent deficiency at steps 2, 3, or 4 of Figure 2, and historically the conjugating deficiency seemed the most likely. Recent investigations with more nearly pure substrates and enzyme preparations demonstrate greater enzyme activity and marked species variation (*32,35,36*). Serial measurements in prematurely born infants showed their lower capacity to conjugate the artificial substrate, umbelliferone, as compared to adults. However, the transferase activity in preterm infants did not increase until they were more than 30 days old, when their neonatal hyperbilirubinemia had long since come and gone (37). In our limited studies (four human fetuses between 20 and 23 weeks gestational age), we found that the fetal liver can conjugate bilirubin at a third the rate for adults. Furthermore the gallbladder bile of these fetuses contained 68 to 136 μmol bilirubin/litre (4–8 mg/100 ml), at least two thirds of which was direct reacting and presumably conjugated. Glucuronosyltransferase activity can evidently vary considerably during fetal and neonatal life, and it is inferred from human studies (39–42)—in which there was either decreased or increased neonatal jaundice—that greater activity can be induced by exposure to phenobarbital and other compounds stimulating synthesis of smooth endoplasmic reticulum and that activity can be depressed by fatty acids and humoral agents.

HEPATIC EXCRETION OF BILIRUBIN

Once bilirubin has been conjugated, it normally is excreted at the canaliculus of the hepatocyte (step 6, Figure 2) into the biliary tree and eventually is delivered into the small intestine. This excretory process is thought to be an energy-dependent (i.e., "active") secretion, because the concentration of bilirubin in bile normally exceeds that of the plasma and liver homogenates by 50- to 100-fold (42). In those diseases listed in Table 1 as undersecretion owing to obstruction or of mixed origin, both conjugated and total bilirubin typically appear in the serum in abnormally high concentrations. Some of the bilirubin that has been conjugated regurgitates from the hepatocyte or canalicular apparatus back into the circulation. The presence of more than 26 μmol of "direct-reacting" bilirubin/litre (1.5 mg/100 ml) of serum provides an important clue that the cause of an infant's jaundice may be hepatic injury, the major exception being infants with marked hemolytic disease, who are forming conjugated bilirubin faster than their hepatocytes can secrete it, which is normally the rate-limiting step for hepatic clearance (43). This has been referred to in the past as "inspissated bile syndrome" (44), a term more appropriately reserved for the regurgitative jaundice seen in cystic fibrosis of the pancreas with hepatic fibrosis and inspissated material in the portal bile ducts.

ENTEROHEPATIC CIRCULATION OF BILIRUBIN

Once it is within the intestinal tract, bilirubin is normally reduced to urobilinogens by the actions of the intestinal bacteria (45,46). The urobilinogens can be reabsorbed and cleared by the liver and secreted into bile or they can be excreted by the renal mechanisms of both glomerular filtration and tubular secretion (47). However, in utero and at birth there are no bacteria in the gut, and urobilinogens are not formed. The gut of the infant does contain β-glucuronidase (EC 3.2.1.31), which can catalyze the deconjugation of bilirubin (48). The resulting unconjugated bilirubin is more readily absorbed from the intestine (49), and it can also be excreted in the feces (step 7, Figure 2). During fetal life, meconium is not evacuated, so it seems essential that bilirubin that reaches the intestine be reabsorbed. Indeed, if bilirubin were being conjugated and excreted at 20 weeks gestation and the enterohepatic circulation and placental clearance of bilirubin were not active, one can imagine that by 40 weeks gestation the infant's intestinal lumen might be filled by one continuous pigmented gallstone.

More than half of the bilirubin in the meconium of newborns is chloroform extractable, and so is thought to be unconjugated bilirubin, which indicates that considerable deconjugation of bilirubin occurs within the intestinal lumen of fetuses and newborns if the fetal liver excretes only conjugated bilirubin. There is about 1 mg bilirubin/g meconium (wet weight) and at term, the infant's intestinal contents contain an estimated 100 to 200 g of meconium; the intestinal tract thus contains a total of 100 to 200 mg of bilirubin, 5 to 10 times the amount produced per day in normal term infants. Delayed passage of meconium after birth and continued enterohepatic circulation will increase the load of bilirubin that requires hepatic clearance. In the intestinal tract, the previously excreted bilirubin that is reabsorbed is likely to exceed the capacity of the liver to clear bilirubin formed at the already accelerated daily rates of production characteristic of newly born infants. That there is enterohepatic circulation of bilirubin in newborns has been indirectly demonstrated by blocking intestinal absorption of bilirubin in both experimental animals and in term infants. Oral feeding of either charcoal, cholestyramine, or agar was associated with decreased serum bilirubin concentrations, and with agar feedings increased fecal excretions of bilirubin in rats and infants were demonstrated (50–53).

Those diseases of neonatal life that are associated with neonatal hyperbilirubinemia because of delayed passage of meconium often herald themselves by either the early appearance of jaundice or of serum bilirubin values exceeding 206 μmol/litre (12 mg/100 ml). Intestinal atresias, meconium-plug syndromes, Hirschsprung's disease, and cystic fibrosis of the pancreas are often associated with pathological neonatal hyperbilirubinemia because of delayed clearance of meconium (3).

DIFFERENTIAL DIAGNOSIS OF NEONATAL HYPERBILIRUBINEMIA

In view of the many pathological entities that manifest their presence either directly or indirectly by their effects on bilirubin metabolism, significant jaundice during neonatal life requires thoughtful inquiry as to its cause and is challenging because of the occurrence of so-called physiological jaundice; those clinical instances of neonatal jaundice that should stimulate concern must be distinguished from those that can be comfortably dismissed as physiological. The guidelines illustrated in Figure 3 have been clinically useful to us in making such a distinction. Serum bilirubin concentrations exceeding those that fall within the idealized curve of maximum values for physiological hyperbilirubinemia of neonatal life warrant further diagnostic evaluation. There are three essential points to the curve:

(*a*) Development of visible icterus before the infant is 36 h old indicates that bilirubin is accumulating excessively, as objectively reflected by serum bilirubin concentrations exceeding 120 μmol/litre (7 mg/100 ml). The early appearance of jaundice usually represents overproduction of bilirubin because of hemolytic disorders of the newborn, and relevant hematologic studies will identify these.

(*b*) Whenever the hyperbilirubinemia exceeds 210 μmol/litre (12 mg/100 ml), diagnostic study is necessary to determine the cause. Milder hemolytic disorders are often encountered that did not cause early icterus as well as the many causes categorized in Table 1 as the result of undersecretion. In the absence of hemolytic disease and hepatitis, we find that the enterohepatic circulation of bilirubin is the most frequent cause of hyperbilirubinemia. Although it is difficult to measure the amount of meconium passed, a record of the time of initial passage has proved to be very useful. Infants with delayed

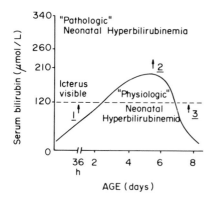

Figure 3. Relation between serum bilirubin concentrations and time during neonatal life that distinguishes physiological from pathological hyperbilirubinemia. *1*, *2*, and *3* refer to the three essential points made in the text.

passage of meconium (>12 h) will frequently develop hyperbilirubinemia during the ensuing days, with values that are greater than 210 μmol/litre (12 mg/100 ml) (*54*).

(*c*)   Persistence of visible icterus beyond the seventh day of life most often implies impaired hepatic excretion of bilirubin. Most commonly, this is seen in infants who are breast fed, and the impairment has been ascribed to high concentrations of pregnane-$3\alpha,20\beta$-diol in the milk of some mothers (*55*), but most such cases are probably caused by excessive amounts of fatty acids in the milk, as well as by environmental chemicals that may be transmitted via milk and inhibit conjugation of bilirubin in the infant (*39,56*). Cessation of breast feeding (or alternate breast-milk and formula feeds) is usually followed within 48 h by a significant decrease in the infant's serum bilirubin. Of importance is the recognition of congenital hypothyroidism—not because of its frequency, but because early diagnosis permits a more optimistic outlook for future mental development. Excessive or persisting neonatal jaundice may be the only physical manifestation of thyroid insufficiency this early in life (*57*).

Increases in the "direct-reacting" fraction of the serum bilirubin usually indicate infections and inflammation of the liver, but infants with galactosemia and tyrosinosis also can show substantial concentrations of conjugated bilirubin in their sera by this time (*3*).

BILIRUBIN ENCEPHALOPATHY

Serum bilirubin values greater than 210 μmol/litre (12 mg/100 ml) during neonatal life not only signal a need for diagnostic study to determine the cause, but create additional concern that such values have been associated with toxicity attributable to the bilirubin itself. In term infants this toxicity—known as "kernicterus"—is clinically manifested by lethargy, a depressed Moro embrace reflex, and opisthotonic posturing. When fatal, there is characteristic yellow staining of neurones of the basal ganglia and hippocampus by bilirubin. The clinical signs of kernicterus are less specific in premature infants, who often exhibit only apneic periods and abnormal withdrawal responses to extension of the extremities. Fetal distress and asphyxia at birth are common in those premature infants whose kernicterus is associated with relatively low antemortem concentrations of bilirubin (*59,60*). The prior hypoxic injury has been postulated to render

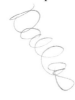

neuronal tissues more susceptible to bilirubin toxicity. Also, secondary precipitation of bilirubin in neurones that were damaged by prior asphyxia would equally reflect the so-called kernicterus seen in the brains of very premature infants with relatively low [<210 μmol/litre (12.0 mg/100 ml)] antemortem concentrations of serum bilirubin (61).

There also are nonlethal forms of bilirubin toxicity of the central nervous system, in which brain damage is manifested by spastic cerebral palsy with choreoathetosis in infants who survived severe neonatal jaundice. More subtle signs of organic brain damage are delayed motor development at nine months of age (62) and cognitive dysfunctions at five years of age in the absence of cerebral palsy (63,64). These subtle lesions ascribed to bilirubin encephalopathy have not been associated with any characteristic physical signs during neonatal life, and the eventual identification of brain damage was not closely correlated to either the mean or maximum concentration of bilirubin during the neonatal period (63). Consequently, the total serum bilirubin concentration does not adequately predict risk of bilirubin toxicity for the identification of the milder forms of bilirubin encephalopathy.

SATURATION OF SERUM ALBUMIN WITH BILIRUBIN AND ITS RELATIONSHIP TO KERNICTERUS

Figure 4 illustrates why data on total serum bilirubin concentration cannot be expected to provide sufficient information to allow them to be used to predict those infants at risk to bilirubin toxicity. In extracellular fluids, bilirubin is attached to albumin; thus very little is actually ultrafiltrable and can appear in the protein-free fluid. Yet only the fraction of the bilirubin that is dissociated from albumin is free to diffuse into cells and be toxic to cell membranes or organelles (65).

Figure 4 also indicates that albumin has two sites at which it can bind bilirubin (66).

On the right of the albumin molecule is an indented site, which has an extremely high affinity for bilirubin ($K = 10^8$) (67). Water-soluble anions such as salicylate and sulfonamides, as well as protons, are weakly competitive in displacing bilirubin from this site (68). The imidazole rings of histidine are believed to be involved in this binding of bilirubin (69,70), and the fluorescence and circular dichroism of albumin-bound bilirubin is related to its binding at this site (71,72).

The second class of binding sites on albumin for bilirubin is shown at the left of the diagram. There are many of these, and apparently they are hydrophilic, because many water-soluble organic anions competitively bind to albumin at these loci. The affinity of albumin for bilirubin at these secondary sites ($K = 10^6$), is considerably less than at the primary one (67). The ϵ-amino groups of lysine are believed to be important in this binding, because prior acetylation of albumin decreases its binding capacity for bilirubin and other organic anions (73). The competitive displacement of bilirubin from albumin by water-soluble organic anions such as benzoate, sulfonamides, and salicylate occurs at this site. In vitro, there is no significant interference with the albumin binding of bili-

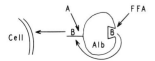

Figure 4. Diagrammatic representation of the protein binding of bilirubin and its dissociation and diffusion into cells. The albumin (*Alb*) has two types of binding sites for bilirubin (*B*).

rubin by organic anions until the molar ratio of bilirubin to albumin exceeds 10, when significant binding of bilirubin at these secondary sites would be expected (68).

Unfortunately, not all of the primary sites of albumin are available in vivo for the binding of bilirubin (66). Both nonesterified fatty acids and hematin can apparently decrease the availability of the primary sites on albumin for binding of bilirubin and force the bilirubin to be transported at the secondary sites (Figure 4). If the binding of bilirubin to albumin is governed by the lower-affinity constant, then greater concentrations of protein-free (diffusible) bilirubin must exist in the extracellular fluids, and the potential risk of bilirubin toxicity becomes greater. Two infants may have identical values for total bilirubin concentrations in their sera, but in one, much more of the bilirubin may be transported by albumin at its secondary binding site because, for example, this infant did not receive sufficient caloric intake to minimize endogenous lipolysis. The consequent elevation in the circulating concentrations of free fatty acids will decrease the capacity of the infant's albumin in extracellular fluids to bind bilirubin at the primary, high-affinity site, and such an infant not only has a greater concentration of diffusible bilirubin, because the amount bound to albumin is governed by the lower association constant, but whenever bilirubin is bound to albumin at its secondary sites it is subject to competitive displacement by exogenously administered anions, as well as by hydrogen (acidemia) (66).

Several laboratory techniques (74) are used to distinguish these two infants in terms of their potential risk to bilirubin encephalopathy. These tests are based on measurements of the relative concentrations of the reactants in the equilibrium between albumin and bilirubin: $Alb + B \rightleftharpoons AlbB$.

(a) The fraction of the bilirubin that is bound by the lower-affinity (hydrophilic) site of albumin can be quantitated by measuring the amount of bilirubin that is displaced after an organic anion, salicylate, is added (75).

(b) The concentration of bilirubin dissociated from albumin in the aqueous phase of plasma can be measured directly by enzymatic analysis (76) or indirectly by Sephadex gel filtration of the plasma (77). In the latter technique, the tightly bound bilirubin is separated from the ultrafiltrable and easily dissociable bilirubin and can subsequently be measured independently.

(c) The potential binding capacity of the serum albumin can be assessed by measuring its ability to bind exogenously administered anions such as 2-(4-hydroxyazobenzene) benzoic acid (78) and bilirubin itself (79).

(d) Another technique is the direct measurement of the concentration of bilirubin in the cell, by determining the concentration of bilirubin in the erythrocytes of jaundiced infants (80).

The avoidance of morbidity associated with neonatal hyperbilirubinemia requires that physicians responsible for the clinical care of neonates understand the distinction between physiological and pathological jaundice and be able to ascertain when further diagnostic study is needed to explain neonatal jaundice. Equally important is that associated laboratory services not only provide accurate measurements of concentrations of conjugated and unconjugated serum bilirubin, but also be prepared to assess the relative risk of bilirubin encephalopathy to which a given infant is liable. The latter requires that the laboratory be able to measure at least one of the reactants involved in the binding of bilirubin to albumin, if the care afforded an infant that develops "pathological" jaundice is to be optimum.

ACKNOWLEDGMENT

This work was supported by Grant HD 02268, NIH, United States Public Health Service.

REFERENCES

1. Hardy, J. B. and Peeples, M. O., Serum bilirubin levels in newborn infants. Distributions and associations with neurological abnormalities during the first years of life, *Johns Hopkins Med. J.* **128**, 265–272 (1971).

2. Davidson, L. T., Merritt, K. K. and Weech, A.A., Hyperbilirubinemia in the newborn, *Am. J. Dis. Child.* **61**, 958–980 (1941).

3. Odell, G. B., Poland, R. L. and Ostrea, E. M. Jr., Neonatal hyperbilirubinemia. In *Care of the High Risk Neonate*. M. H. Klaus and A. A. Fanaroff, Eds. W. B. Saunders Co., Philadelphia, Pa. 1973, p 183.

4. London, I. M., West, E., Shemin, D., and Rittenberg, D., On the origin of bile pigment in normal man, *J. Biol. Chem.* **184**, 351–358 (1950).

5. Robinson, S. H., Lester, R., Crigler, J. F., and Tsong, M., Early-labeled peak of bile pigment in man. Studies with glycine-C^{14} and delta-aminolevulinic acid-^{3}H, *N. Engl. J. Med.* **277**, 1323–1329 (1967).

6. Vest, M., Strebel, L., and Hauenstein, D., The extent of "shunt" bilirubin and erythrocyte survival in the newborn infant measured by the administration of (^{15}N) glycine, *Biochem. J.* **95**, 11c (1965). Abstract.

7. Tenhunen, R., Marver, H. S., and Schmid, R., Microsomal heme oxygenase. Characterization of the enzyme, *J. Biol. Chem.* **244**, 6388–6394 (1969).

8. Maisels, M. J. et al., Endogenous production of carbon monoxide in normal and erythroblastotic newborn infants, *J. Clin. Invest.* **50**, 1-8 (1971).

9. Pearson, H. A., Life-span of the fetal red blood cell, *J. Pediatr.* **70**, 166 (1967).

10. Bennhold, H., Ueber die Vehikelfunktion der Serumeiweisskörper, *Ergeb. Inn. Med. Kinderheilkd* **42**, 273 (1932).

11. Schenker, S., Dawber, N. H., and Schmid, R., Bilirubin metabolism in the fetus, *J. Clin. Invest.* **43**, 32–39 (1964).

12. Lester, R., Behrman, R. E., and Lucey, J. F., Transfer of bilirubin-C^{14} across monkey placenta, *Pediatrics* **32**, 416–419 (1963).

13. Bernstein, R. B. et al., Bilirubin metabolism in the fetus, *J. Clin. Invest,* **48**, 1678–1688 (1969).

14. Ogawa, J., Postnatal circulatory observations of liver and intestine in newborn infants. In *Proceedings of the XI International Congress of Pediatrics*, 1965, p 87.

15. Gersony, W. M., Persistence of the fetal circulation. A commentary, *J. Pediatr.* **82**, 1103–1106 (1973).

16. Cornelius, C. E., Ben Ezzer, J., and Arias, I. M., Binding of sulfobromophthalein sodium (BSP) and other organic anions by rat liver plasma membranes in vitro, *Proc. Soc. Exp. Biol. Med.* **124**, 665–667 (1967).

17. Hammaker, L. and Schmid, R., Interference with bile pigment uptake in the liver by flavaspidic acid, *Gastroenterology* **53**, 31 (1967).

18. Levi, A. J., Gatmaitan, Z., and Arias, I. M., Two hepatic cytoplasmic protein fractions, Y and Z, and their possible role in the hepatic uptake of bilirubin, sulfobromophthalein and other anions, *J. Clin. Invest.* **48**, 2156–2167 (1969).

19. Grodsky, G. M., Kolb, H. J., Fanska, R. E. and Nemechek, C., Effect of age of rat on development of hepatic carriers for bilirubin: A possible explanation for physiologic jaundice and hyperbilirubinaemia in the newborn, *Metabolism* **19**, 246–252 (1970).

20. Reyes, H., Levi, A. J., Gatmitan, Z., and Arias, I. M., Studies of Y and Z, two hepatic cytoplasmic organic anion-binding proteins: Effect of drugs, chemicals, hormones, and cholestasis, *J. Clin. Invest.* **50**, 2242 (1971).

21. Levi, A. J., Gatmaitan, Z., and Arias, I. M., Deficiency of hepatic organic anion-binding protein, impaired organic anion uptake by liver and "physiologic" jaundice in newborn monkeys, *N. Engl. J. Med.* **283**, 1136–1139 (1970).

22. Reyes, H., Levi, A. J., Gatmaitan, Z., and Arias, I. M., Organic anion-binding protein in rat liver drug induction and its physiologic consequence, *Proc. Nat. Acad. Sci. U.S.A.* **64**, 168–170 (1969).

23. Lathe, G. H., the degradation of haem by mammals and its excretion as conjugated bilirubin, *Essays Biochem.* **8**, 107–148 (1972).

24. Heirwegh, K. P. M., Meurirssen, J. A. T. P. and Fevery, J., Critique of the assay and significance of bilirubin conjugation, *Adv. Clin. Chem.* **16**, 239–289 (1973).

25. Dutton, G. J., The biosynthesis of glucuronides. Chap. 3 in *Glucuronic Acid Free and Combined Chemistry, Biochemistry, Pharmacology and Medicine*, G. J. Dutton, Ed., Academic Press, Inc., New York, N.Y., 1966, p 186.

26. Brown, A. K. and Zuelzer, W. W., Studies on the neonatal development of the glucuronide conjugating system, *J. Clin. Invest.* **37**, 332 (1958).

27. Bakken, A. F., Thaler, M. M., and Schmid, R., Metabolic regulation of heme catabolism and bilirubin production, I. Hormonal control of hepatic heme oxygenase activity, *J. Clin. Invest.* **51**, 530 (1972).

28. Pogell, B. M. and Leloir, L. F., Nucleotide activation of liver microsomal glucuronidation, *J. Biol. Chem.* **236**, 293–298 (1961).

29. Dutton, G. J. and Storey, I. D. E., Uridine compounds in glucuronic acid metabolism. I. The formation of glucuronides in liver suspensions, *Biochem. J.* **57**, 275–283 (1954).

30. Lathe, G. H. and Walker, M., The synthesis of bilirubin glucuronide in animal and human liver, *Biochem. J.* **70**, 705–712 (1958).

31. Dutton, G. J., Glucuronide synthesis in foetal liver and other tissues, *Biochem. J.* **71**, 141–148 (1959).

32. Gartner, L. M. and Arias, I. M., The transfer of bilirubin from blood to bile in the neonatal guinea pig. *Pediatr. Res.* **3**, 171–180 (1969).

33. Axelrod, J. Schmid, R., and Hammaker, L., A biochemical lesion in congenital non-obstructive non-haemolytic jaundice, *Nature* **180**, 1426 (1957).

34. Crigler, J. F. and Najjar, V. A., Congenital familial nonhemolytic jaundice with kernicterus, *Pediatrics.* **10**, 169-180 (1952).

35. Strebel, L. and Odell, G. B., Bilirubin uridine diphosphoglucuronyl transferase in rat liver microsomes: Genetic variation and maturation, *Pediatr. Res.* **5**, 548–559 (1971).

36. Dutton, G. J., Langelaan, D. E., and Ross, P. E., High glucuronide synthesis in newborn liver: choice of species and substrate, *Biochem. J.* **93**, 4P (1964). Abstract.

37. Di Toro, R., Lupi, L., and Ansanelli, V., Glucuronation of the liver in premature babies, *Nature* **219**, 265–267 (1968).

38. Maurer, H. M. et al., Reduction in concentration of total serum bilirubin in offspring of women treated with phenobarbitone during pregnancy, *Lancet* **ii**, 122–124 (1968).

39. Bevan, B. R. and Holton, J. B., Inhibition of bilirubin conjugation in rat liver slices by free fatty acids, with relevance to the problem of breast milk jaundice, *Clin. Chim. Acta* **41**, 101–107 (1972).

40. Arias, I. M., Wolfson, S., Lucey, J. F., and McKay, R. J., Jr., Transient familial neonatal hyperbilirubinaemia, *J. Clin. Invest.* **44**, 1442–1450 (1965).

41. Gartner, L. and Arias, I. M., The hormonal regulation of hepatic bilirubin excretion. In *Bilirubin Metabolism*, I. A. D. Bouchier and B. H. Billing, Eds. Oxford, 1967. Blackwell Scientific Publications, p. 175.

42. Odell, G. B., Natzschka, J., and Storey, G. B. N., The distribution of bilirubin in liver and kidney in jaundiced rats, *Am. J. Dis. Child.* **112**, 351–359 (1966).

43. Arias, I. M., Johnson, L., and Wolfson, S., Biliary excretion of injected conjugated and unconjugated bilirubin by normal and Gunn rats, *Am. J. Physiol.* **200**, 1901–1094 (1961).

44. Hsia, D. Y. et al., Prolonged obstructive jaundice in infancy. 1. General survey of 156 cases, *Pediatrics* **10**, 243–252 (1952).

45. Watson, C. J., Campbell, M., and Lowry, P. T., Preferential reduction of conjugated bilirubin to urobilinogen by normal fecal flora, *Proc. Soc. Exp. Biol. Med.* **98**, 707–711 (1958).

46. Troxler, R. F., Dawber, N. H., and Lester, R., Synthesis of urobilinogen by broken cell preparations of intestinal bacteria, *Gastroenterology* **54**, 568–574 (1968).

47. Levy, M., Lester, R., and Levinsky, N. G., Renal excretion of urobilinogen in the dog, *J. Clin. Invest.* **47**, 2117 (1968).

48. Brodersen, R. and Hermann, L. S., Intestinal reabsorption of unconjugated bilirubin: A possible contributing factor in neonatal jaundice, *Lancet* **i**, 1242 (1963).

49. Lester, R. and Schmid, R., Intestinal absorption of bile pigments. II. Bilirubin absorption in man, *N. Engl. J. Med.* **269**, 178–182 (1963).

50. Lester, R., Hammaker, L., and Schmid, R., A new therapeutic approach to unconjugated hyperbilirubinaemia, *Lancet* **ii**, 1257 (1962).

51. Ulstrom, R. A. and Eisenklam, E., The enterohepatic shunting of bilirubin in the newborn infant. 1. Use of oral activated charcoal to reduce normal serum bilirubin values, *J. Pediatr.* **65**, 27–37 (1964).

52. Poland, R. L. and Odell, G. B., Physiologic jaundice: The enterohepatic circulation of bilirubin, *N. Engl. J. Med.* **284**, 1–6 (1971).

53. Odell, G. B. et al., Protection from bilirubin nephropathy in jaundiced Gunn rats, *Gastroenterology* **66**, 1218–1224 (1974).

54. Rosta, J., Makoi., and Kertész, A., Delayed meconium passage and hyperbilirubinaemia, *Lancet* **ii**, 1138 (1968).

55. Arias, I. M., Gartner, L. M., Seifter, S., and Furman, M., Prolonged neonatal unconjugated hyperbilirubinaemia associated with breast feeding and a steroid, pregnane-3(α),20(β)-diol, in maternal milk that inhibits glucuronide formation in vitro, *J. Clin. Invest.* **43**, 2037–2047 (1964).

56. Odell, G. B., unpublished observations.

57. Akerren, Y., Early diagnosis and early therapy in congenital critinism, *Arch. Dis. Child.* **30**, 254–256 (1955).

58. Odell, G. B. The biologic basis of pediatric practice. In *Postnatal Care*, R. E. Cooke et al., Eds. McGraw-Hill, New York, N.Y., 1968, chap. 154, p 1500.

59. Stern, L. and Denton, R. L., Kernicterus in small premature infants, *Pediatrics* **35**, 483–485 (1965).

60. Keenan, W. J., Perlstein, P. H., Light, I. J. and Sutherland, J. M., Kernicterus in small sick premature infants receiving phototherapy, *Pediatrics* **49**, 652–655 (1972).

61. Gartner, L. M., Snyder, R. N., Chabon, R. S., and Bernstein, J., Kernicterus: High incidence in premature infants with low serum bilirubin concentrations. *Pediatrics* **45**, 906–917 (1970).

62. Boggs, T. R., Jr., Hardy, J. B., and Frazier, T. M., Correlation of neonatal serum total bilirubin concentrations and developmental status at age eight months, *J. Pediatr.* **71**, 553–560 (1967).

63. Odell, G. B., Storey, G. N. B., and Rosenberg, L. A., Studies in kernicterus. III. The saturation of serum proteins with bilirubin during neonatal life and its relationship to brain damage at five years, *J. Pediatr.* **76**, 12–21 (1970).

64. Johnson, L. and Boggs, T. R., Jr., Bilirubin-dependent brain damage: Incidence and indications for treatment. In *Phototherapy in the Newborn: An Overview*. National Academy of Sciences, Washington, D.C., 1975.

65. Odell, G. B., The dissociation of bilirubin from albumin and its clinical implications, *J. Pediat.* **55**, 268–279 (1959).

66. Odell, G. B., Influence of binding on the toxicity of bilirubin, *Ann. N.Y. Acad. Sci.* **226**, 225 (1973).

67. Jacobsen, J., Binding of bilirubin to human serum albumin—determination of the dissociation constants, *Fed. Eur. Biochem. Soc. Lett.* **5**, 113 (1969).

68. Odell, G. B., The distribution of bilirubin between albumin and mitochondria, *J. Pediatr.* **68**, 164–180 (1966).

69. Odell, G. B., Brown, R. S., and Holtzman, N. A., Dye-sensitized photooxidation of albumin associated with a decreased capacity for protein-binding of bilirubin. *Birth Defects: Original Article Series*. VI, 31–36 (1970). Williams and Wilkins Co., Baltimore, Md. 1970.

70. Jacobsen, C., Chemical modification of the high affinity bilirubin-binding site of human-serum albumin, *Eur. J. Biochem.* **27**, 513–519 (1972).

71. Roth, M., Dosage fluorimetrique de la bilirubine, *Clin. Chim. Acta* **17**, 487-492 (1967).

72. Blauer, G., Harmatz, D., and Snir, J., Optical properties of bilirubin-serum albumin complexes in aqueous solution. 1. Dependence on pH, *Biochim. Biophys. Acta* **278**, 68–88 (1972).

73. Martin, N. H., Preparation and properties of serum and plasma proteins. XXI. Interactions with bilirubin, *J. Am. Chem. Soc.* **71**, 1230 (1949).

74. Odell, G. B., Methods for measurement of the relative saturation of serum albumin with bilirubin in the management of neonatal hyperbilirubinemia. In *Phototherapy in the Newborn: An Overview*. National Academy of Sciences, Washington, D.C., 1975.

75. Odell, G. B., Cohen, S. N., and Kelly, P. C., Studies in kernicterus. II. The determination of the saturation of serum albumin with bilirubin, *J. Pediatr.* **74**, 214–230 (1969).

76. Jacobsen, J. and Wennberg, R. P., Determination of unbound bilirubin in the serum of newborns, *Clin. Chem.* **20**, 783 (1974).

77. Kaufmann, N. A., Kapitulnik, J., and Blondheim, S. H. The adsorption of bilirubin by Sephadex and its relationship to the criteria for exchange transfusion, *Pediatrics* **44**, 543–548 (1969).

78. Porter, E. G. and Waters, W. J. A rapid micromethod for measuring the reserve albumin binding capacity in serum from newborn infants with hyperbilirubinemia, *J. Lab. Clin. Med.* **67**, 660–668 (1966).

79. Schiff, D., Chan, G., and Stern, L. Sephadex G-25 quantitative estimation of free bilirubin potential in jaundiced infants' sera: A guide to the prevention of kernicterus, *J. Lab. Clin. Med.* **80**, 455–462 (1972).

80. Bratlid, D., Reserve albumin binding capacity, salicylate saturation index, and red cell binding of bilirubin in neonatal jaundice, *Arch. Dis. Child.* **48**, 393–397 (1973).

Clinical and Biochemical Aspects
of the Infant
of the Diabetic Mother

ANNE B. FLETCHER, M.D.

The infant of the diabetic mother has continued in part to live up to the words of Farquhar (*1*) who said, "their trembling anxiety seems to speak of intrauterine indiscretions of which we know nothing." We have learned a great deal of what happens after delivery, but very little is known of what happens to the infant in the uterus.

WHAT PREGNANCY DOES TO NORMAL AND DIABETIC WOMEN

To understand the problems of the infant of the diabetic mother, one should consider carbohydrate metabolism during a normal pregnancy. The normal pregnant woman has an increased incidence of renal glycosuria, a lower tolerance to an oral glucose load, increased concentrations of free fatty acids, increased insulinlike activity in the serum, and accelerated insulin breakdown during fasting (*2*). These changes have been attributed to increasing prolactin (mammatropic hormone) concentrations, beginning in the second trimester and continuing to near term, and they appear to facilitate transfer of glucose, fatty acids, and amino acids as required for growth of the fetus. In short, pregnancy is diabetogenic.

In the pregnant diabetic, prolactin concentrations are even higher than in the normal pregnant woman, and thus—if this hypothesis is correct—one would expect to see a worsening of the disease (*3*). Clinically, an early improvement in glucose tolerance is seen in the first trimester, and it lasts for two to three months. Insulin requirements decrease by 30 to 34%, and hypoglycemia may ensue. Between the 24th and 28th weeks, however, insulin requirements increase by as much as 75%. An abrupt decrease near term may be ominous for the health of the infant. During lactation, insulin concentrations decrease somewhat, but do not become normal. Six to nine months after delivery, the severity of the diabetes reverts to what it was before pregnancy. Aside from changes in

285

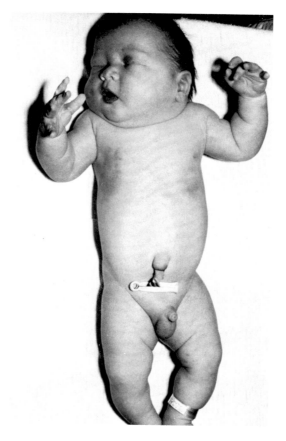

(*A*)

Figure 1A. Typical features of large-for-gestational-age infant of a diabetic mother. **B.** Close-up of facial features of an infant of a diabetic mother.

carbohydrate metabolism, the diabetic pregnancy is fraught with other problems, including increased incidence of stillbirths, toxemia, polyhydramnios, pyelonephritis, and urinary tract infection, as well as an increased likelihood of premature birth.

All complications in the mother and infant vary with the classification of the diabetic condition in the mother, progressing in severity from A to F (Table 1) (4).

CLASSIFICATION OF INFANTS

Typically, one thinks of the diabetic mother's infant as fat, plethoric, jittery, and large for gestational age (Figure 1, *A* and *B*). However, some of these infants are small for gestational age, most commonly those of the more severely diabetic mothers. Others will have a more nearly normal appearance. The infants of gestational diabetic women (those who exhibit symptoms of diabetes only during pregnancy) tend to have far fewer problems.

Most of the remaining discussion will center around the infant of the diabetic mother. About one in every 1000 live-born infants will fit into this category and be a problem to the practicing neonatologist.

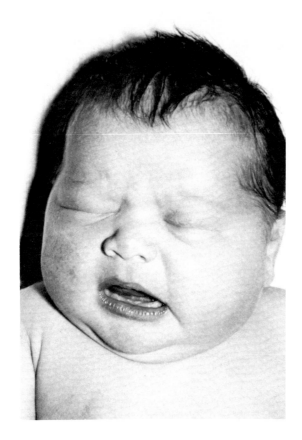

(B)

Figure 1. (*Continued*)

Table 1. White's Classification of Diabetes[a]

Class	Onset	Duration	Insulin	Other criteria
	Years			
A	Any	Any	0	0
B	>20	<10	+	0
C	10–19	10–19	+	0
D	<10 or	>20	+	Calcified, arteries, benign retinopathy
E	Any	Any	+	Calcified pelvic arteries
F	Any	Any		Benign retinopathy, nephropathy

[a] Modified from Table 14–2, p. 588 of ref. 4.

BODY COMPOSITION

For many years, it was thought that the large size of such infants reflected excessive body water, but an increased amount of fat is now known to be the principal cause, although visceral enlargement of the liver, heart, pancreas, adrenal glands, and kidneys also contributes. The brain does not share this excess; in fact, it is smaller than in control infants of similar weight and gestational age (5). Another characteristic finding in these infants is the β-cell hypertrophy and hyperplasia found in the pancreas along with an unusual infiltration of eosinophils of unknown etiology.

PATHOPHYSIOLOGY AND METABOLIC DERANGEMENTS

Four theories have been proposed to explain the pathological findings in these infants:

Hyperadrenocorticism. This was proposed because the appearance of these infants resembled that of individuals with Cushing's syndrome, but this theory was discarded because serum cortisol concentrations were normal.

Excessive secretion of somatotropin (growth hormone). The excessive growth of the infant of the diabetic mother suggested to others that somatotropin (growth hormone) might be involved. This idea, too, was discarded, because somatotropin concentrations in the cord serum were found to be normal. It is also well known that somatotropin is not required for normal growth in utero.

Hyperinsulinism. Many authors (6–8) have attempted to assess insulin concentrations in cord plasma and in the infant's plasma. Methods used measured insulinlike activity and immunoreactive insulin, both of which measure insulin antibodies, which pass easily across the placenta from mother to infant. Thus, much of such work is necessarily done on infants whose mothers were not on insulin or on infants of gestational diabetics (6). Results are therefore inconclusive. In general, insulin concentrations in cord blood have been found to be normal. A newer method, which measures immunoreactivity of the C-peptide part of proinsulin, may prove useful in the future for infants whose mothers are receiving insulin (9).

The response to a glucose load by these infants is interesting. Normal infants respond by delayed glucose utilization (the glucose utilization constant, $K_t = 0.77\%$ per min), and they have two temporal peaks of insulin secretion, a small early peak followed by a larger one at 1 h. Infants whose mothers have been on insulin have only a large early peak and utilize glucose much more rapidly ($K_t = 2.57\%$ per min) (10). One could infer from these data that the infant of the diabetic mother does have hyperinsulinism in response to glucose loads, and this, in fact, is what is generally accepted.

Hyperinsulinism combined with epinephrine depletion. The theory of McCann et al. (11), is the most recent one (Figure 2). According to it, the infant in utero responds to maternal hyperglycemia with an increased secretion of insulin. At times, the infant could become hypoglycemic and, in turn, would release epinephrine to counteract this. Eventually, epinephrine would be depleted. When the infant is faced with extrauterine existence, this lack of epinephrine results in decreased peripheral and pulmonary perfusion and decreased cardiac output and leads to hypoxia, acidosis, and respiratory distress. Some,

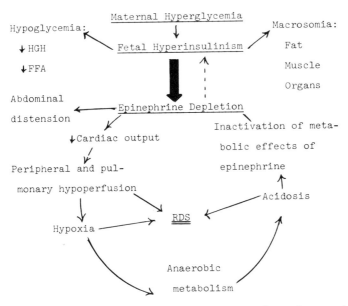

Figure 2. Hyperinsulinism-epinephrine depletion theory (modified from reference 11).

but not all, infants of diabetic mothers show subnormal concentrations of epinephrine in their serum, but this theory could explain the excessive size of these infants and many of the other postnatal problems.

SPECIAL PROBLEMS OF THE INFANT OF THE DIABETIC MOTHER

Hypoglycemia

The infant of the diabetic mother exhibits most of the problems seen in the premature infant. One of the more common and occasionally difficult problems is a rapid decrease in blood sugar to less than 1.7 mmol/litre (30 mg/100 ml) shortly after delivery. This early hypoglycemia is thought to be due to maternal hyperglycemia causing increased insulin secretion by the infant, an increase that is unopposed after the cord is clamped. It is much less frequently seen in the well-controlled mother, but varies a great deal among reported series (2,12). Symptoms include jitteriness, apnea, cyanosis, respiratory distress, and, more rarely, convulsions. These symptoms must be differentiated from other difficulties that can affect these infants at birth. Blood glucose must be measured frequently, particularly if feedings cannot be started promptly.

Hypocalcemia

A serum calcium of less than 1.75 mmol/litre (7.0 mg/100 ml) occurs frequently enough in the infant of the diabetic mother that it usually is checked routinely, especially if the infant shows any signs of neuromuscular irritability or hypotonia. Hypocalcemia during the first postnatal day is more prevalent in infants with a history of difficult deliveries, resuscitation, or respiratory distress, and in those whose mothers have had repeated abortions (13). The infant of the diabetic mother frequently fits into these categories.

The subnormal calcium is thought to be the result of a transient secondary hypoparathyroidism because of the increased values for serum calcium observed in the mother during pregnancy (14) and also due to a lack of calcium intake shortly after birth.

Hyperbilirubinemia

Above-normal bilirubin values [greater than 205–260 μmol/litre (12–15 mg/100 ml)] occur more frequently in infants of diabetic mothers than in other infants of either similar weight or similar gestational age. Increased erythrocyte incompatibilities have not been reported, and thus these values evidently are the result of one or more of the following: greater immaturity of the infant; slower passage of meconium, and, therefore, recirculation of bilirubin pigments through the enterohepatic shunt; polycythemia; or a slightly decreased extracellular fluid volume that results in hemoconcentration. None of these has been proved to be the cause.

Hyaline Membrane Disease

Infants of diabetic mothers have a slightly increased incidence of hyaline membrane disease when compared with premature infants of similar gestational age or full-term infants. Until recently, it was presumed that a greater degree of prematurity was associated with a particular gestational age. However, Gluck and Kulovich (15), who used lecithin/sphingomyelin ratios of 2:1 or greater as a criterion of maturity, showed that infants whose mothers were class A-C diabetics did have a decreased rate of lung maturation. In normal infants, the lung usually matures at 35 to 36 weeks of gestation, while lung maturity in the diabetic mother's infant is delayed until 37 to 38 weeks. In fetuses of class D-F diabetics, the maturation of the lung may be accelerated, most likely as a result of intrauterine distress from chronic hypoperfusion of the uterine circulation. Once the disease is present, tachypnea, retractions, grunting, and cyanosis are symptoms similar to those seen in other infants with hyaline membrane disease. Severity varies inversely with gestational age.

Infection

Newborn infants, particularly if premature, though not immunologically incompetent, do have an increased risk of infection. They have been shown to have delayed cellular immunity and decreased complement concentrations, opsonin activity, and chemotaxis (16). Although it has not been investigated in infants of diabetic mothers, one would expect them to have similar difficulties. Additional factors that place these infants at risk are the high incidence of urinary tract infection and the intermittent hyperglycemia, which causes blood to act as a better-than-usual culture medium. Sepsis may be more difficult to diagnose because of the pre-existing tendency of these infants to lethargy, neuromuscular irritability, jaundice, and abdominal distention. Thus it must be looked for if its presence is at all suspected.

Renal-Vein Thrombosis

First described by Avery et al. (17), renal-vein thrombosis occurs more commonly in the infants of diabetic mothers than in the normal newborn population. It has been seen in the stillborn as well. Causes contributing to this abnormality may be decreased extracellular volume, polycythemia, or transient dehydration. The presence of flank masses, hematuria, and disseminated intravascular coagulation defects suggests the diagnosis.

Congenital Malformations

The infant of the diabetic mother is also subject to an increased incidence of congenital anomalies, which varies with classification of diabetes in the mother (Table 2) (*18*). The most common defects seen include congenital heart disease (particularly ventricular septal defect and transposition of the great vessels) and spinal anomalies varying from hemivertebrae to the syndrome of caudal regression or sacral agenesis.

Table 2.   Percentage of Congenital Malformations in 853 Infants of Diabetic Mothers and Normal Controls[a]

Source	Total	Major	Multiple
Total cases	6.4	5.2	1.6
Class:			
A—C	4.4	—	—
D—F	10.7	—	—
Controls	2.1	1.2	0.2

[a] Modified from ref. *18*.

The most popular explanations for these defects have included the maternal environment (hypoglycemia, vascular compromise), genetic influences, and exogenous substances (insulin, oral hypoglycemia agents). None has been proved unequivocally.

TREATMENT OF THE INFANT OF THE DIABETIC MOTHER

Treatment of the infant of the diabetic mother begins first and foremost with careful management of the mother, which, in turn, begins with early classification of her diabetic state and frequent prenatal visits. Hospitalization at 34 weeks' gestation will ensure strict control thereafter and monitoring of various indexes of maturity of the infant by amniocentesis. Delivery at 38 to 39 weeks, when the lungs are known to be mature, will give the best possible chances for the infant. Should the infant be very large, delivery should be by cesarean section.

Other treatment includes frequent and careful attention to the values for blood sugar, calcium and both conjugated and unconjugated bilirubin. Laboratory studies needed are summarized in Table 3. If hypoglycemia of 1.7 mmol/litre (30 mg/100 ml) or less is present, early feedings or an intravenous infusion of dextrose (100–150 g/litre) should be instituted. Dextrose in a concentration of 500 g/litre is contraindicated, as it may lead to rebound hypoglycemia. Steroids may be required when the blood glucose concentration is unresponsive to other therapy. Serum calcium concentrations of less than 1.75 mmol/litre (7.0 mg/100 ml) are usually treated with intravenous or oral calcium gluconate, 200 mg/kg body weight. Hyperbilirubinemia of greater than 100 to 120 μmol/litre (6.0–7.0 mg/100 ml) may be treated with the "bilirubin light" (Model PT-53-1; Air Shields, Photo Therapy Unit, Hatboro, Pa. 19040) once a basic hemolytic work-up is done. There is danger of kernicterus when the molar ratio of bilirubin/albumin exceeds 1. This can be estimated by using a number corresponding to 3.7 times the total protein as the concentration of bilirubin at which exchange transfusion is mandatory, when the protein concentration is expressed in g/100 ml and the bilirubin concentration in mg/100 ml (*19*). If citrate-phosphate-dextrose or acid-citrate-dextrose blood is used, blood sugars must be monitored after the transfusion since "rebound" hypoglycemia may result. When heparinized blood is used, however, the blood sugar should be monitored during the transfusion because such blood is low in glucose and may cause further hypoglycemia. Hyaline membrane disease is managed similarly both in infants of diabetic mothers and in other prematures: strict monitoring of inspired oxygen and blood gases and the judicious use of small blood transfusions to maintain the hematocrit at greater than 0.45 (45%) or a mean blood pressure greater than 3.9 kPa (40 cm of H_2O, or 29 mmHg). Sodium bicarbonate or more rarely tris(hydroxymethyl)aminomethane (THAM) are used to maintain the pH of the blood between 7.30 and 7.35. In using the latter, one must monitor the serum sodium, to be sure its concentration does not exceed 150 mmol/litre (150 mEq/litre). If infection is suspected, it is vigorously treated with broad-spectrum antibiotics such as ampicillin and gentamicin, once cultures of the blood, cerebrospinal fluid, and urine have been obtained. With careful treatment, the mortality and morbidity of these infants are low.

Table 3. Laboratory Studies Frequently Done on the Infant of a Diabetic Mother

Problem	Laboratory study to be followed
Hypoglycemia	Blood sugar
Hypocalcemia	Serum calcium
Hyaline-membrane disease	Serial hemoglobin, hematocrit, blood gases, pH, electrolytes
Hyperbilirubinemia	Blood type, mother and infant Coombs test (direct and indirect), total protein, bilirubin (direct and indirect), hemoglobin, hematocrit, blood smear
Infection	Blood, urine, CSF culture
Congenital malformations	Whatever is indicated
Renal vein thrombosis	Urinalysis, intravenous pyelogram

PROGNOSIS

There are few long-term follow-up studies of these children, but those that have appeared are encouraging (*20–22*). Development and intelligence quotient appear to be normal. When maternal acetonuria is present during pregnancy, the intelligence quotients are decreased slightly but significantly as compared to normal controls (*23*). These children generally tend to be obese and may show excessive growth spurts during the adolescent years, for reasons that are unclear. Mortality during the first year is slightly greater than for normal children, because of the congenital cardiac malformations. Perhaps of most concern is the increased incidence of manifest diabetes (0.7–10.5%) and abnormal glucose tolerance tests (up to 38%) in this population in 9- to 30-year follow-ups, thus increasing the diabetic gene in the population. Yet at this time the diabetic woman should, if she desires, be encouraged to have at least a limited family.

SUMMARY

The infant of a diabetic mother presents fascinating problems in neonatal medicine, both clinically and biochemically. The typical infant is fat, plethoric, and jittery. There are other categories of newborns that exhibit biochemical abnormalities and appearance that resemble those of the infant of a diabetic mother, and will be a potential problem to the physician and the clinical laboratory. Several theories have been proposed in past years to explain their pathophysiology: (*a*) excess somatotropin, (*b*) excess steroid production, (*c*) hyperinsulinism, and (*d*) hyperinsulinism combined with epinephrine depletion.

Clinical problems to which the infant of the diabetic mother is prone include prematurity, respiratory distress syndrome, hypoglycemia, hypocalcemia, hyperbilirubinemia, increased incidence of malformations, and predilection for infections. Medical care begins in utero with careful control of the mother's diabetic condition and continues after birth with bacterial cultures and strict monitoring of the infant's vital signs and of his blood gases and the concentrations of glucose, calcium, and bilirubin in the serum.

With modern management, the probability that these infants will survive is excellent, varying mainly with the severity of the maternal condition. Nine- to thirty-year follow-ups show a 10- to 200-fold increase in the incidence of diabetes and a tendency toward obesity. The children usually have normal intelligence.

REFERENCES

1. Farquhar, J. W., The child of the diabetic woman, *Arch. Dis. Child.* 34, 76 (1959).

2. Pedersen, J., *The Diabetic and Her Newborn*. Williams and Wilkins, Baltimore, M d. 1ᶜ67, p 22.

3. Silenkow, H. A. et al., Patterns of serum immunoreactive human placental lactogen (IR-HPL) and chorionic gondaotropin (IR-HCG) in diabetic pregnancy, *Diabetes* 20, 696 (1971).

4. White, P., Pregnancy and diabetes. In *Joslin's Diabetes Mellitus*, 2nd ed., A. Marble et al., Eds. Lea and Febiger, Philadelphia, Pa., 1971, p 588.

5. Naeye, R. L., Infants of diabetic mothers: A quantitative morphologic study, *Pediatrics* 35, 980 (1965).

6. Cornblath, M., Studies in insulin secretion: A comparison of normal infants and infants of gestational diabetic mothers, *Pediatr. Res.* 2, 301 (1968). Abstract.

7. Baird, J. D. and Farquhar, J. W., The insulin secreting capacity of the pancreas in the newborn infants of normal and diabetic women, *Lancet* i, 71 (1962).

8. Obenshain, S. S. et al., Human fetal insulin response to sustained maternal hyperglycemia, *N. Engl. J. Med.* 284, 566 (1970).

9. Block, M. B. et al., C-Peptide immuno-reactivity (CRP): Method for studying infants of insulin treated diabetic mothers, *Pediatrics* 53, 923 (1974).

10. McCann, M. L. et al., The prevention of hypoglycemia in infants of diabetic mothers, *Proc. Soc. Pediatr. Res.*, May 5, 1965.

11. McCann, M. L. et al., A new therapeutic rationale for the infant of the diabetic mother, *Mo. Med.* 65, 275 (1968).

12. Cornblath, M. and Schwartz, R., Infant of the diabetic mother. In *Disorders of Carbohydrate Metabolism in Infancy*, W. B. Saunders, Philadelphia, Pa., 1966, p 65.

13. Tsang, R. C. and Oh, W., Neonatal hypocalcemia in low birth weight infants, *Pediatrics* 45, 773 (1970).

14. Tsang, R. C., Kleinman, L. I., Sutherland, J. M., and Light, I. J., Hypocalcemia in infants of diabetic mothers, *J. Pediatr.* **80,** 384 (1972).

15. Gluck, L. and Kulovich, M. V., Lecithin/sphingomyelin ratios in amniotic fluid in normal and abnormal pregnancy, *Am. J. Obstet. Gynecol.* **115,** 539 (1973).

16. Dossett, J. H., Microbial defenses of the child and man, *Pediatr. Clin. North Am.* **19,** 355 (1972).

17. Avery, M. E., Oppenheimer, E. H., and Gordon, H. H., Renal vein thrombosis in newborn infants of diabetic mothers, *N. Engl. J. Med.* **256,** 1134 (1957).

18. Pederson, L. M., Tygstrup, I., and Pedersen, J., Congenital malformations in newborn infants of diabetic women, *Lancet* **i,** 1124 (1964).

19. Odell, G. et al., Studies in kernicterus, II. The determination of the saturation of serum albumin with bilirubin, *J. Pediatr.* **74,** 214 (1969).

20. Pedersen, J., Follow-up examinations of children of diabetic mothers. *Acta. Paediatr. Scand.* (Suppl.) **77,** 208 (1948). (Abstract).

21. White, P., Koshy, P., and Duckers, J., The management of pregnancy complicating diabetes and of children of diabetic mothers, *Med. Clin. North Amer.* **37,** 1481 (1953).

22. Farquhar, J. W., Prognosis for babies born to diabetic mothers in Edinburgh, *Arch. Dis. Child.* **44,** 36 (1969).

23. Churchill, J. A., Berendes, H. W., and Nemore, V., Neuropsychological defects in children of diabetic mothers, *Am. J. Obstet. Gynecol.* **105,** 257 (1969).

Acid-Base, Fluid, and Electrolyte Disturbances in the Newborn

WILLIAM C. HEIRD, M.D.

Most newborn infants can adapt competently to the usual physiological stresses of extrauterine life. However, their immature homeostatic mechanisms make successful contention with undue stress virtually impossible, especially for the prematurely born infant. The homeostatic mechanisms most often taxed by undue stress are those governing acid-base, fluid, and electrolyte homeostasis. In this chapter, I discuss some of the disturbances that result from interference with these homeostatic mechanisms, along with some of the general principles for dealing with these disturbances. Both of these specific aspects will be discussed within the framework of the principles underlying the maintenance of acid-base as well as fluid and electrolyte equilibrium.

REGULATION OF ACID-BASE EQUILIBRIUM

The newborn is subject to many disease states that are manifest by acid-base disturbances—for example, respiratory distress syndrome, drug-induced central nervous system depression, congenital renal disorders, and organic or functional gastrointestinal disorders. Essential to proper diagnosis and treatment of these disorders is an understanding of the principles of acid-base regulation. In general, this regulation can be viewed as a complex interaction between physicochemical mechanisms on the one hand and physiological mechanisms on the other (1–3).

Physicochemical mechanisms. The physicochemical mechanisms for regulating acid-base equilibrium primarily are the various buffer systems of body fluids, buffers being defined as substances that can minimize a change in pH when acid or base is added to the system. In biological systems, buffers are composed of weak acids (HB) and their conjugate bases (B^-):

$$HB \rightleftharpoons H^+ + B^- \qquad [1]$$

weak acid   conjugate base

Each such acid with its conjugate base is called a buffer pair.

Two examples will remind the reader how buffers operate. Strong acid added to a buffer system is converted to a weak acid by reaction with the conjugate base:

$$\underset{\text{strong acid}}{H^+X^-} + \underset{\text{conjugate base}}{Na^+B^-} \rightarrow \underset{\text{neutral salt}}{Na^+X^-} + \underset{\text{weak acid}}{HB} \qquad [2]$$

Strong base, on the other hand, reacts with a weak acid to generate the conjugate base and water:

$$\underset{\text{strong base}}{Na^+OH^-} + \underset{\text{weak acid}}{HB} \rightarrow \underset{\text{conjugate base}}{Na^+B^-} + \underset{\text{water}}{H_2O} \qquad [3]$$

The pH of a buffered solution is defined by the Henderson-Hasselbalch equation (which is simply a special case of the general equation for dissociation; the Michaelis-Menton equation used in enzymology is another):

$$pH = pK' + \log \frac{[\text{conjugate base}]}{[\text{weak acid}]} \qquad [4]$$

This equation states that the pH is equal to a constant, pK', which is characteristic of the particular buffer system, plus the logarithm of the ratio of the concentrations (signified by the brackets) of the conjugate base and the undissociated acid.

Many substances in the various body-water compartments behave as buffers, those in blood being the best characterized. Buffers in the blood are usually grouped into the bicarbonate system and the nonbicarbonate system (Table 1). The bicarbonate system is

Table 1. Quantitative Importance of Each Component of Blood Buffers[a]

Buffer system	% buffering in whole blood
Nonbicarbonate buffers	
Hemoglobin and oxyhemoglobin	35
Organic phosphate	3
Inorganic phosphate	2
Plasma protein	7
Total nonbicarbonate buffers	47
Bicarbonate buffers	
Plasma bicarbonate	35
Erythrocyte bicarbonate	18
Total bicarbonate buffers	53

[a] Reproduced, with permission, from Winters and Dell (1).

present chiefly in the plasma. In this system, HCO_3^- is the conjugate base and H_2CO_3 is the weak acid. The nonbicarbonate system, present chiefly in the erythrocyte, consists largely of hemoglobin, with smaller contributions from plasma proteins and from organic and inorganic phosphates. The nonbicarbonate buffers are collectively designated by the symbols HBuf (the weak acid) and Buf⁻ (the conjugate base). If the erythrocyte membrane is disregarded and all blood buffers are assumed to exist in a homogeneous medium, the following equation holds:

$$\text{pH} = \text{pK}'_{\text{H}_2\text{CO}_3} + \log \frac{[\text{HCO}_3^-]}{[\text{H}_2\text{CO}_3]} = \text{pK}'_{\text{HBuf}} + \log \frac{[\text{Buf}^-]}{[\text{HBuf}]} \tag{5}$$

This equation says that the pH of blood is a function of the ratio of the two sets of buffers, which in turn gives rise to the following implications: (*a*) any strong acid or base that is added will be buffered by both systems; (*b*) primary changes in the bicarbonate buffer pair can be buffered only by the nonbicarbonate buffers; and (*c*) the physiological mechanisms for pH regulation need regulate only one buffer pair—i.e., if one pair is regulated, all others will be regulated automatically.

Physiological regulation. The bicarbonate buffer system possesses several unique advantages as a physiological pH regulator.

First, the weak acid of the system (H_2CO_3) is in equilibrium with the dissolved carbon dioxide of the plasma:

$$\text{H}_2\text{CO}_3 \rightleftharpoons \text{H}_2\text{O} + (\text{CO}_2)_\text{d} \tag{6}$$

At equilibrium, the amount of dissolved CO_2 exceeds that of H_2CO_3 by a factor of 810 to 1; thus for practical purposes H_2CO_3 and $(CO_2)_\text{d}$ can be treated interchangeably.

Secondly, the dissolved CO_2 of pulmonary capillary blood achieves equilibrium with the partial pressure of CO_2 (p_{CO_2}) in the alveolar gas phase of the lung, a relationship given by Henry's law:

$$\text{H}_2\text{CO}_3 + (\text{CO}_2)_\text{d} = \text{S} \cdot p_{CO_2} \tag{7}$$

where S is the solubility constant for CO_2 in plasma and has a value of 0.0301 mmol of $(CO_2)_\text{d}$ per litre of plasma for each unit (mmHg) of p_{CO_2}. In health, $S \cdot p_{CO_2}$ (0.0301 × 40 mmHg) equals 1.2 mmol/litre.

A third biological advantage of this buffer system in physiological control is the almost unlimited supply of CO_2 available from metabolism.

Finally, the plasma concentration of the conjugate base of the bicarbonate buffer system (i.e., $[\text{HCO}_3^-]$) can be regulated by the renal tubule. When this concentration is excessive, renal tubular reabsorption of bicarbonate can be decreased; when it is too low, bicarbonate reabsorption can be increased and "new" bicarbonate can be synthesized by the renal tubular epithelium.

As expressed by the Henderson-Hasselbalch equation, blood pH is equal to a constant plus the log of the ratio of the concentrations of bicarbonate and dissolved CO_2:

$$\text{pH} = 6.1 + \log \frac{[\text{HCO}_3^-]}{(\text{S} \cdot p_{CO_2})} \tag{8}$$

Thus if the ratio of $[\text{HCO}_3^-]/(\text{S} \cdot p_{CO_2})$ is decreased, pH decreases; if it is increased, pH increases. In maintaining normal acid-base equilibrium, as well as in countering disorders of the equilibrium, it is apparent that the body strives to maintain the ratio (rather than the amounts) so as to give a normal pH.

Plasma p_{CO_2} is controlled through changes in alveolar ventilation, which are mediated through the respiratory center of the central nervous system. The stimulus triggering increased alveolar ventilation seems to be an increase in arterial p_{CO_2} or a decrease in the arterial pH or p_{O_2}, while decreased alveolar ventilation is triggered by opposite changes of these stimuli. The exact mechanism by which these stimuli bring about changes in alveolar ventilation is not known.

Physiologically, plasma bicarbonate concentration is regulated through three possible renal tubular actions: (*a*) reabsorption of all filtered bicarbonate, (*b*) synthesis of new bicarbonate, or (*c*) reabsorption of less bicarbonate than is filtered. The normal tubule reabsorbs practically all the glomerular filtrate; thus the first of these actions scarcely affects plasma bicarbonate concentration. However, this mechanism coupled with synthesis of new bicarbonate can produce an increased plasma bicarbonate concentration. "New" bicarbonate is produced by the tubules from carbonic acid. But hydrogen ion must be excreted in the urine for the reabsorbed bicarbonate to be effective, and because the lower limit of urinary pH is 4.0, hydrogen ion must be buffered to be excreted. This buffering is accomplished by excretion of the hydrogen ion, either as NH_4^+ or as titratable acid. Thus, for every millimole (milliequivalent) of either ammonium or titratable acid excreted, 1 mmol (mEq) of bicarbonate is returned to the extracellular fluid. Neither of these two mechanisms may be fully developed in the newborn or pre-term infant. In addition, the mechanism for bicarbonate reabsorption may also be impaired. Thus the newborn infant has a diminished physiological renal reserve for dealing with acid-base disorders. This fact, coupled with the fact that none of the physiological mechanisms for acid-base control ever functions at maximum efficiency (i.e., to completely prevent pH changes), makes the newborn infant's position in the face of acid-base disturbances even more precarious.

DISTURBANCES OF ACID-BASE EQUILIBRIUM

Acid-base disorders are classified primarily by the number and type of etiological factors giving rise to the disturbance (3). A "simple" acid-base disturbance is one in which only one etiological factor is involved; a "mixed" disturbance is one in which more than one primary etiological factor is present. Based on etiological factors, acid-base disturbances are classified as either metabolic disturbances or respiratory disturbances. Metabolic disturbances result from either gain or loss of strong acid or base by the extracellular fluid; respiratory disturbances are due to a gain or loss of CO_2. Once a primary disturbance has been produced, secondary physiological mechanisms are set in motion to ameliorate the blood pH deviation caused by that disturbance. These secondary adjustments, called compensation, in turn effect an adjustment of the component of acid-base equilibrium not primarily affected by the primary etiological factor. Thus, for a metabolic disorder, compensation is respiratory and for a respiratory disorder, compensation is renal (metabolic). Correction of an acid-base disturbance, as opposed to compensation, involves those physiological mechanisms that fully correct the primary abnormality.

Metabolic acidosis. Metabolic acidosis is defined as the condition resulting from accumulation of acid other than carbonic acid by the extracellular fluid or loss of bicarbonate from the extracellular fluid (Table 2). The response of the blood buffers to the gain of strong acid (HA) is depicted as follows:

$$HA + HCO_3^- \rightarrow A^- + H_2CO_3 \rightarrow H_2O + CO_2 \qquad [9]$$

$$HA + Buf^- \rightarrow A^- + HBuf \qquad [10]$$

These reactions are prompt, and compensatory hyperventilation begins almost immediately. Later, buffering by the tissues—visualized as exchange of H^+ for cellular cations—also assumes a significant role.

Because bicarbonate loss can be buffered only by the nonbicarbonate buffers, the buffer reactions in response to a loss of bicarbonate are different:

$$CO_2 + H_2O \rightarrow H_2CO_3 + Buf^- \rightarrow HBuf + HCO_3^- \qquad [11]$$

After an immediate adjustment of ventilation with respect to CO_2 production, the more sustained respiratory compensation, as just shown, plays a role. So far as is known, the compensatory mechanisms against metabolic acidosis are fully operative in the newborn—provided, of course, that pulmonary function is adequate.

Metabolic alkalosis. Metabolic alkalosis results from a loss of hydrogen ions from the extracellular fluid or from a gain of exogenous bicarbonate (Table 2). Because water is the source of the hydrogen ions that are being lost, the immediate consequences of this loss may be visualized as a gain of hydroxyl ions. The immediate buffer responses are as follows:

$$OH^- + H_2CO_3 \rightarrow HCO_3^- + H_2O \qquad [12]$$

and

$$OH^- + HBuf \rightarrow Buf^- + H_2O \qquad [13]$$

As a result of consumption of carbonic acid, p_{CO_2} decreases. This decrease in turn results in decreased ventilation until a normal plasma p_{CO_2} is again reached. Although this response can be sustained, resulting in increased plasma p_{CO_2} values, plasma p_{CO_2} values higher than 6.0 to 6.7 kPa (45–50 mmHg) are rarely seen.

Respiratory acidosis. Respiratory acidosis results from a decrease in alveolar ventilation relative to CO_2 production (Table 3). The immediate consequence is an increased alveolar p_{CO_2} and thus an increased arterial p_{CO_2} and carbonic acid. The buffer response to increased carbonic acid occurs via the nonbicarbonate buffers:

$$CO_2 + H_2O \rightarrow H_2CO_3 + Buf^- \rightarrow HBuf + HCO_3^- \qquad [14]$$

Secondary renal compensatory responses, which require several days under the best conditions, consist of reabsorption of all filtered bicarbonate and generation of new bicarbonate through hydrogen ion excretion—processes that are probably limited in the newborn infant.

Respiratory alkalosis. Respiratory alkalosis results from increased alveolar ventilation relative to CO_2 production (Table 3) so that alveolar and arterial p_{CO_2} decrease. This decreased arterial carbonic acid is replaced exclusively by the nonbicarbonate buffers:

$$HCO_3^- + HBuf \rightarrow Buf^- + H_2CO_3 \rightarrow (CO_2)_d + H_2O \qquad [15]$$

Tissue buffering also contributes by exchange of hydrogen ion for extracellular cations. If hyperventilation causing metabolic alkalosis is sustained, renal compensation occurs as excretion of bicarbonate.

Other acid-base disturbances. Two other disorders of acid-base equilibrium should be classified as simple disturbances. These are dilution acidosis and contraction alkalosis. In these disturbances, the primary etiological factors are expansion and contraction of

Table 2.   General Causes of Metabolic Acid–Base Disturbances

General cause	Specific cause	Example
	Metabolic Acidosis	
Gain of strong acid by extracellular fluid	Gain of exogenous acid (HCl)	NH$_4$Cl acidosis
	Incomplete oxidation of fat	Diabetic or starvation ketoacidosis
	Incomplete oxidation of carbohydrate	Organic acidosis
	Gain of H$_2$SO$_4$, H$_3$PO$_4$, and (?) organic acids	Uremic acidosis
Loss of HCO$_3^-$ from extracellular fluid	Via the kidney	Renal tubular acidosis
	Via gastrointestinal tract	Diarrheal acidosis
	Metabolic Alkalosis	
Gain by HCO$_3^-$ by extracellular fluid	Gain of exogenous HCO$_3^-$	Ingestion of infusion of HCO$_3^-$
	Oxidation of organic acids	Ingestion of infusion of lactate, citrate, etc.
Loss of acid from extracellular fluid	Loss of HCl	Vomiting of gastric juice
	Loss of H$^+$ via the kidney	Diuretic therapy; K$^+$ depletion
	? Extrarenal transfer of H$^+$ to intracellular fluid	?K$^+$ depletion

the extracellular fluid volume, respectively, without affecting the total amount of buffer in the compartment. For example, dilution of bicarbonate through infusion of saline results in dilution acidosis, whereas diuresis of edema fluid induced by diuretic administration, which results in a decreased extracellular fluid volume without bicarbonate diuresis, causes contraction alkalosis. Either of these may occur from time to time in the newborn infant.

Perhaps the most common disturbance of acid-base equilibrium in the newborn period is a mixed disturbance, respiratory acidosis and metabolic acidosis, as commonly seen in patients with the idiopathic respiratory distress syndrome. Of course, other mixed disturbances can occur and are encountered occasionally in the newborn infant.

LABORATORY FINDINGS IN ACID-BASE DISORDERS

The bicarbonate buffer system is the traditional base of reference for characterization of acid-base equilibrium as expressed in the Henderson-Hasselbalch equation (equation 8). This equation contains three unknowns (pH, HCO$_3^-$, and p_{CO_2}) and two constants (pK$'$ and S). Obviously, two of these three unknowns must be measured to solve the

Table 3. General Causes of Respiratory Acid–Base Disturbances

General cause	Site in respiratory system	Mechanisms
	Respiratory Acidosis	
Decrease in alveolar ventilation	Central nervous system	Depression of respiratory center (disease, certain drugs)
	Airways and (or) lungs	Decreased ventilation or diffusion (intrinsic lung or airway disease)
	Chest wall	Loss of bellows action (structural or functional abnormalities of chest wall or muscles)
	Respiratory Alkalosis	
Increase in alveolar ventilation	Central nervous system	Primary stimulation of respiratory center (emotion, certain drugs)
	Peripheral chemoreceptors	Reflex stimulation of respiratory center (hypoxemia)
	Intrathoracic stretch receptors	Reflex stimulation of respiratory center (localized pulmonary disease)

equation. One method involves measuring the pH of blood or plasma and the total CO_2 content of plasma $(CO_2)_t$, which is defined as $HCO_3^- + (S \cdot p_{CO_2})$. Other methods involve electrometric measurement of plasma p_{CO_2} and blood pH or measurements of blood pH and plasma p_{CO_2} by the equilibration, or Astrup, method.

Whole-blood buffer base, defined as the sum of all conjugate bases of both the bicarbonate and the nonbicarbonate buffer systems (i.e., HCO_3^- and Buf^-) in whole blood, is an additional variable for characterization of acid-base equilibrium in blood. The difference between the observed buffer base of any blood sample and the normal buffer base of that sample is called the base excess. Thus the base excess gives an accurate measure of the amount of strong acid or strong base that has been added to whole blood. For example, a base excess of 10 mmol/litre (mEq/litre) indicates addition of 10 mmol/litre (mEq/litre) of base (or loss of 10 mmol/litre (mEq/litre) of hydrogen ion), whereas a base excess of −10 mmol/litre (mEq/litre) indicates addition of a similar amount of strong acid (or loss of base).

One further laboratory measurement is of importance in characterizing clinical acid-base disturbances: the R fraction, or anion gap, which is calculated as follows:

$$R = plasma[Na^+] - (plasma[Cl^-] + plasma[HCO_3^-]) \qquad [16]$$

In the newborn, the normal value for R is about 10 to 15 mmol/litre (mEq/litre). In metabolic acidosis that is a result of accumulation of strong acid other than hydrochloric acid, the value of R increases; in metabolic acidosis that is a result of accumulation of hydrochloric acid or of a loss of bicarbonate, the R fraction remains normal.

GENERAL PRINCIPLES OF TREATMENT OF ACID-BASE DISORDERS

In any acid-base disorder, there are three general principles of treatment: (*a*) control the process producing the primary disorder, if possible, (*b*) augment any deranged physiological corrective mechanisms, and (*c*) attack the displacement of blood pH directly with acidifying or alkalinizing therapy. Some of these principles will be illustrated here.

Treatment of metabolic acidosis. In some instances, therapy of metabolic acidosis aimed at control of the primary cause of the acidosis is possible—for example, control of diarrhea in diarrheal acidosis, adequate oxygenation in lactic acidosis, and insulin therapy in diabetic ketoacidosis. Nearly all patients with metabolic acidosis have concomitant deficits of sodium and water, and such deficits impair the urinary acidification mechanisms. Thus, rehydration with attendant restoration of renal function is important in correcting acidosis, because it allows maximal excretion of hydrogen ions (as NH_4^+ or titratable acid, or both), thereby returning bicarbonate to the plasma.

Despite these measures, severe degrees of metabolic acidosis may require that the low blood pH be attacked directly. There are several formulas for computing the amount of bicarbonate necessary to restore plasma bicarbonate to normal. All of these take the following general form:

$$HCO_3^- \text{ needed} = HCO_3^- \text{ deficit (or base excess)} \times \text{"}HCO_3^- \text{ space"} \qquad [17]$$

Use of these formulas is limited by lack of an accurate estimate of the value for the "HCO_3^- space" (*i.e.*, the volume in which bicarbonate is distributed). The various values recommended for this space range from 20 to 60% of the body weight. Thus, rather than rely on this rather uncertain approach, it is preferable simply to administer 2 to 4 mmol (2–4 mEq) of sodium bicarbonate intravenously per kilogram body weight over a 4 to 6 h period, and then reassess the acid-base status. Further dosage can then be planned on the basis of this experience. With this approach, the patient, in effect, is titrated serially according to feedback information from blood acid-base analyses.

Metabolic alkalosis. Treatment of metabolic alkalosis should be aimed at control of the primary disorder (e.g., vomiting, overzealous diuretic therapy). In addition, adequate amounts of sodium chloride and potassium chloride must be provided so as to allow the corrective renal mechanism for excretion of bicarbonate to operate maximally. Occasionally, the administration of acidifying salts such as arginine hydrochloride, which yield HCl when metabolized, may be necessary. The dosage of this agent can be calculated from the following equation:

$$\text{Dose of arginine HCl} = (\text{normal plasma } [Cl^-] - \text{observed plasma } [Cl^-])$$

$$\times 0.3 \text{ body weight (kg)} \qquad [18]$$

Arginine hydrochloride should be given slowly (over a 6–12 h period) with serial monitoring of blood acid-base status.

Respiratory acidosis. Therapy for respiratory acidosis should be directed primarily toward the cause of decreased alveolar ventilation, which in the neonate often means intermittent or continuous respiratory assistance. Supportive bicarbonate therapy to increase the blood pH may be undertaken in severe acidosis (plasma pH < 7.20). Tris(hydroxymethyl)-aminomethane, because it buffers carbon dioxide, has been advocated as a superior agent for treatment of severe respiratory acidosis. This effect, at best, provides only a transient decrease in plasma p_{CO_2}; amounts of it far exceeding its LD_{50} would be necessary to buffer all the carbon dioxide produced by metabolism over any sustained period of time. However, a transient improvement in blood pH might be important if intracardiac or intrapulmonary shunts, thought to be contributors to the decreased oxygenation, could be influenced favorably. Even so, there is no evidence for a superiority of tris(hydroxy-methyl)aminomethane over sodium bicarbonate. Certainly, it exerts as much or more osmotic effect per unit of buffering as does sodium bicarbonate (4).

Respiratory alkalosis. Therapy for respiratory alkalosis should also be directed toward the primary cause of increased alveolar ventilation. Most instances of respiratory alkalosis in the newborn period are secondary to drug administration either to the mother or to the baby; thus the period of hyperventilation might be prolonged, depending on the infant's ability to metabolize or excrete the particular drug that was administered. In any case, severe disturbances are rare, and the usual so-called physiological metabolic acidosis seen in the first hours of life helps offset the elevated pH in this condition. Increasing the p_{CO_2} of the inspired air might be of very transient benefit, but prolonged breathing of CO_2 will only increase the arterial p_{CO_2} and further stimulate the respiratory center.

PHYSIOLOGICAL CHARACTERISTICS OF BODY FLUIDS

Body-fluid compartments. Figure 1 depicts the traditional representation of the total body water and its two major subdivisions, the extracellular and intracellular compartments. About 75% of the total weight of the normal newborn infant consists of water, whereas only 60% of the total weight of the older child or adult is water. When distribution of the total body water is considered (Figure 2), the difference between infants and older children or adults is even more apparent. In the newborn about half of the total body water is extracellular fluid, whereas in the adult it comprises at most only 20% to 25% of the total body water (5). Thus with increasing age, the proportion of the total body weight that is water and the proportion of this water that is extracellular fluid decrease and the proportion that is intracellular fluid increases. The fraction of total body water that is extracellular fluid is even greater in the fetus than in the term infant. Thus, the younger the infant, the "wetter" he is, and this increased "wetness" is due primarily to an increased fraction of extracellular fluid.

Composition of body fluids. In contrast to distribution, the composition of the body fluids remains nearly constant throughout life. The composition of plasma, interstitial fluid, and intracellular fluid is compared in Figure 1. In plasma, sodium is the principal cation and the anions are mainly chloride and bicarbonate, with protein contributing a small but significant fraction. Interstitial fluid is an ultrafiltrate of plasma; thus its composition is similar to that of plasma except that it has a lower protein content, which means that the concentration of diffusible inorganic anions must be slightly higher. In the intracellular fluid, the principal cations are potassium and magnesium, while the principal anions consist of cellular proteins plus inorganic and organic phosphates.

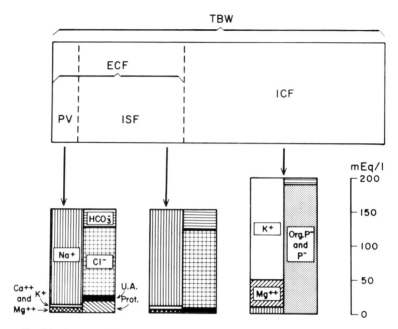

Figure 1. Total body water (*TBW*) and its subdivision, extracellular fluid (*ECF*) and intracellular fluid (*ICF*). The *ECF* in turn, is subdivided into plasma volume (*PV*) and the interstitial fluid (*ISF*). From Heird, William C., Grebin, Burton, and Winters, Robert W.: The stabilization of disorders of water, electrolyte, and acid-base metabolism in newborn infants under intensive care. In Abramson, Harold, editor: Resuscitation of the newborn infant and related emergency procedures in the perinatal center special care nursery, ed. 3, St. Louis, 1973, The C. V. Mosby Co.

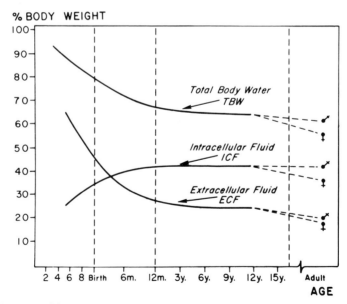

Figure 2. Changes in *TBW*, *ECF*, and *ICF* as a function of age. Data represent smoothed curves from the original data of Friss-Hansen (5).

304

Osmotic characteristics of body fluids. The total body water can be thought of as two solutions (the intracellular and extracellular fluids, each with its dissolved constituents) separated by a semipermeable membrane (the cell membrane). This membrane allows free passage of the solvent (water) but restrains movement of the electrolytes. Net movements of water across such a membrane reflect the chemical potential of water in each of the two compartments. Although the chemical potential of water can be altered in a number of ways, change of solute concentration is the most relevant with regard to discussion of the body fluids. For example, when a nonpenetrating solute such as sodium chloride is added to the extracellular fluid, the chemical potential of water in the compartment is decreased, while the chemical potential of intracellular water is unchanged, at least initially (Figure 3). Thus, less water moves from the extracellular to the intracellular compartment, whereas movement in the opposite direction is unchanged, resulting in a net water movement from the intracellular to the extracellular space. This movement ceases when the chemical potential of the water in the two compartments again becomes equal. The degree to which a solute decreases the chemical potential of water represents the osmotic pressure imparted to the solvent by the solute. The effect of a solute on osmotic pressure is a colligative property—i.e., it depends only on the number (and not the kind, size, or charge) of nonpenetrating solute particles present in the solution. In quantitating the osmotic effect of a given solute, the unit of osmole is used. It is defined as:

$$\text{osmole} = n(\text{moles}) \qquad [19]$$

where n is the number of particles produced by dissociation of 1 mole of solute. For example, 1 mmol of sodium chloride in solution dissociates into 1 mmol of sodium ion and 1 mmol of chloride ion, and thus represents 2 mosmol of osmotic activity (i.e., n = 2, assuming "ideal" behavior). Urea and glucose, on the other hand, are nondissociable solutes (n = 1) and represent only 1 mosmol of osmotic activity per millimole. The total osmolarity of either compartment of body fluids is the sum of the individual contributions of *all* solutes, the nonpenetrating ones (electrolytes) as well as those that can penetrate the cell membrane (such as urea). The effective (actual) osmotic pressure,

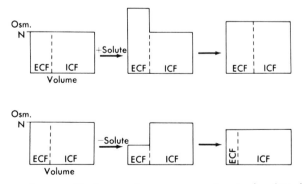

Figure 3. Internal exchanges of body water in response to solute load or loss. [Reproduced, with permission, from Heird et al. (21).] From Heird, William C., Grebin, Burton, and Winters, Robert W.: The stabilization of disorders of water, electrolyte, and acid-base metabolism in newborn infants under intensive care. In Abramson, Harold, editor: Resuscitation of the newborn infant and related emergency procedures in the perinatal center special care nursery, ed. 3, St. Louis, 1973, The C. V. Mosby Co.

on the other hand, is determined by only the nonpenetrating solutes, because only these can differentially affect the chemical potential of water and thus differentially affect osmotic pressure.

For most purposes the effective osmolarity of the plasma and of the extracellular fluid can be approximated by the following rule (which will not hold if the plasma is either hyperlipemic or hyperglycemic):

$$\text{Effective osmolarity} = 2 \times \text{plasma } [Na^+] \tag{20}$$

In a steady state, with free passage of water across the cell membrane, the osmolarity of all phases of the body fluids is equal. Thus, the response of the body to a solute load (L_{osm}) can be predicted by the following equation:

$$\underset{\substack{\text{(initial total} \\ \text{body solute)}}}{(TBW)_1 \times (osm)_1} + \underset{\substack{\text{(load of} \\ \text{solute)}}}{L_{osm}} = \underset{\substack{\text{(final total} \\ \text{body solute)}}}{(TBW)_2 \times (osm)_2} \tag{21}$$

where TBW is total body water, and osm is effective osmolarity. Because TBW remains constant ($TBW_1 = TBW_2$) with "pure" solute load or "pure" solute loss (i.e., negative L_{osm}), equation 21 can be rewritten as follows:

$$L_{osm} = TBW\,(osm_2 - osm_1) \tag{22}$$

Furthermore, because of the relationship between plasma $[Na^+]$ and effective osmolarity:

$$L_{Na}^+ = TBW\,([Na^+]_2 - [Na^+]_1) \tag{23}$$

This expression is useful in correction of hyponatremic states and will be referred to when fluid and electrolyte replacement is discussed.

The osmotic effects of both a water load and a water loss are shown in Figure 4. A similar expression dealing with loads or losses of water can be derived. In these cases total body solute is constant:

$$\underset{\substack{\text{(initial total} \\ \text{body solute)}}}{(TBW_1 \times [osm]_1)} = \underset{\substack{\text{(final total} \\ \text{body solute)}}}{(TBW_2 \times [osm]_2)} \tag{24}$$

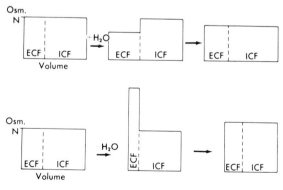

Figure 4. Internal exchanges of body water in response to fluid load or loss. *Osm* N is normal osmolarity. Reproduced, with permission, from Heird et al. (*21*) (see legend to Fig. 3).

with addition of water (L_{H_2O}):

$$TBW_2 = TBW_1 + L_{H_2O} \qquad [25]$$

Thus:

$$(TBW_1 \times [osm]_1) = (TBW_1 + L_{H_2O}) \times [osm]_2 \qquad [26]$$

or

$$L_{H_2O} = \frac{TBW_1([osm]_1 - [osm]_2)}{[osm]_2} \qquad [27]$$

This last expression is also useful in dealing with problems of water replacement.

Physiological regulation of volume and osmolarity of body fluids. Both the effective osmolarity and the volume of the body fluids are regulated within narrow limits by a complex neuro-endocrine system. Osmolarity is regulated through control of the plasma sodium concentration; the volume of the extracellular fluid is regulated by control of the amount of sodium and water in that compartment. The overall action of this complex system, conceived as two interrelated feedback loops, is depicted schematically in Figure 5 (6).

The operation of the system may be illustrated by an example. With delivery of a "pure" solute load (i.e., without water), the body fluids become hyperosmolar. Hypothalamic receptors, in turn, are triggered by this hyperosmolarity, giving rise to the sensation of thirst, and water, if available, will be ingested by the organism. In addition, other receptors cause secretion of vasopressin (antidiuretic hormone) by the posterior pituitary gland. This hormone acts on the renal tubule to increase reabsorption of water, producing a decreased volume of more concentrated urine. Hypo-osmolarity of the extracellular fluid, on the other hand, sets an opposite series of events into motion.

Although this mechanism can regulate osmolarity of the body fluids, it cannot regulate the absolute volume of the extracellular fluid. This regulation is accomplished by control of renal sodium excretion mediated by the adrenal salt-retaining hormone aldosterone (and probably other factors as well). The exact stimulus to the so-called volume receptor is not known, but a decrease in extracellular fluid volume is known to cause an augmented secretion of aldosterone, as well as activation of other responses, all of

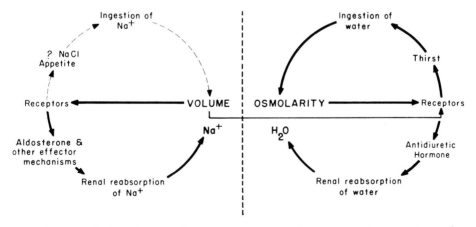

Figure 5. Overall view of neuroendocrine-renal system regulating osmolarity and volume of the ECF. [Adapted from Winters (6).]

which promote reabsorption of sodium by the renal tubule. Expansion of extracellular volume, on the other hand, leads to a decrease in aldosterone secretion and thus to increased renal excretion of sodium (along with water).

Little evidence is available concerning the quantitative operational limits of this system in the newborn. It has been thought for some time that glomerular filtration rate is low in the newborn period (7–10) and evidence is accumulating to suggest that tubular active-transport mechanisms may be even more limited (11). Thus, functionally, the kidney of the newborn infant is characterized by a state of glomerulotubular imbalance. However, this state may be transient; both glomerular filtration and tubular transport can be enhanced by appropriate stimuli (12). The newborn infant rarely shows the expected diuretic response to a water load during the first three days of postnatal life (13), but maximal urine dilution can be achieved by about five days of age (13,14). Even then the rate of water excretion in response to a water load is limited compared to the response of the more mature kidney (14). The maximum concentrating ability of the kidney in the newborn appears to be about half that of the adult (15,16), but feeding either urea or a high-protein diet (16) restores this function toward that of the normal adult. Some evidence suggests that vasopressin is decreased in the newborn period (17) and that the renal tubules do not respond maximally to the available vasopressin. The status of the aldosterone mechanisms in the newborn period is even less clear. Thus, it would appear that the same general regulatory mechanisms for volume and osmolarity that are operative in the adult are present in the newborn, but that they function on a somewhat limited basis, especially with respect to the renal effector mechanisms. The most significant defect from a clinical point of view seems to be limitation in handling a water load, with the ability to dispose of a solute load being limited to a somewhat lesser extent.

DISORDERS OF HYDRATION

Hydration disorders may involve either a net gain or a net loss of water in association with either gain or loss of solute. Net gain of pure water (i.e., without gain or loss of solute)—so-called water intoxication—is usually induced iatrogenically by overly generous administration of fluids containing insufficient solute. On the other hand, loss of body water, with or without solute, may accompany many disease states. These losses may result from either decreased intake or an increased output of solute and water.

Types of dehydration. The relationship between the deficit of water and the deficit of solute determines the type of dehydration produced. Thus, if these two deficits occur in the same relationship as exists in the normal body fluids, the osmolarity of the extracellular fluid remains normal and a state of isotonic dehydration is produced. On the other hand, when the deficit of solute in relation to water is hyposmotic, the osmolarity of the extracellular fluid is increased, resulting in hypertonic dehydration. The third type of dehydration, hypotonic dehydration, results from loss of water containing solute in hyperosmotic proportions; in this case the plasma osmolarity and sodium concentration are decreased.

Signs of dehydration. The clinical signs of dehydration seem to be related to the degree of reduction in extracellular fluid volume. Classically, these signs include dryness of the skin and mucous membranes, diminished skin turgor, depression of the anterior fontanel, and decreased intraocular tension. Acute change in body weight is the most reliable index of the degree of dehydration in older children and adults. This index, however, is less reliable in the newborn infant because of the abrupt "normal" loss of weight (i.e., of body water) that occurs in the first days of life. Nevertheless, weight change remains the most accurate means of determining the degree of dehydration. Generally, when dealing with isotonic dehydration, a loss of 5% (50 ml/kg) of the initial body weight is associated with mild clinical signs of dehydration, a loss of 10% (100 mg/kg) produces moderate clinical signs of dehydration, and a loss of 15% (150 ml/kg) results in peripheral vascular collapse, with the usual clinical signs of shock. For any given degree of change in extracellular fluid volume, these signs tend to be more pronounced in infants with hypotonic dehydration and less pronounced in those with hypertonic dehydration.

Laboratory data in dehydration. Because of the relationship between plasma osmolarity and plasma sodium concentration (equation 20), the initial sodium concentration determines the type of dehydration. Thus, plasma sodium concentration is increased in hypertonic dehydration, decreased in hypotonic dehydration, and normal in isotonic dehydration. The concentrations of other electrolytes vary, depending on acid-base status and body potassium stores. Plasma potassium concentration may be normal or elevated in acidosis, even when total body potassium is decreased. Plasma chloride concentration tends to vary with plasma sodium concentration, but is also affected by changes in bicarbonate concentration. Obviously, plasma bicarbonate concentration depends on whether acidosis or alkalosis accompanies dehydration. Hemoconcentration—as evidenced by increased hemoglobin concentration, increased packed-cell volume, or increased plasma protein concentration—occurs in states of dehydration; because of changing normal values in the newborn period, however, these changes are often difficult to discern. Prerenal azotemia, a rather consistent accompaniment of significant dehydration in older infants and children, may not be present in the newborn infant because of his limited sources of urea production.

REQUIREMENTS FOR MAINTAINING FLUID AND ELECTROLYTES

Fluid and electrolytes. Physiologically, caloric expenditure is the most relevant basis for estimating maintenance fluid requirements, because it focuses attention on the factors likely to modify maintenance requirements—*i.e.*, changes in body temperature, ambient temperature, ambient humidity, activity, and respiratory rate. Holliday and Segar (*18*) have published a smoothed curve of the available data relating caloric expenditure to body weight. Based on these data, the estimated caloric expenditure is 100 cal/kg body weight (1 cal = 4.18 J) for a child weighing up to 10 kg. During the neonatal period, the value of 100 cal/kg is probably too high, because metabolic rate is lower during the first few days of life and because the activity of the newborn infant is characteristically decreased. Figure 6 depicts a reasonable estimate for caloric expenditure of a newborn infant in the resting state versus that for a healthy growing infant (*19*).

In general, 100 ml of water is required for each 100 cal (*19*). This water allotment replaces that lost through the lungs and skin (as "insensible" water loss), through the kidneys (as urine), and through the gastrointestinal tract (as stool). The deposition of new body water accompanying growth can be neglected in infants who are receiving the

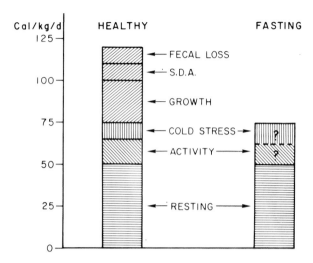

Figure 6. Caloric requirements of healthy and fasting newborn infants. [Adapted from data of Sinclair et al. (*19*).]

usual parenteral fluids. Insensible water loss varies considerably (±15%), depending primarily on the ambient humidity. Urinary water loss is even more difficult to estimate precisely; even during the newborn period, the kidney can vary the volume of urine excreted according to the solute load (obligatory water excretion) and the available water. Generally, an allotment for urinary volume of 55 ml/100 cal will allow excretion of the usual range of solute load within a urine concentration range of 150 to 450 mosm/litre, values that unduly tax neither the diluting nor the concentrating ability. Under usual circumstances of parenteral fluid therapy, gastrointestinal fluid losses are minimal.

Maintenance electrolyte requirements are even more difficult to estimate. Generally, daily provision of 1 to 3 mmol (1–3 mEq) of sodium, potassium, and chloride per 100 cal is satisfactory. These amounts tax neither the maximum excretory capacity nor the maximum conservation capacity of the newborn's kidney for these ions. Thus, an aqueous solution of glucose (50 g/litre) containing 25 mmol of both NaCl and KCl per litre, when given in amounts equivalent to 100 ml/100 cal expended, would probably meet all electrolyte and water requirements for maintenance purposes.

One of the most perplexing problems of fluid therapy during the newborn period is to decide when maintenance fluids should be provided. For instance, both term and preterm infants lose weight during the first few days of life, due chiefly to loss of extracellular fluid. This phenomenon has been assumed to be "physiological," and even with adequate intake sodium loss usually exceeds sodium intake during the first week of life (*20*). Nonetheless, clinical signs of dehydration are seen during the first few days of life. Thus it seems logical that the goal of maintenance fluid therapy during the neonatal period should be to attain zero balance with respect to water, sodium, and chloride, and any recommendation obviously must be varied according to any specific infant's clinical response and the subsequent laboratory findings.

Caloric maintenance.   Although desirable, full caloric maintenance generally is unnecessary for short-term maintenance fluid therapy. Rather, about 20 Cal/100 ml of fluid (5 g glucose/100 ml) is provided in these situations. Although some tissue catabolism can be prevented with this caloric intake, growth and positive nitrogen balance certainly cannot be expected. Obviously, if an infant's condition precludes provision of adequate calories and protein by the oral route for a prolonged period, intravenous provision of these substances should be considered. (See chapter on *Total Intravenous Nutrition.*)

GENERAL PRINCIPLES FOR TREATING FLUID AND ELECTROLYTE DISORDERS

Formulation of therapy. The aim of therapy in dehydration is to restore to the body fluids the amounts of water and solute that have been lost. Before a rational plan for fluid therapy can be formulated, four things must be assessed: the total water deficit, the solute deficit, the distribution of the solute deficit between sodium and potassium, and the type and severity of the accompanying acid-base disorder.

Water deficit is estimated by the observed change in body weight or by the severity of the clinical signs of dehydration or both.

Solute deficits can be estimated as the difference between the expected normal total body solute and that present after the deficit has occurred (Δ TBS):

$$\Delta \text{ TBS} = ([\text{TBW}]_1 \times [280 \text{ mosm/litre}]) - ([\text{TBW}]_2 \times [\text{osm/litre}]_2) \quad [28]$$

or

$$\text{Solute deficit} = \text{normal TBS} - \text{observed TBS}$$

This calculation gives the total solute deficit in milliosmoles per kilogram of body weight.

The next step is to estimate the partition of the cation losses between sodium and potassium. In most states of dehydration, about equal proportions of sodium and potassium can be assumed to have been lost (an obvious exception being adrenal insufficiency, in which no appreciable potassium is lost). All solute deficits obviously include anions, primarily chloride and bicarbonate, and the proportions of these that have been lost depend on the acid-base abnormality present.

The calculation to determine the solute deficit can be illustrated in a dehydrated patient who has lost 0.10 litre water/kg body weight, and who has a plasma sodium concentration of 129 mmol/litre and an assumed normal total body water of 0.65 litre/kg:

$$\Delta \text{ TBS} = ([0.65 \text{ litre/kg}] \times [280 \text{ mmol/litre}])$$

$$- ([0.55 \text{ litre/kg}] \times [258 \text{ mmol/litre}]) \quad [29]$$

$$\Delta \text{ TBS} = 182 - 142 = 40 \text{ mmol/kg} \quad [30]$$

Of this solute deficit, half the total cation loss of 20 mmol is assumed to be sodium and the other half potassium, with the proportion of chloride to bicarbonate loss being determined by the patient's acid-base status.

General scheme of replacement therapy. Once these estimates have been made, restoration of water and solute deficits can begin and should proceed in three phases: (*a*) treatment of shock, if present, (*b*) restoration of extracellular deficits of sodium and water, and (*c*) restoration of intracellular potassium losses.

Shock is best treated by transfusing whole blood (10 ml/kg body weight) or by infusing plasma (20 ml/kg). In usual practice, however, 20 ml/kg of an isotonic sodium solution (Figure 7) is given during 1 to 2 h. After restoration of adequate circulatory

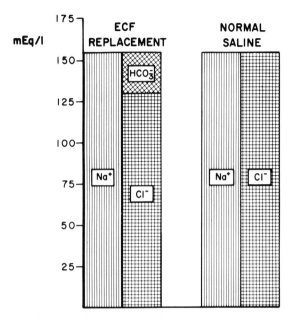

Figure 7. Composition of isotonic replacement fluids. Extracellular replacement fluid (*left*) should be used in patients with acidosis or no acid-base disorder, whereas normal saline (*right*) should be used in alkalotic patients. [Reproduced, with permission, from Heird et al. (*21*).] From Heird, William C., Grebin, Burton, and Winters, Robert W.: The stabilization of disorders of water, electrolyte, and acid-base metabolism in newborn infants under intensive care. In Abramson, Harold, editor: Resuscitation of the newborn infant and related emergency procedures in the perinatal center special care nursery, ed. 3, St. Louis, 1973, The C. V. Mosby Co.

status, the next phase of therapy can begin. This phase is designed to replace the remainder of the sodium deficit and about half to three fourths of the water deficit over a period of 8 to 24 h, depending on the severity of dehydration. If a concomitant acid-base disturbance is present, the anionic composition of the sodium salts given during this phase should be designed so as partially or completely to restore the acid-base status to normal. During the third phase of therapy, the remainder of the water deficit can be replaced. Potassium replacement can begin any time after adequate urine flow is established, but potassium deficits should be replaced no faster than 3 mmol/kg/day, with the concentration of potassium in the infusion fluid not exceeding 40 mmol/litre. Complete replacement of potassium deficits generally takes several days.

In addition to deficit therapy, appropriate amounts of water, electrolytes, and calories should be provided for maintenance purposes as well as adequate water and electrolyte to match any continuing losses. Obviously, serial laboratory and clinical monitoring of the progress of therapy should be carried out and the therapy adjusted appropriately.

SUMMARY

Acid-base equilibrium is regulated by complex interactions between physiochemical and physiological mechanisms. The physiochemical mechanisms consist of various buffer systems, usually grouped into the bicarbonate and the nonbicarbonate systems. The bicarbonate system is the best characterized of these and can be expressed by the familiar Henderson-Hasselbalch equation:

$$pH = pK + \log \frac{[HCO_3^-]}{0.03 \, p_{CO_2}}$$

The physiological mechanisms consist of pulmonary control of p_{CO_2} and renal control of the bicarbonate concentration. Failure of these mechanisms results in aberrations of acid-base equilibrium. Such disorders include metabolic acidosis and alkalosis, as well as respiratory acidosis and alkalosis. The general principles of treatment of acid-base disorders include: (*a*) control of the process producing the primary disorder, (*b*) augmentation of any deranged physiological corrective mechanism, and (*c*) an attack on the displacement of blood pH directly with acidifying or alkalinizing therapy.

Fluid accounts for up to 80% of the body weight at birth, a percentage that decreases with age so that, in adults, fluid accounts for only 60 to 65% of the total body weight. This fluid consists of intracellular and extracellular compartments, both of which have characteristic solute compositions. The volume and content of the fluid spaces of the body are regulated to some extent by osmometric principles and through complex physiological (neuroendocrine) mechanisms. These mechanisms, however, are not always adequate to prevent fluid and electrolyte disorders, especially in the newborn infant. The most common disorder is dehydration, or loss of total body water. Dehydration can be classified as: (*a*) isotonic, or loss of isotonic fluid with the plasma remaining isotonic; (*b*) hypotonic, or a loss of a hypertonic fluid with the plasma remaining hypotonic; and (*c*) hypertonic, or a loss of a hypotonic fluid with plasma remaining hypertonic. These states of dehydration are defined by the plasma sodium concentration, which is normal in isotonic dehydration, below normal in hypotonic dehydration, and above normal in hypertonic dehydration.

The aim of therapy for dehydration is to restore to the body fluids the amounts of water and solute that have been lost. The general scheme of this replacement therapy should proceed in three phases: (*a*) treatment of shock, if present, (*b*) restoration of the extracellular deficit of sodium and water, and (*c*) restoration of intracellular potassium losses. In addition to this deficit therapy, appropriate amounts of water, electrolytes, and calories for maintenance purposes should be provided, as well as adequate water and electrolyte to match ongoing losses.

REFERENCES

1. Winters, R. W. and Dell, R. B., Regulation of acid-base equilibrium. In *Physiological Controls and Regulation*. W. S. Yamamota and J. R. Brobeck, Eds., W. B. Saunders Co., Philadelphia, Pa., 1965, pp. 181–238

2. Winters, R. W., Engel, K., and Dell, R. B., *Acid-base Physiology in Medicine: A Self-instruction Program*, 2nd ed., The London Co., Westlake, Ohio, 1969.

3. Dell, R. B., Normal acid-base regulation. In *The Body Fluids in Pediatrics*, R. W. Winters, Ed., Little, Brown, Boston, Mass., 1973, pp. 23–45

4. Heird, W. C., Dell, R. B., and Winters, W. R., Osmotic effects of THAM, *Pediatr. Res.* **6**, 495, 1972.

5. Friis-Hansen, B., *Changes in Body Water Compartments during Growth*, Munksgaard, Copenhagen, 1956, p. 50.

6. Winters, R. W., Disorders of electrolyte and acid-base metabolism. In *Pediatrics*, 14th ed., H. L. Barnett, Ed., Appleton-Century-Crofts, New York, N.Y., 1968, pp. 336–368.

7. Barnett, H. L., Renal physiology in infants and children. I. Method for estimation of glomerular filtration rate, *Proc. Soc. Exp. Biol. Med.* **44,** 654 (1940).

8. Dean, R. F. A. and McCance, R. A., Inulin, diodone, creatinine and urea clearances in newborn infants, *J. Physiol.* **106,** 431 (1947).

9. Barnett, H. L., Hare, K., NcNamara, H., and Hare, R., Measurement of glomerular filtration rate in premature infants, *J. Clin. Invest.* **27,** 691 (1948).

10. West, G. R., Smith, H. W., and Chasis, H., Glomerular filtration rate, effective renal blood flow, and maximal tubular excretory capacity in infancy, *J. Pediatr.* **32,** 10 (1948).

11. Edelmann, C. M., Jr. and Spitzer, A., The maturing kidney, *J. Pediatr.* **75,** 509 (1969).

12. Nash, M. A. and Edelmann, C. M., Jr., The developing kidney, *Nephron* **2,** 71 (1973).

13. Ames, R. G., Urinary water excretion and neurohypophysial function in full term and premature infants shortly after birth, *Pediatrics* **12,** 272 (1953).

14. McCance, R. A., Naylor, N. J. B., and Widdowson, E. M., The response of infants to a large dose of water, *Arch. Dis. Child.* **29,** 104 (1954).

15. Calcagno, P. L., Rubin, M. A., and Weintraub, D. H., Studies on the renal concentrating and diluting mechanisms in the premature infant, *J. Clin. Invest.* **33,** 91 (1954).

16. Edelmann, C. M., Jr. and Barnett, H. L., Role of the kidney in water metabolism in young infants, *J. Pediatr.* **56,** 154 (1960).

17. Janovsky, M., Martinek, J., and Stonicova, V., Antidiuretic activity in the plasma of human infants after a load of sodium chloride, *Acta Pediatr. Scand.* **54,** 543 (1965).

18. Holliday, M. A. and Segar, W. E., The maintenance need for water in parenteral fluid therapy, *Pediatrics* **19,** 823 (1957).

19. Sinclair, J. C., Driscoll, J. M., Jr., Heird, W. C., and Winters, R. W., Supportive management of the sick neonate: Parenteral calories, water, and electrolytes, *Pediatr. Clin. North Am.* **17,** 63 (1970).

20. Butterfield, J., Lubchenco, L. O., Bergstedt, J., and O'Brein, D., Patterns in electrolyte and nitrogen balance in the newborn premature infant, *Pediatrics* **26,** 777 (1960).

21. Heird, W. C., Grebin, B., and Winters, R. W., The stabilization of disorders of water, electrolyte, and acid-base metabolism in newborn infants. In *Resuscitation of the Newborn Infant*, H. Abramson, Ed., C. V. Mosby, Saint Louis, Mo., 1973, pp. 240–261.

Intravenous Alimentation
of the Low-Birth-Weight Infant

JOHN M. DRISCOLL, JR., M.D.

WILLIAM C. HEIRD, M.D.

ROBERT W. WINTERS, M.D.

Standard feeding of newborns has long been a subject of nutritional controversy. Points of discussion have been the content of the formula, the time of initial feedings, and the volume of feedings. Current practice generally consists of attempting to feed infants as early as possible, with the infant's physical and neurologic status being the factor determining when feedings begin. This approach circumvents reported problems associated with delayed feedings such as hypoglycemia (1), hyperkalemia (2), hyperbilirubinemia (3), and azotemia (4).

In healthy, vigorous infants, this approach presents no problem. However, in sick, debilitated, or premature infants, the successful institution of early oral feeding may be difficult. A poor or unsustained suck (5), an uncoordinated swallowing mechanism (6), delayed gastric emptying (7), or some combination of these are pathophysiological factors common to many of these infants. Each of these neurophysiological deficiencies predisposes the infant to vomiting or aspiration, or both. Early therapy with intravenous fluids has been used in attempting to avoid these additional hazards, but during the neonatal period, these infusions are limited by the infant's altered renal function (8,9). Gordon (10) previously has established 120 Cal/kg body weight/day (500 kJ·kg⁻¹/24 h) as the premature infant's caloric requirements, allowing a daily weight gain of 15 g/kg. Thus, physicians have often been forced to compromise by meeting the sick infant's fluid requirements with dextrose solutions while simultaneously failing to meet his caloric needs.

Compounding this problem is the fact that recent human and animal investigations have shown that there is a critical period for brain growth and subsequent physical and functional brain development (11,12). This interval covers the antenatal period and the early postnatal period. Nutritional deficiency during these periods results in altered brain growth. Animal experiments have clearly demarcated the duration of this critical neonatal

315

period and have also delineated the functional, chemical, and physical results of under-nutrition during this time (*11,12*). Human studies suggest similar results (*13,14*), but further investigation to document the exact duration of this critical time period is still required.

Until recently, there was not much experience with alternative methods of intravenous nutrition. In the past, many investigators recorded their experience with intravenous feeding of concentrated carbohydrate solutions, hydrolyzed protein, fat emulsions, and alcohol as sources of intravenous nutrition in both animals and humans. Complications often negated the potential benefits of such infusions.

In 1968, Wilmore and Dudrick demonstrated the feasibility and nutritional effective-ness of intravenous alimentation (*15*). By placing an indwelling catheter in a major vessel (Figure 1), where rapid flow quickly dilutes the hyperosmolar infusate, they successfully maintained both human and animal subjects in positive nitrogen balance, and in younger subjects sustained growth while the subjects were receiving only intravenous nutrients. With these methods, Wilmore and Dudrick successfully limited the risks of intravenous alimentation and presented clinicians with an alternative therapeutic approach that satis-fies fluid, nutritional, and caloric requirements.

CLINICAL MATERIALS AND METHODS

Composition of the Intravenous Fluid

Table 1 lists the requirements for any parenteral fluid mixture that is to provide enough fluid, calories, and minerals to promote growth. The nitrogen source must provide both essential and nonessential amino acids; at present it is derived from either a hydrolysate of fibrin or casein or is a mixture of pure amino acids. Neither of these sources provides

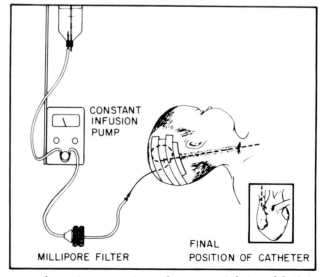

Figure 1. Placement of central venous catheters for constant infusion of fluid through a Millipore filter.

an ideal amino acid mixture, but until present testing of new mixtures is further advanced, we are limited to these nitrogen sources. At present, we use 2.5 g/kg body weight/day in low-birth-weight infants, though some investigators have used 4.0 g/kg/day. With the lower intake, we have been able to achieve positive nitrogen balance and weight gain without the risk of azotemia.

Table 1. Requirements for Total Parenteral Nutrition

Requirement	Source
Amino acids	Hydrolysates (fibrin, casein)
	Crystalline amino acid mixtures
Calories	Glucose, fructose (lipid, alcohol)
Electrolytes (Na, K, Cl)	Additives
Minerals (Ca, Mg, P)	Additives
Fat and water soluble vitamins	Additives
Essential fatty acids	(iv lipid)
Trace minerals (Zn, Cu, etc.)	Additives

In this country, glucose is the most commonly used nonprotein source of calories, although fructose, maltose, and alcohol have also been infused. In Canada and Europe, intravenous preparations of fat have been extensively used, but FDA regulations presently prohibit its use in this country. Ethanol has had limited use because of potential hepatic toxicity (*16*) and differing tolerance of it by infants (*17*). We use glucose, 25 to 30 g/kg/day to meet full caloric requirements.

Minerals and vitamins are added to the mixture at pre-established maintenance requirements. Obviously, these requirements are based on oral intakes, although parenteral needs may be significantly different.

Table 2 shows the usual final composition of the mixture that we are infusing. Obviously, it is a chemically complex mixture with a high osmolality. Figure 2 shows the contributions of the various components of the presently used mixture to the total osmolality. This osmolality required continuous slow infusion of the solution into a large central vein if it is to be tolerated both chemically and locally by the vessel and blood cells.

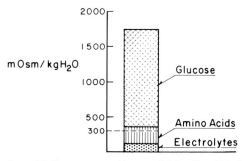

Figure 2. Osmolality of usual infusate to provide 110 Cal/kg/day (460 kJ·kg^{-1}/day) at a rate of 125 ml/kg/day.

Table 2.   Usual Composition of Infusate

Nitrogen source	2.5 g/kg/day
Glucose	25–30 g/kg/day
NaCl	3–4 mmol/kg/day
KH_2PO_4	2–3 mmol/kg/day
Ca gluconate	0.25 mmol/kg/day
	(0.5 mEq/kg/day)
$MgSO_4$	0.125 mmol/kg/day
	(0.25 mEq/kg/day)
Multiple vitamins with iron	1 ml/day
Vitamin B_{12}	50 μg/day
Folic acid	50–75 μg/day
Vitamin K_1	250–500 μg/day
Total volume	130 ml/kg per day

In the low-birth-weight infant, the initial infusate generally contains 10 g/kg of glucose, with the remainder of the mixture as previously cited. The glucose content is gradually increased to 25 to 30 g/kg/day in accordance with the patient's tolerance of glucose as assessed by serial determinations of sugar in the blood and urine.

The infusate is prepared daily in a laminar-flow hood by a registered pharmacist under the direction of one of the investigators, who carefully assesses the infant's clinical status and laboratory data before specifying the amount and content of the next day's infusate. A 0.22 μm (average pore size) Millipore filter is placed in the infusion line as a final filter, to remove debris and microorganisms.

Monitoring

Inexperience with the technique and lack of information regarding the metabolic responses of the premature infant necessitate frequent chemical monitoring (Table 3), which is done by microchemical methods. All urine and stool passed are saved and their nitrogen content is determined by the micro-Kjeldahl method.

Table 3.   Chemical Monitoring Schedule

Variable	Initial period	Later period
Plasma Na^+, K^+, Cl^-, glucose, urea nitrogen	daily	3 times/week
Blood acid–base status	daily	3 times/week
Plasma Ca^{2+}, P, and Mg^{2+}	3 times/week	1-2 times/week
Blood NH_3	3 times/week	weekly
Hemogram	2 times/week	2 times/week
Total protein, alb./glob. ratio	weekly	weekly
Urinary glucose	4 times/day	daily

After the first two or three weeks of total intravenous alimentation, the clinical status of each infant is assessed with respect to feasibility and safety of oral feedings. As oral feedings are begun, the intravenous alimentation solution is proportionately decreased and finally discontinued when adequate fluid and calories can be provided by oral feedings alone.

Limitations

The requirements for essential fatty acids and trace minerals are unknown at the present time, but both are necessary for total parenteral nutrition (*18*). At present in this country, the infusates that we use do not contain either fatty acids or trace minerals. Attempts by some investigators to meet these requirements through periodic transfusions are inadequate, particularly with respect to essential fatty acids.

Patients

Fourteen infants weighing less than 1200 g at birth were studied during periods of intravenous alimentation. Five of the infants were boys and the rest girls. Four were small for gestational age; the others were not. The birth weights ranged from 720 to 1150 g, with a mean of 863 g. None of the infants had idiopathic respiratory distress syndrome, but six infants had pulmonary insufficiency of prematurity and four infants had recurrent apnea. Intravenous alimentation was begun within 2 days for eight of the infants and between 8 and 15 days in the others. The average duration of therapy was 17.7 days (range, 5 to 24 days).

RESULTS

Weight Gain

With one exception, all patients gained weight, ranging from 1.1 to 14.7 g per day. The pattern of weight change was similar to that expected in conventionally managed infants: an initial weight loss followed by a persistent weight gain. The time required to regain initial body weight after institution of intravenous nutrition varied but still represented a marked improvement over that expected in conventionally managed infants of similar weights. A substantial part of this time could be attributed to inadequate caloric intake because hyperglycemia [blood glucose > 13.9 mmol/litre (250 mg/100 ml)] had made it necessary to temporarily decrease the glucose concentration of the infusate.

The caloric intake of 10 of the infants exceeded 100 Cal/kg per day (420 kJ·kg^{-1}/24 h) over a period averaging between five and six days. In this group of infants, the average time to regain their initial weight was seven to eight days. The main factor that determines the time required to gain initial weight appears to be the time required to achieve a caloric intake exceeding 100 Cal/kg per day (420 kJ·kg^{-1}/24 h) (Figure 3).

At first we hesitated to use insulin, but in the most recent infants we have administered small (0.25 to 0.50 unit) doses of insulin, to control the initial hyperglycemia. The use of insulin may decrease the interval needed to achieve a caloric intake greater than 100 Cal/kg per day (420 kJ·kg^{-1}/24 h), but our experience is as yet very limited.

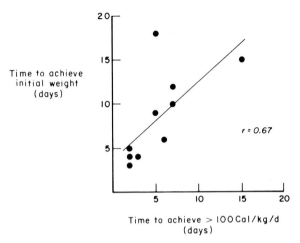

Figure 3. Relationship of time to achieve a caloric intake greater than 100 Cal/kg/day (420 kJ·kg^{-1}/ 24 h) to time to regain initial weight.

Nitrogen Balance and Weight Gain

Figure 4 shows the average nitrogen balances of eight infants over periods of 9 to 21 days (average, 15.5 days) during which caloric intake was at least 100 Cal/kg per day (420 kJ·kg^{-1}/24 h). Over this interval the average daily gain in body weight for all eight infants was 15.2 g/day (range, 11.0–19.3 g), and all showed positive nitrogen balances (average, 0.22 g/day; range, 0.20–0.28 g/day).

The probable quality of the weight gain observed in these infants can be inferred from the data on nitrogen balance for these eight infants. Deposition of 1 g of nitrogen corresponds to about 30 g of lean body mass, so the average nitrogen balance of 0.22 g/day is equivalent to 6.6 g of lean body tissue. The average weight gain of these infants was 15.2 g/day; thus the remaining 8.6 g must be explained. It is unlikely that all of this unexplained weight gain represents an accumulation of additional water; it would amount to about 150 g of water, or about 15% of body weight in these infants. Because none of our infants were edematous, we conclude that the weight gain not attributable to a change in lean body mass was due largely if not entirely to fat, amounting to an average gain in fat of about 8.3 g/day.

Blood Acid-Base Status

Nearly all infants developed a chronic respiratory acidosis, with plasma p_{CO_2} values above the upper limit of normal, defined as 5.6 kPa (42 mmHg). None of these acid-base

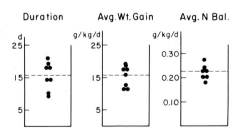

Figure 4. Duration of intravenous alimentation, average daily weight gain, and average daily nitrogen balance of eight low-birth-weight infants receiving more than 100 Cal/kg/day (420 kJ·kg^{-1}/ 24 h).

changes were believed to be related to the infusate, but rather they were attributed to the pulmonary insufficiency commonly seen in such low-birth-weight infants.

Because it is widely believed that hypercapnea or acidemia, or both, exert a catabolic effect on nitrogen metabolism, we compared the daily nitrogen balances of eight patients with the daily values observed for blood pH and plasma p_{CO_2}. Figure 5 shows that there was no clear relationship between the degree of either hypercapnea or acidemia and the degree of positive nitrogen balance achieved. Furthermore, positive nitrogen balances were achieved despite p_{CO_2} values as high as 10.3 kPa (85 mmHg) and blood pH values as low as 7.15.

Complications

Complications related to total parenteral nutrition can be divided into three groups: septic, catheter related, and metabolic (*19*). Because the infusate promotes the growth of certain organisms and fungi, meticulous aseptic technique must be used, not only in placing the catheter but also in its subsequent care. With strict control of technique, the risk of sepsis can be minimized. Likewise, catheter-related complications can be prevented by the development of a team that is well-trained, dedicated, and expert in the placement and maintenance of the central catheters. Metabolic complications of many types have been reported with intravenous alimentation (*19*) (Table 4).

In our series of 14 low-birth-weight infants, one infant died of candida sepsis after five days of infusion. The diagnosis was not suspected clinically. No other septic or catheter-related complications occurred. Episodes of hyperglycemia were the most common problems in our early experience; with more careful monitoring, these can be minimized.

Two infants who had received no inorganic phosphate in their infusate developed hypercalcemia and hypophosphatemia. Deletion of calcium from the infusate did not alter these abnormalities, but addition of inorganic phosphate (2 mmol/kg body weight/day) promptly corrected both abnormalities.

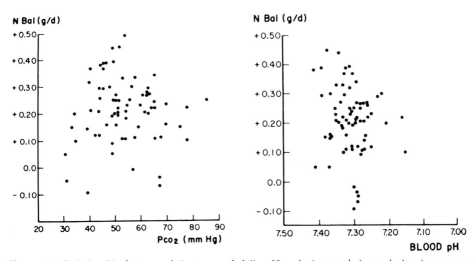

Figure 5. Relationship between daily p_{CO_2} and daily pH and nitrogen balance during intravenous alimentation.

Table 4.   Metabolic Complications of Total Parenteral Nutrition

Glucose disorders:	Hyperglycemia (osmotic diuresis, hyperosmolarity), hypoglycemia
Electrolyte disorders:	Hyper- or hypo-natremia, -kalemia, -chloremia
Mineral disorders:	Hyper- or hypo-calcemia, -phosphatemia, -magnesemia
Acid–base disorders:	Hyperchloremic metabolic acidosis
Disorders of N metabolism:	Azotemia
	Hyperammonemia
	Abnormal plasma aminograms
Vitamin disorders:	Hyper- or hypo-vitaminoses
Fatty acid disorders:	Essential fatty-acid deficiency
Trace mineral disorders:	Zn, Cu deficiencies
Hepatic disorders:	Abnormal activity of alanine and aspartate aminotransferase in serum, hepatomegaly, aspartate and alanine aminotransferases (SGOT and SGPT).

Blood urea nitrogen concentrations exceeding 7.1 mmol/litre (20 mg/100 ml) mostly occurred in the first week of intravenous alimentation and most often in infants receiving 4 g of protein/kilogram body weight/day. No value exceeding 17.9 mmol/litre (50 mg/100 ml) was noted. In all instances, decreasing the protein content of the infusate was accompanied by a decreased blood urea nitrogen concentration.

Outcome

Table 5 describes our results for these 14 infants. Six of them died, five of causes unrelated to the technique. The one death from candida sepsis was obviously related to the procedure.

Table 5.   Summary of Course for 14 Infants on Intravenous Alimentation (I.A.)

Age at which I.A. was begun	
0—2 days:	8 infants
8—15 days:	6 infants
Duration of I.A.	
Average:	17.7 days
Range:	5–24 days
Time required to:	
Achieve 100 Cal/kg/day:	5.6 days (n = 10)
Regain initial weight:	7.8 days (n = 10)

Of the eight survivors, one has been lost to follow-up and another was subsequently readmitted with bacterial meningitis and died. The six infants being followed range in age from 18 to 40 months. Three are neurologically normal, two are suspect, and one is abnormal. Obviously, a longer and larger follow-up of both the neurological and behavioral development of more low-birth-weight infants is indicated before any conclusion can be reached regarding the long-term positive or negative effect of intravenous nutrition on subsequent growth and function of the central nervous system.

SUMMARY

Intravenous alimentation can produce satisfactory growth and positive nitrogen balance without undue risk. The long-term developmental results require a much larger experience than is presently available. Until such evidence is available, intravenous alimentation has no place in the routine management of the low-birth-weight infant. Clearly, however, the technique can be used with adequate precaution without significant risk in selected infants and deserves cautious exploration in these infants.

ACKNOWLEDGMENT

The original research of the authors was supported by grants PM-HL-14218 and HD-08434 from NIH, USPHS.

REFERENCES

1. Smallpiece, V. and Davies, P. A., Immediate feeding of premature infants with undiluted breast milk, *Lancet* ii, 1349 (1964).

2. Auld, P. A. M., Byangananda, P., and Mehta, S., The influence of an early caloric intake with intravenous glucose in catabolism of premature infants, *Pediatrics* 37, 592 (1966).

3. Hubbell, J. P. Jr., et al., "Early" versus "late" feeding of infants of diabetic mothers, *N. Engl. J. Med.* 265, 835 (1961).

4. Hansen, J. D. and Smith, C. A., Effects of withholding fluid in the immediate postnatal period, *Pediatrics* 12, 99 (1953).

5. Crumb, E. P., Gore, P. M., and Horton, C. P., The sucking behavior in premature infants, *Hum. Biol.* 30, 128 (1958).

6. Ardran, G. M. and Kemp, F. H., A correlation between sucking pressures and movements of tongue, *Acta Pediatr. Scand.* 48, 261 (1959).

7. Keller, A., Studies of motility relations of the infant's stomach, *Nord. Med.* 38, 1141 (1948).

8. McCance, R. A. and Widdowson, E. M., Normal renal function in the first two days of life, *Arch. Dis. Child* 29, 488 (1959).

9. Ames, R. G., Urinary water excretion and neurohypophysial function in full term and premature infants shortly after birth, *Pediatrics* 12, 272 (1953).

10. Gordon, H. H., Levine, S. Z., Deamer, W. C., and McNamara, H., Respiratory metabolism in infancy and childhood, *Am. J. Dis. Child.* 59, 1185 (1940).

11. Winick, M. and Noble, A., Cellular response in rat during malnutrition at various ages, *J. Nutr.* 89, 300 (1966).

12. Winick, M., Malnutrition and brain development, *J. Pediatr.* 74, 667 (1969).

13. Winnick, M. and Rosso, P., The effect of severe early malnutrition on cellular growth of human brain, *Pediatr. Res.* 3, 181 (1969).

14. Cravioto, J., DeLicardie, E. R., and Birch, H. G., Nutrition, growth and neurointegrative development: An experimental and ecologic study, *Pediatrics* 38, 319 (1968).

15. Wilmore, D. W., and Dudrick, S. J., Growth and development of an infant receiving all nutrients exclusively by vein, *J. Am. Med. Assoc.* 203, 140 (1968).

16. Rubin, E. and Lieber, C. S., Fatty liver, alcoholic hepatitis cirrhosis produced by alcohol in primates, *N. Engl. J. Med.* 290, 128 (1974).

17. Peden, V. H., Sammon, T. J., and Downey, D. A., Intravenously induced infantile intoxication with ethanol, *J. Pediatr.* 83, 490 (1973).

18. Holman, R. T., Essential fatty acid deficiency in humans. In *Dietary Lipids and Postnatal Development.*, C. Golle, G. Jacini, and A. Pecele, Eds., Raven Press, New York, N.Y., 1973, p 127.

19. Heird, W. C. and Winters, R. W., Total parenteral nutrition: The state of the art, *J. Pediat.* (to be published).

20. Goldman, D. S., Microbiological safety of solutions and delivery to the patient. In *Symposium on Total Parenteral Nutrition*, June 17–19, 1972, Council on Foods and Nutrition of American Medical Association, 535 N. Dearborn St., Chicago, Ill. 60610, p 32.

Obligations of the
Pediatric Clinical Laboratory

JOCELYN M. HICKS, Ph.D.

DONALD S. YOUNG, M.B., Ph.D.

OBLIGATIONS OF THE PEDIATRIC CLINICAL LABORATORY

Many of the problems of the pediatric clinical laboratory are unrecognized by hospital administrators and physicians. These problems are probably most difficult for the director of the clinical laboratory in a general hospital catering to both infants and adults, because two entirely different types of laboratory service must be maintained if first-class service is to be provided for all patients.

In many respects, the responsibility of the director of the pediatric laboratory and of the typical general hospital laboratory are similar. They include service, teaching, research and administration. In this paper, these obligations will be considered as they affect the pediatric laboratory and the general laboratory; situations that require special consideration in the pediatric laboratory will be identified.

SERVICE

The major difference between a pediatric and general hospital clinical laboratory is in the service they provide. Despite the wide variety of diseases found in the adult hospital population, and the typical mixture of medical, surgical, and obstetrical patients in the general hospital, the patient population is quite homogeneous in the way it affects the clinical laboratory. In the pediatric hospital, the patient population is much less uniform. It includes premature infants, other newborns, and children in all stages of development, including adolescents.

Problems that are of particular concern to the director of the pediatric laboratory include the proper collection of specimens, the lack of availability of suitable instrumentation for the mechanization of test procedures, and the need to use only a small quantity of specimen for each test. The pediatric laboratory staff must be capable of performing many tests that are not done in the general hospital laboratory. Many more tests have to be run on an emergency basis in the pediatric hospital than in the hospital for adults. Some of these tests are for constituents that are never measured on an emergency basis in the general hospital laboratory.

Because of the difficulties in collection of blood specimens in the pediatric hospital, it is difficult to process tests in the laboratory on a batch basis, which has become one of the essential tenets in the general hospital laboratory to improve efficiency and achieve greater reproducibility of data. Each specimen may have to be processed separately and the test performed by hand. The instruments that enable the mechanization of different tests on the same sample such as the Dupont *aca* or the Instrumentation Laboratory Clinicard require too much sample to allow their use in the pediatric laboratory. This lack of batch processing and mechanization of tests necessitates a larger staff than in the general hospital to perform the same number of tests.

The Special Committee on Pediatric Clinical Chemistry of the American Association for Clinical Chemistry has obtained data on the staffing patterns of some laboratories of its own members. These are summarized in Table 1. The data are illustrated for one month. These figures do not take into consideration the different types of patients in the various hospitals and can only give a superficial indication of the staffing needs. In the typical general hospital, technologists would be expected to perform at least twice the number of analyses performed by their counterparts in the pediatric laboratory. Inevitably the actual cost per test must be higher in the pediatric laboratory, because labor accounts for about 70% of all costs of the laboratory.

While screening of an adult population is widely accepted and frequently used, appropriate "battery" testing in children is used very little. However, if it can be justified that a certain number and frequency of tests are required for the diagnosis and treatment of a disease in an adult, then the pediatric laboratory should accept the responsibility of performing the same tests with the same frequency when a child has the same disease. Because disease manifestations fluctuate more frequently and to a greater extent in the child than in the adult, there is perhaps a correspondingly greater justification for more tests to be performed on a sick child.

Specimen Collection

Although venipunctures are practical in older children, heel or finger puncture is the most efficient and least traumatic procedure for obtaining blood from infants and young children. A well-performed heel prick is much simpler than a venipuncture in infants and may be repeated at frequent intervals. Heel pricks must be performed carefully, and a free flow of blood is essential to avoid contamination with tissue fluid and to prevent hemolysis of the specimen. Other acceptable but less desirable sites for obtaining capillary blood are the great toe and the earlobe. Considerable errors may be introduced into laboratory data if specimens are not properly collected. When laboratory data are interpreted, it is essential to recognize the influence of different types of specimens on results. Although Kaplan et al. (1) have shown that there is essentially no difference between results for venous and capillary blood for most tests (although the analytical techniques that were used were inferior to those currently available), there are real differences in blood pH and glucose. Venous blood reveals the action of tissue metabolism as indicated by lower pH and glucose. Because values for both blood pH and glucose are less in venous blood than in capillary blood, the laboratory must establish the interrelationship between data

Table 1. Work Load and Staffing of Nine Pediatric Laboratories

	1	2	3	4	5	6	7	8	9
Number of pediatric beds	125	250	301	167	184	100	776	250	164
Number of tests on outpatient and as "stats" (in thousands)	41	3.2	152	38	78	—	204	126	85
Total number of tests including standards and controls (in thousands)	12.7	20.2	17.5	7.4	19.6	1.9	70.8	20.2	24.6
Total daytime laboratory staff	14.5	9	13	5	18	3	24	14	19
Total number of tests per staff member per month	876	2244	1346	1488	1089	633	2950	1442	1294

obtained on venous and capillary blood so that results may be meaningful on one individual even though different types of specimen were used. The relationship between lead in whole blood, determined in both capillary and venous blood, is illustrated in Figure 1. Figure 2 shows the relationship between serum thyroxine determined simultaneously in capillary and venous blood.

Variability attributable to collection factors may be minimized by reducing the number of individuals who are allowed to collect blood. At present, there is no mechanical device that can ensure reproducibility of specimen collection. It is our experience that a blood-drawing team is essential in a pediatric laboratory, because the experience of such persons allows collection of good nonhemolyzed specimens. It also allows routine specimens to be drawn at one time and while the patient is in the fasting state. We advocate the collection of specimens at 0600 hours.

Before the blood is collected, the heel should be warmed to increase blood flow. It then is cleaned well with povidone-iodine (Betadine). A careful and deep puncture is made with a Redi-Lance blood lancet (Clay Adams Division, Becton-Dickinson Co., Parsipanny, N.J. 07054) or its equivalent. The blood is allowed to drip freely into the collection tube, which is preferably made of glass if determinations are to be performed on serum, because there is little tendency for the clot to adhere to the wall. If a glucose analysis is required, the specimen for this test should be collected directly into a tube containing an anticoagulant with an antiglycolytic agent. We use ethylenediaminetetra-acetate with sodium fluoride. During collection of the specimen, at no time should the skin surface be allowed to come into contact with the tube, lest hemolysis occur. After the collection, a cotton ball is pressed over the wound for a short time to stop the bleeding.

It is particularly difficult to collect urine specimens from babies. For casual specimens, urine is usually collected by attaching a plastic bag directly to the skin. Collection of 24-h specimens is much more difficult than in the adult. It is necessary to ensure that the bladder is empty at the start of the collection, because residual urine may contribute a large error to the generally small volume produced by an infant during a day. A series of

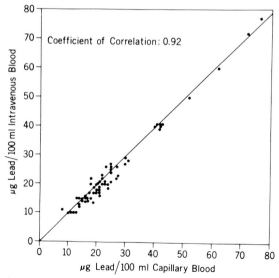

Figure 1. Relation between concentrations of lead in venous and capillary blood.

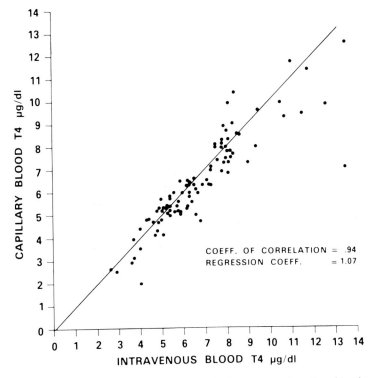

Figure 2.   Relation between serum thyroxine in venous and capillary blood.

collection bags may be used to collect urine, with the contents mixed and preserved as required for the requested test. A metabolic bed may be used for the collection of 24-h specimens when the use of disposable bags is impractical.

Volume of Specimens

The total blood volume of a child is very much less than that of an adult; that of the healthy newborn is about 275 ml (2), and in the premature infant it is even less. The figure of 80 ml/kg body weight may be used to estimate the blood volume. The hematocrit in the infant at birth is about 0.56 (56%), so the volume of plasma or the serum for analysis is even less than might be anticipated from the blood volume (3). DeMarsh et al. (4) have also shown that the erythrocyte count (and hence the hematocrit) of capillary blood is greater than that of central venous blood. An infant's hematocrit does not decline to the adult value until almost a month after birth.

Careful monitoring of the volume of blood removed from an infant is essential and a record of the quantity removed should be maintained in the neonatal nursing unit or in the clinical laboratory. Blood hemoglobin and hematocrit should be monitored, and re-placement transfusion may be necessary to maintain these.

It is essential that the quantity of blood required by the clinical laboratory be kept to a minimum. It is now possible to perform most tests in a pediatric clinical laboratory on less than 25 μl of serum for each test. Indeed, less than 10 μl is required for most of the commonly requested tests. To ensure most efficient use of the infant's blood, several tests should be performed on the same specimen rather than on different specimens.

Tests Performed in the Pediatric Laboratory

The pediatric laboratory must be capable of performing almost all the tests performed in the general hospital laboratory, as well as several others not requested in adult patients. In the pediatric laboratory there is frequently a greater need for a rapid turnaround of results. The neonatal unit, especially its intensive care section, places great demands on the laboratory. The respiratory distress syndrome is, fortunately, rare in the newborn, although it is considerably more prevalent in premature infants. These babies must be monitored closely and blood-gas determinations must be made several times a day. Initially, at least, serum calcium, bilirubin, and electrolytes must be measured daily. To avoid delay in the transport of specimens to the laboratory for analysis, we recommend placing the blood-gas laboratory in the nursery area; this ensures a close working relationship between the nursery staff and the technologist who is committed full time to the tests for the neonatal unit.

The infant of the diabetic mother also requires many laboratory tests during the newborn period. These include not only blood glucose determinations but also serum electrolytes, bilirubin, calcium, and osmolality. Results of tests should be made available to the physician with as little delay as possible.

A very important part of a pediatric laboratory's work is the diagnosis of metabolic errors. In our laboratory, we routinely screen the urine of newborn infants to detect abnormal amounts of reducing substances, cystine, phenylketones, and acid mucopolysaccharides. We also screen for the presence of keto compounds and perform a ferric chloride test on the urine of all newborn infants. If there is clinical suspicion of a neuroblastoma, the urine is spot tested for the presence of increased amounts of 4-hydroxy-3-methoxymandelic acid (vanillylmandelic acid). If there is a strong suggestion of an aminoacidopathy, the laboratory must be prepared to perform a screening test and quantitative chromatographic analysis for amino acids in both serum and urine. The laboratory should also be able to measure serum phenylalanine and tyrosine specifically for the diagnosis of phenylketonuria and the monitoring of its treatment.

It is necessary to be able to measure UTP:α-D-galactose-1-phosphate uridylyltransferase (EC 2.7.7.10), to detect galactosemia, and urinary hydroxycorticosteroids and ketosteroids, to assist physicians in diagnosing the adrenogenital syndrome. All of these tests must be performed well and rapidly so that appropriate treatment may be instituted to avoid irreversible damage of developing organs, especially the brain. Many additional tests may also be required to make the diagnosis of specific metabolic diseases, because essentially all of these are made, or confirmed, from clinical laboratory data. If it is impossible to perform these tests within the laboratory, it is essential that the laboratory director have available a list of laboratories that are prepared to perform the determinations at short notice. Many of these tests are so complex that they are usually performed in only a few specialized laboratories. Among such tests we include those for the diagnosis of organic acidurias, such as methylmalonic aciduria. Even more specialized laboratories may perform the tissue enzyme assays that are essential for confirming the diagnosis of an error of metabolism. It is probably desirable that only a few of these very specialized laboratories exist, so that the highest standards of quality control for the diagnosis of specific diseases may be maintained.

Laboratory Instrumentation and Methodology

In the general hospital laboratory, mechanization of analytical tests has improved the precision of results as well as increased the efficiency of the laboratory. To be beneficial in the pediatric laboratory, instruments must also be capable of performing satisfactorily with a small volume of sample. They must also make use of methods that are specific for the major analyte, to avoid interferences from endogenous or exogenous compounds. In the pediatric laboratory, the work is not readily adaptable to batch-processing procedures, and generally the number of specimens for any test is small. Neeley (5), among others, has demonstrated the adaptability of the continuous-flow (AutoAnalyzer) concept to processing the small volumes of specimens available from children. Even the large Technicon SMAC system is theoretically suitable for analyzing specimens from a pediatric hospital, because it consumes 350 μl of serum for 20 of the most common tests. However, one seldom needs 20 tests done at any one time on an infant, and this would involve drawing a millilitre of blood. The Ortho "Accuchem" is similar in its requirements and will perform 17 different determinations on 250 μl of serum. Both of these systems are still undergoing field evaluation and their performance in a critical routine environment is uncertain. The expense of these systems and their great rate of analysis militate against their acceptance in anything other than the largest pediatric hospitals.

The Abbott ABA-100 has found considerable application in pediatric laboratories. A small volume of sample is required for most tests (as little as 5 μl for some), and it can be readily switched from one test procedure to another. The bichromatic spectrophotometric measurement procedure minimizes interferences from endogenous or exogenous materials without the need for performing separate blank determinations. Specific enzymatic procedures are available for measuring glucose, uric acid, cholesterol, and triacylglycerols (triglycerides). The various commercial models of the centrifugal analyzer developed at Oak Ridge National Laboratories (6) can perform most of the tests required in the pediatric laboratory with adequate accuracy, precision, and specificity. The miniature version of the same instrument (7) appears to be even more appropriate for processing the pediatric laboratory's work load at a lower cost while still maintaining adequate standards of performance. If fluorescence were incorporated into the system as a measuring technique, it would increase the sensitivity and specificity attainable.

Several modular analytical systems have been developed for handling pediatric samples. These include the Beckman Spinco, developed from the early work of Sanz (8) and still in common use, and the Micromedics system, which is being developed from Sanz's more recent work. The Eppendorf system is similar in its modular design to the Beckman Spinco apparatus, although a different principle is used for pipetting the sample and reagents. A competent laboratory director can devise his own system by coupling a precise mechanical pipet with a sensitive measuring system.

Fluorometry is appropriately sensitive, although it requires considerable care in the cleaning of glassware to eliminate analytical interferences. The chemist should be aware of possible quenching effects that may also occur. Radioimmunological procedures generally have even greater sensitivity and specificity and, thereoretically at least, are very suitable for use in the pediatric laboratory.

Some tests may be performed in instruments initially developed for use in the general laboratory. Examples are the Beckman Glucose, BUN, and System One Analyzers, which only require 10 μl serum for a glucose determination and 10 μl of serum for a urea nitrogen determination, both of which can be completed within a couple of minutes.

Certain requirements are common to all systems for the analysis of specimens in the pediatric laboratory: (*a*) The precision of pipetting a sample, in particular, must be well controlled. Less than 1% error is desirable, to minimize the analytical variability of the results. (*b*) There must be precautions to minimize evaporation of specimen, such as the use of narrow and deep containers to reduce surface area from which evaporation can take place, or the creation of a barrier between the specimen and the air, for example, with "Seraseal" (Abbott Diagnostics Division, South Pasadena, Calif. 91030) or a similar solution that may be layered over the serum. Throughout the laboratory, tubes containing serum should be kept cool and covered. (*c*) The methods used must withstand a high concentration of bilirubin, which may occur as a result of physiological jaundice of the newborn or of Rh, ABO, or other blood-group incompatibilities or because of sepsis or biliary atresia. As far as possible, results should not be influenced by the presence of hemoglobin, as hemolysis is more likely to occur in specimens of capillary blood than in venous blood specimens.

The clinical state of infants in the nursery often has to be monitored several times within a day. On each of these occasions, as many as eight tests may have to be performed. This poses problems of specimen identification. It is impossible to attach a label directly to a capillary blood tube, and specimens are best identified by being placed in a test tube that is appropriately labeled. However, when a sample is removed from a test tube, as must be done in the clinical laboratory, there must be considerable vigilance if errors are not to occur. Within the laboratory, profile cards on which all laboratory data are entered chronologically for each individual enable unexpected changes in laboratory data to be identified rapidly. If large changes are noted, the results are checked and the nursery unit is notified immediately. Information about any change in therapy is elicited from the nursing staff. This is especially important to know for correct interpretation of data on serum calcium and potassium. Because of the rapidity with which the concentration of these constituents can change in the blood of newborns, all results should be called to the attention of the nursing unit as soon as they are obtained.

The clinical state of sick children is frequently more labile than in adults so that more laboratory tests may be required on an emergency basis. For example, uric acid determinations may be required "stat" in children with acute leukemia, or serum iron determinations in children who accidentally ingest iron tablets. Laboratory staff must be prepared to do these tests at any time of the day. Because of the risk of meningitis during the first two months of postnatal life, spinal taps are performed as a diagnostic procedure more often than in the adult population, and the laboratory must determine protein and glucose during any of the daily work shifts. Indeed, in many pediatric laboratories, the evening and night shifts are almost as busy as the day shift. It is therefore imperative that the staff be well trained, to assure that the quality of work is the same for all shifts.

Quality Assurance and Quality of Work

Quality assurance is as important in the pediatric laboratory as it is in any other type of laboratory. Control samples should be analyzed with each batch of tests, even though a batch may consist of only one or two blood specimens. Standards must be analyzed with every unknown. While most control samples measure a concentration in the typical normal range, the wide spread of results that may occur with the pediatric population often necessitates checks outside the normal range to verify that the concentration of substances is indeed outside that range, for example, for high serum bilirubin or low blood-glucose concentrations.

It is possible to obtain precise laboratory data in a pediatric laboratory, although most tests are performed manually by different technologists. In our laboratory, the coefficient of variation for day-to-day analyses for serum sodium, potassium, and chloride is less than 1%, for cholesterol it is 2.5%, and for glucose and urea nitrogen it is 5%. A pediatric laboratory should be able to meet all the proficiency standards of the regulatory agencies without difficulty.

Toxicology

It is essential to provide at least a limited toxicological service in a pediatric clinical chemistry laboratory. Accidental overdosage with iron or salicylate is the most common problem, and the laboratory must be prepared to measure these substances in serum at any time of the day or night. It is also important to be able to monitor the concentration of certain drugs, such as phenobarbital and diphenylhydantoin in epileptic patients and theophylline in asthmatic patients. The concentration of salicylate should also be monitored in patients with rheumatic problems. Only by doing this is it possible to guarantee that adequate doses of drugs are administered. In urban areas, it is important that a reliable technique for screening for lead poisoning is available with quantitation to assist the monitoring of treatment. Screening programs make it necessary for a laboratory to handle large numbers of blood-lead and blood-erythrocyte-protoporphyrin analyses. In some areas of the country, it may be necessary to perform morphine analysis for young narcotic addicts.

Reference Values

Correct interpretation of laboratory data depends on an appropriate yardstick being available to which the data may be compared. In the pediatric laboratory, the reference values (normal ranges) must be adjusted with the development of the child. Laboratory data obtained for serum from cord blood often approximate those for the mother's serum, but thereafter change rapidly—for example, serum calcium may change from 2.35 mmol/litre (4.7 mEq/litre) at birth to 2.00 mmol/litre (4.0 mEq/litre) 48 to 72 h later. Serum proteins undergo considerable change also, especially the concentration of immunoglobulins. Many other constituents are also affected, yet little information is available on the concentration of many constituents in the blood of healthy infants. An understanding of the different reference values in children will help the clinical chemist play an active role in the proper management and diagnosis of the patients.

TEACHING

One of the most important aspects of good service is linked with the teaching responsibilities of the laboratory director. It is useful for both the pediatricians and the senior laboratory staff for the latter to attend and participate in rounds, to find out why tests have been ordered, to learn how the results are applied, and to suggest alternative or additional tests that should be performed. This is especially useful when the child fails to thrive without obvious cause. It is essential that the clinical chemist discuss the case with the physician and attempt to assist him in understanding the possible underlying biochemical abnormalities.

The staff of all good laboratories should become involved in teaching. They should attend rounds, lectures, and seminars in the hospital. Initially, the laboratory director must ensure that his own staff has a thorough understanding of why particular tests are requested, so that they understand why certain methods have been chosen to perform them and what the results may mean. The director should discuss case histories of the patients with both his technical and professional staffs, to enable them to understand their role in the health-care team.

Pediatric laboratories should participate in the teaching of medical technology students so that these trainees may be exposed to the exacting and challenging type of work that is performed in a pediatric laboratory. In this training, the students should also be exposed to the elucidation of metabolic errors in problems that are unique to the pediatric laboratory.

A clinical chemist should also become involved in the teaching of medical students. Directors of laboratories should consider setting up elective programs in laboratory medicine to teach students during their senior year, the time when they are most interested in understanding the biochemistry of disease. This is not only useful to the student but also has benefits to the laboratory, because an in-depth appreciation of the laboratory's capabilities and limitations will enable the physician to use the laboratory more effectively. Clinical chemists should not limit their teaching to students but should present new developments in laboratory medicine at grand rounds and should become actively involved in other forms of postgraduate training of medical staff.

The pediatric clinical chemists should teach their colleagues in clinical pathology and clinical chemistry the importance of microchemical techniques and their potential application throughout the clinical laboratory. They should encourage their colleagues to foster the same relationship with their clinical staff that frequently exists between pediatric clinical chemists and pediatricians. The pediatric clinical chemist should become involved in the postdoctoral training of analytical or physical chemists in pediatric clinical chemistry.

RESEARCH AND DEVELOPMENT

Research is one of the responsibilities most often neglected by the clinical chemist. Yet the pediatric laboratory, like other clinical laboratories, provides great opportunities for research by the chemist, biochemist, and physician.

Opportunities exist for the scaling down of existing test procedures to make them suitable for pediatric use and to develop alternative methods to measure the same constituents with use of smaller volumes of sample. It is also necessary to develop new tests such as a quick and reliable method for determining the quantity of bilirubin bound to albumin and the bilirubin-binding capacity of the albumin. A method for determining the concentration of ionized calcium is needed for which less than 50 μl of serum should be used. Appropriate "batteries" of tests need to be developed for screening newborns to determine their health.

Instrumentation is required that will, in effect, mechanize the laboratory tests in the pediatric laboratory. The apparatus should have the same flexibility as the Dupont *aca*, which allows either many different tests on the same specimen to be performed or the same test on different specimens, yet should require no more than 10 μl of serum for each test. The system should be capable of being calibrated with pure chemicals and should make use of methods that are specific for the major analyses. The precision of the system should equal that obtainable with the most precise methods and systems in use in the general laboratory.

The abnormal biochemical processes underlying many diseases are still not understood. In spite of the very extensive studies done on patients with cystic fibrosis and the many biochemical abnormalities that have been determined, the underlying cause is uncertain. The culture and analysis of cells from amniotic fluid is an area that should be developed to enable more metabolic errors to be diagnosed early, in utero. While many disorders of amino acid metabolism have already been identified, there are probably many additional aminoacidurias yet to be recognized because the compounds that are in excess are ninhydrin negative. Gas-liquid chromatography may have considerable potential usefulness for identifying and elucidating such disorders. There are probably metabolic defects associated with disordered organic acid metabolism that have not yet been described. There are probably identifiable causes of the failure-to-thrive syndrome, which is very difficult to treat in the newborn when the underlying cause cannot be determined. The metabolic consequences of therapeutic regimens such as hyperalimentation used to treat infants failing to thrive still have not yet been determined. It is possible, for example, that trace-metal deficiencies may result (9).

It is important that the clinical chemist become actively involved in the fundamental biochemical research opportunities that abound in the pediatric clinical laboratory. The pediatric clinical chemist has a real opportunity to advance clinical chemistry as a scientific discipline.

ADMINISTRATION

The pediatric clinical laboratory director is, by virtue of his job, an administrator in addition to his other responsibilities. As in most administrative positions, the director's prime responsibility is to obtain enough staff of adequate caliber to ensure that the laboratory is staffed 24 hours a day, seven days a week, with skilled and responsible technologists, so that the quality of work performed constantly exceeds minimally acceptable standards.

Staffing patterns are much different in a pediatric laboratory from those in other laboratories. The number of emergency-basis requests is always very large in proportion to the total work load, and the quantity of work at night and on weekends is also very large. It is therefore important to set up work schedules in such a way that there is always continuity between staff on different shifts and to set up correct priorities for handling work, so that the most important tests are always performed first, especially if not enough blood is available to do all the requested tests of a specimen.

The laboratory director should participate in meetings with his own technical staff and his laboratory supervisors, but he must also participate actively in discussions with clinical and nursing staffs to ensure that he is informed of pending changes in hospital procedures or practices to enable him to act before changes in work load occur.

Future planning is of great importance, both to decide which test to implement, which equipment to replace or purchase, and how to modify the design of the laboratory to meet new demands. The public-relations aspect of a laboratory director's job is often overlooked. It is important that he communicate with the hospital staff by personal contact and through manuals and the like that document the laboratory's requirements, to ensure, for example, that specimens are properly collected. He should provide background information in these manuals for the correct interpretation of laboratory data.

The laboratory director is responsible for preparing a realistic budget. In this, he must consider salaries of his staff and general operating expenses, as well as expenditure for capital equipment. He must also consider the charges to be made for performing laboratory tests.

The laboratory director must keep good records, in order to monitor changes in total work load and the number of different tests that are ordered. He must always have enough background evidence to justify his request for additional resources.

Above all, the laboratory director must ensure that the needs of the hospital patients are met by providing the best possible service to their physicians. He must meet their needs efficiently, well, and economically.

REFERENCES

1. Kaplan, S. A., Yucloglu, A. M., and Strausse, J., Chemical microanalysis: Analysis of capillary and venous blood, *Pediatrics* 24, 270 (1959).

2. Castle, W. B., Disorders of the blood and blood-forming tissues. In *Pathologic Physiology: Mechanics of Disease*, 4th ed., W. A. Sodeman and W. A. Sodeman, Jr., Eds. W. B. Saunders, Philadelphia, Pa., 1967, p 751.

3. Glaser, K., Blood erythroycyte, hematocrit, hemoglobin and thrombocyte values, birth to maturity: Man. In *Standard Values in Blood*, E. C. Albritton, Ed. W. B. Saunders Co., Philadelphia, Pa. 1952, p 38.

4. DeMarsh, Q. B., Alt, A. L., and Windle, W. F., The effect of depriving the infant of its placental blood: On the blood picture duridg the first week of life, *J. Am. Med. Assoc.* 116, 2568 (1941).

5. Neeley, W. E., Wardlaw, S. C., and Sing, H. D., Design and performance of a minaturized high speed continuous-flow analyzer, *Clin. Chem.* 20, 424 (1974).

6. Anderson, N. G., Analytical techniques for cell fractionations XII. A multiple cuvette rotor for a new microanalytical system, *Anal. Biochem.* 28, 545 (1969).

7. Scott, C. D. and Burtis, C. A., A minature Fast Analyzer system, *Anal. Chem.* 45, 327A (1972).

8. Sanz, M. C., Ultramicro methods and standardization of equipment, *Clin. Chem.* 3, 406 (1957).

9. Hambridge, M. and O'Brien, D., *On developmental nutrition: Trace metals.* (No. 7 in a series of reviews on neonatal problems.) Ross Laboratories, Columbus, Ohio 43216.

Index

A